W9-BBZ-721

Men's Health THE BIG BOOK OF Uncommon Knowledge

Men'sHealth THE BIG BOOK OF Uncommon Knowledge

Clever Hacks for Navigating Life with Skill and Swagger

EDITED BY JEFF CSATARI

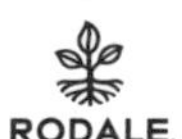
RODALE

Portions of this book were previously published in *Men's Health*.

Rodale books may be purchased for business or promotional use or for special sales.
For information, please write to: Special Markets Department, Rodale Inc., 733 Third Avenue, New York, NY 10017

Men's Health is a registered trademark of Rodale Inc.
Printed in the United States of America
Rodale Inc. makes every effort to use acid-free ♾, recycled paper ♻.

Book design by Joanna Williams

Library of Congress Cataloging-in-Publication Data is on file with the publisher.

ISBN 978-1-62336-515-8 hardcover

Distributed to the trade by Macmillan

2 4 6 8 10 9 7 5 3 1 hardcover

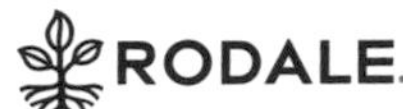

We inspire and enable people to improve their lives and the world around them.

rodalebooks.com

What's Inside . . .

Introduction: How to Know Everything About Anything viii

Chapter 1: 100 Things Every Man Should Know 1

HOW TO . . .

Open a beer without a bottle opener; spin a basketball on a finger; save a life; block a haymaker; cradle a baby; whistle with your fingers; hone a knife; launch a snot rocket; pour a black & tan; make a signature drink; make a toast; change spark plugs; throw a curveball; steer a horse; delivery a eulogy; catch a snake; flirt like a player; tie a trucker's hitch; save for anything; kick in a door; build a bone-crushing handshake; useful rules; and much more.

Chapter 2: Survive in the Wild 35

HOW TO . . .

Start a fire with a flashlight; paddle a canoe; eat a pine tree; survive a bear attack; swim with sharks; make a life preserver from your trousers; catch a fish; clean a fish; flip campfire flapjacks; shit in the woods; find north without a compass; avoid stinging bees; know a crappie from a brownie; stay warm in a sleeping bag; remove a tick; scale a boulder; and ID a big bird.

Chapter 3: Muscle and Fitness 61

HOW TO . . .

Blast belly fat; build massive biceps; scale a rope; become a human flag; lose 10 pounds; banish back pain; punch a speed bag; pound a heavy bag; escape a botched bench press; make a workout sandbag; turn a towel into a barbell; put your spare tire to work; massage sore muscles; choose a four-legged running partner; swing a kettlebell; run faster; make the perfect protein shake; and master the swimmer's flip turn.

Chapter 4: Stealth Health 87

HOW TO . . .

Play doctor; clear a stuffy nose; soothe a smashed thumb; relieve a blow to the groin; beat a bad mood; improve your posture; go to sleep faster; give yourself the Heimlich; grow your brain; pump up your penis; erase a black eye; and diagnose your aches and pains.

Chapter 5: Style and Grooming 103

HOW TO . . .

Stock the perfect wardrobe; look great in a suit; fold a shirt; shine shoes like a soldier; trim gnarly nose hairs; look younger and leaner with clothes; remove stains on a shirt; unstick a stuck zipper; match a shirt collar to your face; match a tie to your suit; break in a baseball cap; tie a half-Windsor knot; dimple your tie; whiten your teeth; fix a bad haircut; and make a statement with eyewear.

Chapter 6: Women 131

HOW TO . . .

Pick up women; date out of your league; choose the perfect gift; tell if she digs you; give her a great massage; use your manners; pass her Google exam; make the first move; deliver a hot French kiss; make her your centerfold; buy lingerie; argue and win; read her signals; survive the spoon; speak her language; and understand hormones.

Chapter 7: Work 157

HOW TO . . .

Train your boss like a dog; give an award-winning presentation; find the safest stall in the men's room; ask for a raise; outsmart your office rival; master the art of small talk; bounce back from a screwup; land the best seat on an airplane; write a kick-ass recommendation; score a hotel upgrade; spin a pen in your fingers; land a job by voicemail; know when to shut up; raise your profile at work; drink with the boss and remain employed; work a room; and retire rich.

Chapter 8: Eat like a Man 175

HOW TO . . .

Make incredible French toast; crack an egg with one hand; MacGyver a walnut; roll your own sushi; cook like a subcontractor; steam the perfect lobster; grow your own salsa; cook the perfect burger and pasta; pan-sear a juicy steak; make chicken soup from scratch; cook a turkey in a trash can; spring-clean your grill; mix incredible sangria; burn your tongue with real Texas chili; shuck an oyster with a screwdriver; roll the perfect burrito; and make to-die-for guacamole.

Chapter 9: How to Win at Everything ... 199

HOW TO . . .

Kick butkus in flag football; win an argument; rule a pool table; win a bar fight; punt a football high and deep; pull off an epic April Fools' joke; triumph in arm wrestling; beat a speeding ticket; win at Scrabble; shred air guitar; learn a great bar trick; blast clay pigeons out of the sky; dominate pub darts; improve your golf score; be a foosball wizard; ace your fantasy football draft; bowl more strikes; win your date a stuffed bunny; crash the front row of a concert; score a spot on a game show; and pick stocks that soar.

Chapter 10: Your Cave ... 227

HOW TO . . .

Break into your own home; paint a room; build a workbench; thaw frozen water pipes; hang drywall; declog a sink; fix a lawn mower; build a kegerator; split a log; stack firewood; replace a door; drown slugs; build a tree house; kick squirrels out of your house; build a crib for Cujo; move furniture like a pro; clean up a grime scene; and craft an Adirondack chair out of an old pallet.

Chapter 11: Big Fun ... 259

HOW TO . . .

Rig a rope swing; build your own water park; teach your dog to fetch a beer from the fridge; build ladder golf; carve a smashing pumpkin; fly a stunt kite; teach your dog to play dead; host an epic poker game; paddle a dragon boat; earn your pilots' wings; dig a horseshoe pit; build a backyard ice rink; scare the hell out of trick-or-treaters; carve an ice sculpture; shred a terrain park; and plan the perfect getaway.

Thanks to Everyone In the Trenches ... 284

Photo and Illustration Credits ... 285

Index ... 286

Introduction

How to Know Everything About Anything

Do you know it all?

I didn't think so. And that makes you pretty smart, according to Socrates, who said:

"The only true wisdom is knowing you know nothing."

When I first read that line, it made me feel a lot better about my ignorance. The older I get, the more often I encounter experiences that demonstrate how very little I really know.

Talking with my teenage daughters, for example.

But there are many, many other instances where I've felt that "I should really know how to do this" only because I'm a man and men are suppose to know this stuff. Stuff like calculating a pitcher's earned run average (it's earned runs divided by innings pitched x 9), changing spark plugs, or hanging drywall. Have you ever tried to hang drywall on a ceiling? It's not easy unless you're privy to a critical carpenter's trick. I wasn't when our upstairs shower leaked in the house and the water soaked the ceiling of the downstairs half-bath. The drywall swelled, then burst, creating a real mess. I called a plumber to fix the leak, but since it's a smallish bathroom, I figured I could replace the ceiling with new drywall myself. How hard could it be? I removed the soggy bits, yanked out the old nails, cut new Sheetrock to fit, and then called my Uncle Rog to give me a hand.

Rog pressed the Sheetrock against the floor joists as I drove in drywall screws. That was a plan, at least. It didn't work so well. The drywall was larger and heavier than I had anticipated, and it sagged even though Uncle Rog spread his hands wide and I used my free hand to hold up one end. As the blood rushed from our outstretched arms, our hands became numb and useless. And we laughed, which made everything much worse.

"We need more hands," I laughed. "Or . . . a deadman," Rog said. "We should have made a deadman."

In carpentry parlance, a deadman is a T-shaped brace made from scrap lumber that leans against a wall and supports the drywall ceiling on one end so you can fasten the other end.

I had never heard of a deadman before, but this tidbit of uncommon knowledge made all the difference. We nailed together a deadman, and my new ceiling went up in minutes without a hitch.

When it comes to hanging overhead drywall, I know next to nothing. But at least now I know what a deadman is and how to construct one, and I can manage to use one right. And now you know, too, or you will when you turn to page 237.

I think that's what Socrates had in mind: No one is an expert at everything, especially guys like me who didn't have an older brother or a father who liked to tinker with hammers/cars/guns/electronics/musical instruments/baseball bats/etc.

The point is that there's so much to know and so much we do not know. A wise guy is one who realizes this and embraces it. A smart man will keep his mouth shut—or not attempt to hang drywall overhead—until he has gathered the facts and explored the empirical evidence to know what he's talking about.

A wise man admits, "I don't have a friggin' clue, so I will find out."

Men's Health magazine was founded on that notion more than 25 years ago by a bunch of guys who weren't too proud to admit that they didn't know jack shit about staying healthy, keeping fit, grooming or dressing themselves, reducing stress in their lives, wooing women, cooking a decent meal, training pets, rearing children, and about a zillion other things a guy should know how to do. So they set out to learn and then to pass that learning on to tens of millions of readers in, now, 60 countries.

Over the years this "uncommon knowledge" has appeared in various places in *Men's Health*—in sections titled Malegrams, How to Do Everything Better, Advantage, Real Life, and, yup, Uncommon Knowledge—reported and written by a slew of people who possess the curiosity to search for the uncommon answers to uncommon questions and present them in a way that is useful and fun to read. This book is an amalgamation of many of those tips, hints, tricks, and strategies curated to provide you with the ultimate handbook for navigating life's challenges and opportunities with skill and swagger like you know what you're doing.

There's tons of useful stuff inside—check out "What's Inside . . . " on page v. Then go sit under a shady tree and start reading. You'll become a better, smarter, more useful man almost instantly.

Jeff Csatari
Executive Editor
Men's Health Books

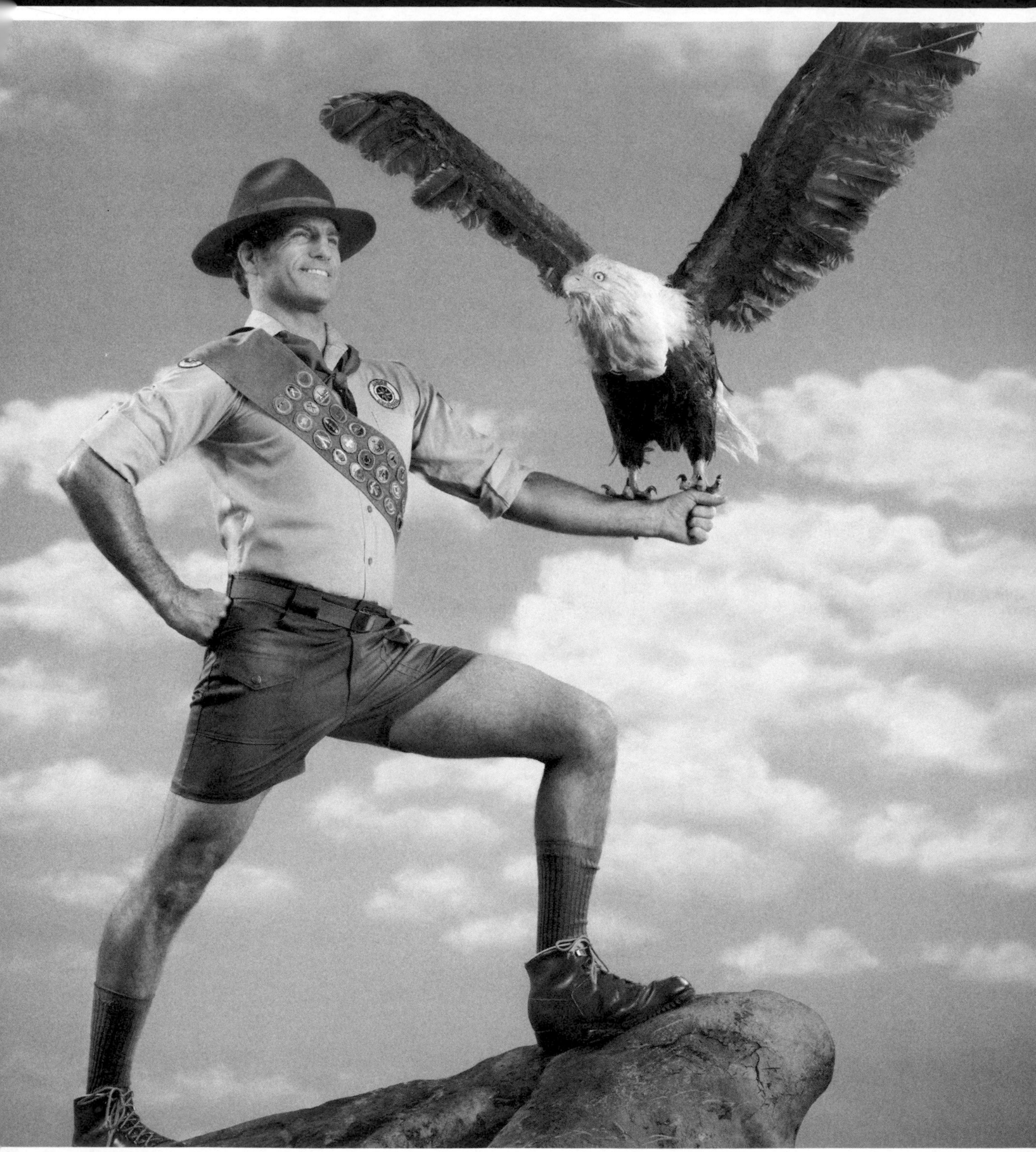

100 Things Every Man Should Know

You Don't Have to Be an Expert. Just Act Like One.

You are expected to know and do certain things in life simply by virtue of having an X and a Y chromosome and the critical SRY gene on the tip of your Y that turned you into a boy way back when. Important things like breaking in a baseball mitt or launching a snot rocket, and dead-serious stuff like handling a chain saw or delivering a moving eulogy. This is not to say that females shouldn't know how to do these things, too. But when you're a man (or want to become a better one), these are required skills. Need to learn quickly how to cradle a baby, make a toast, troubleshoot a car engine, flirt more effectively, or tie a trucker's hitch (not related to flirting)? You're in a good place. We begin *Men's Health: The Big Book of Uncommon Knowledge* with a chapter of critical guy wisdom—hints, tips, tricks, and secrets that'll help you embrace life with skill, confidence, and a little more moxie than you had yesterday.

HOW TO OPEN BOTTLED BEER WITHOUT A BOTTLE OPENER

Use your keys. Choose the longest key on your keychain. Grab the bottle around the neck with your left hand, allowing the neck of the bottle to extend above your index finger and thumb. Align the shaft of the key so that the left edge is just under the cap of the bottle. The tip of the key should lie across the bottom half of your left index finger. Tip: The key should extend far enough onto your left finger that you don't pierce your skin. While levering off your left index finger, use your right hand to pop the top off of the bottle.

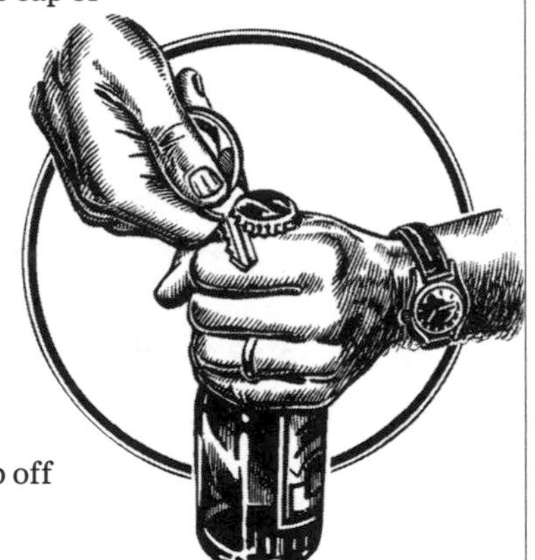

How to Drag an Unconscious Person Out of a Fire

If you need to get an unconscious person out of a dangerous place and he's too heavy to lift, tie his wrists together with your necktie or a piece of sheet and loop your head through his arms. Use your body weight to back him out of harm's way. Step two: Rehearse your "I'm-no-hero" line for the local papers.

RULE #1 **Never put on bagpipe music at a party.**

HOW TO BREAK IN A *Baseball Glove*

Atlanta Braves outfielder Jonny Gomes says the leather of a new glove is too stiff for diving catches. With this method, heat and moisture soften the leather fast.

1. Fill a mug with water and microwave it on high for 30 seconds. Now place your glove in the microwave with the water and nuke both for another 30 seconds.

2. Remove the glove and sit in a chair holding an "uncupped" baseball bat (that is, one with a rounded top) between your knees. Repeatedly slam the glove's pocket onto the top of the bat. Do this 20 to 30 times, until a deep recess forms.

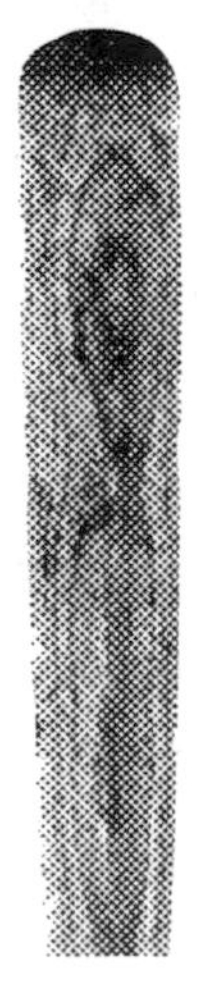

Bonus:

Repair sun damage: If your glove's leather has gone crispy, rub in shaving cream that contains lanolin, a moisturizer. (Try Barbasol Beard Buster Skin Conditioner.) Let it dissolve and wipe off excess.

Spin a Basketball on Your Finger

Practice these steps for at least 6 minutes a day. Within a week you'll stop wobbling and start wowing, says Joseph Odhiambo, the world record holder for fingertip basketball spinning.

1. Do Some Prep

Deflate the ball slightly. This creates more surface area touching your finger, making the ball easier to control.

2. Set Up Your Spin

Hold the ball (seams vertical) with your dominant hand on the far side and your other hand on the side facing you. Keep your elbows bent and tucked close to your body. The ball should be about 4 inches from your chin.

3. Let 'Er Rip

Snap both wrists to start the ball spinning; slower is better at first. The seams should pass by without wobbling. Quickly catch the ball with the pad of your index finger. Count to one. Then try again until you can last for a count of two, then three, and so on. Be sure to stop when you reach each count; this helps build confidence and control.

4. Keep It Up

In 8 seconds, the ball will slow. Bend your finger slightly toward you and try to move the ball to your fingernail, keeping your elbow tucked to your body. This reduces friction between ball and finger, helping maintain spin. Now start lightly batting the ball with all four fingers of your free hand. Whistle "Sweet Georgia Brown."

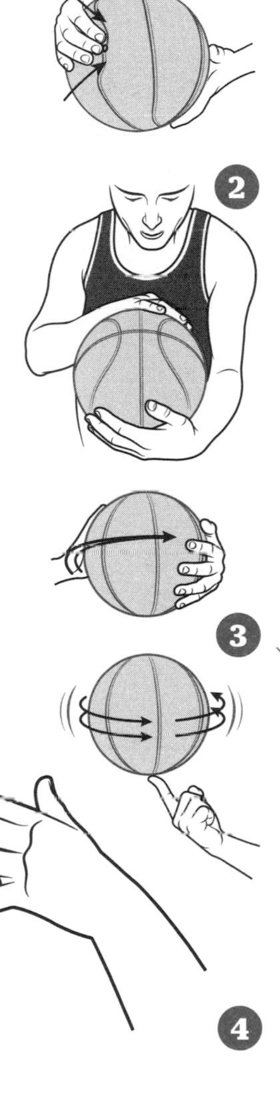

How to Pick Up the Check

The more discreet you are about your act of generosity, the classier you'll look, says etiquette expert Diane Gottsman. Quietly hand your credit card to the host or server when you first enter the restaurant. If you miss your chance, wait until the server delivers the check, reach for it casually, and slip your card in without stopping the conversation. Don't worry about looking the bill over for errors—you can take a copy and do that later. If your guest offers to chip in, wave him or her off once, but if he or she presses further, accept. "Don't let it become a tug-of war," says Gottsman.

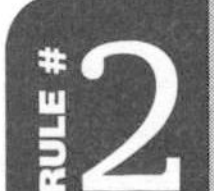

Never underline passages in a book someone has loaned you, especially sex passages.

BLOCK A HAYMAKER

IF YOU CAN'T BACK AWAY FROM A FIGHT, PROTECT YOURSELF. BOXING TRAINER SAM COLONNA AND 2004 OLYMPIC LIGHT-HEAVYWEIGHT GOLD MEDALIST ANDRE "SON OF GOD" WARD SAVE YOUR BUTT.

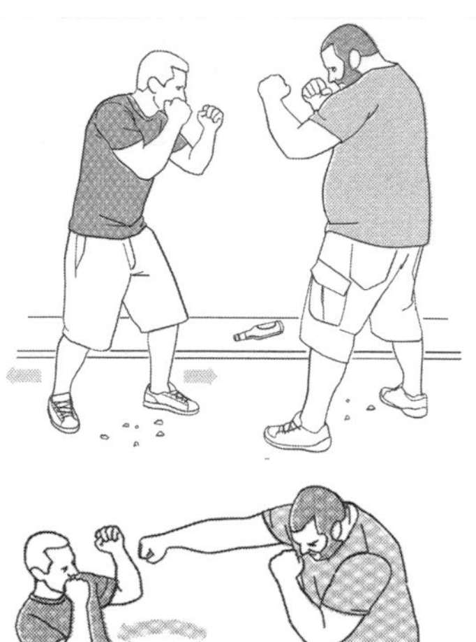

1. Set Your Defense

Strike a slim profile so you'll be harder to hit. Stand sideways, knees bent slightly and legs 2 feet apart. Have your left leg forward if you're right-handed; reverse the stance if you're a southpaw.

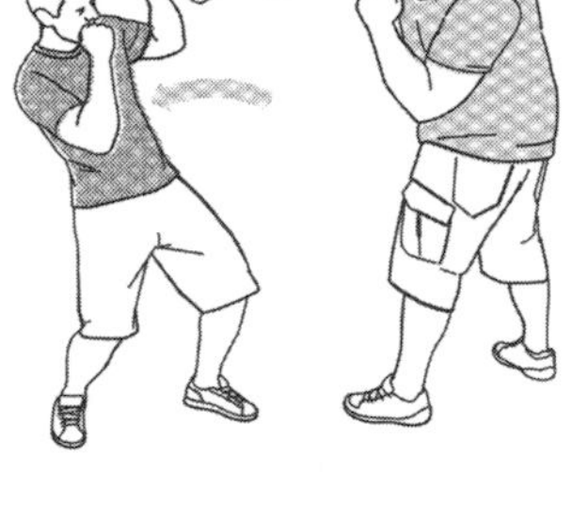

2. Put 'Em Up, Keep 'Em Up

With your chin down, keep your arms in front of you, knuckles facing upward and fists loosely clenched. Tuck your elbows to your ribs. If you're a righty, your right hand should be beside your right cheek and your left hand 5 inches in front of your left cheekbone. Now you're set up to deflect a punch and counter with your own.

3. Find an Escape

Don't be baited into losing your cool. Keep your opponent at arm's length to avoid a jab, and back toward an exit.

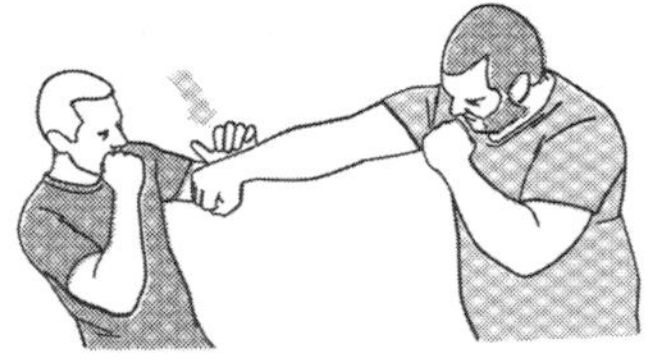

4. Intercept an Assault

No escape? Deflect a punch by slapping it away with your open palm. Reset your defense and use your forearms to fend off additional punches, using your upper body to push your opponent's fists away.

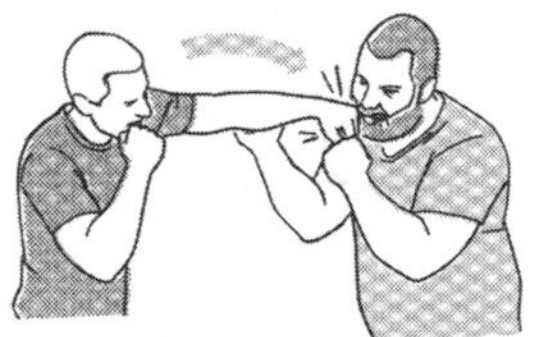

5. Follow Through

If you see an opening, strike with a jab that lands between his chin and ear. Rotate your hips for power and connect with the knuckles of your index and middle fingers. You'll leave him stunned.

RULE # 3

Make your best tip the first one of the night, not your last (you'll get a clean glass for sure).

Play Harmonica

Piano is hard; harmonica is easy. All you need is a starter's harp—the Hohner Special 20, key of C—a sense of rhythm, and patient friends. Right is up the scale, left is down. Match a simple song, breathing with the beat. Once you master "Midnight Rambler," it's okay to don shades and stomp your feet.

How to Cradle a Baby

WITH EIGHT KIDS OF HIS OWN, BILL SEARS, MD, COAUTHOR OF *THE BABY BOOK*, SWEARS BY THE FOOTBALL HOLD TO KEEP A BAMBINO QUIET IN YOUR ARMS.

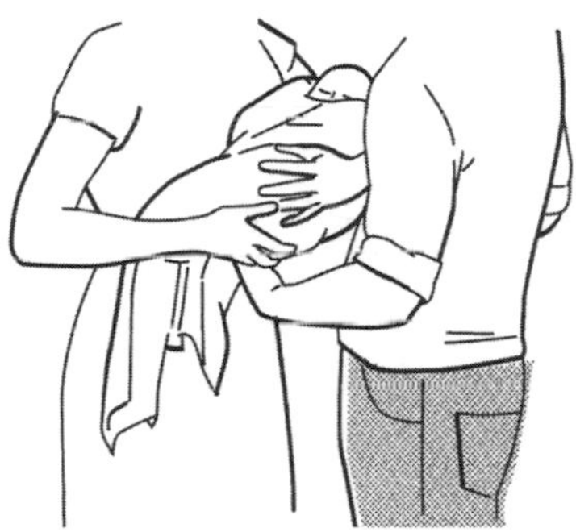

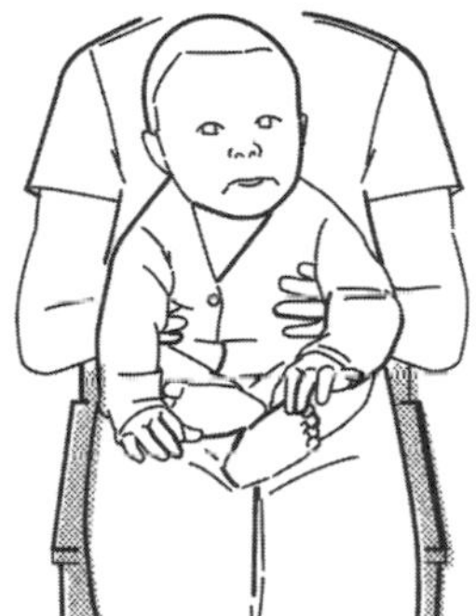

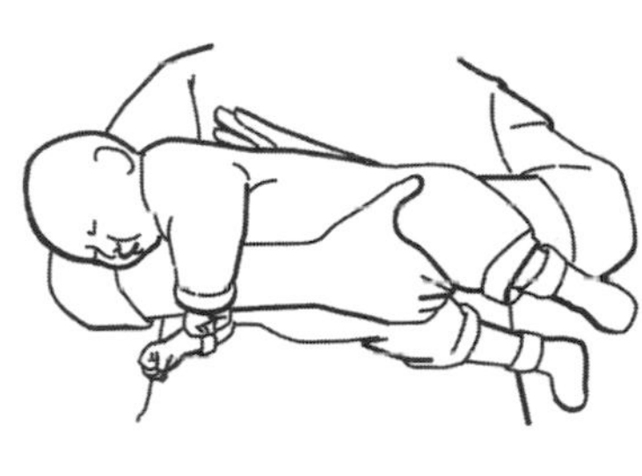

A. Run the Handoff

Stand with your arms cradled in front of your torso so the person with the baby won't have to extend his or her arms. Slip your dominant hand under the infant's head (to provide neck support) and the other under his hips, lifting toward you.

B. Ease Up

Babies often cry while being held because they're uncomfortable. The most common problem: They're being held too tightly. If the baby seems antsy, loosen your grip slightly—you should feel the child's tensed abdomen relax.

C. Soothe Sobs

Sit and gently turn the baby so that his stomach lies along your dominant hand's forearm and his head rests in the crook of your arm. Support the leg on top with your hand. Your forearm's pressure helps him relax his body.

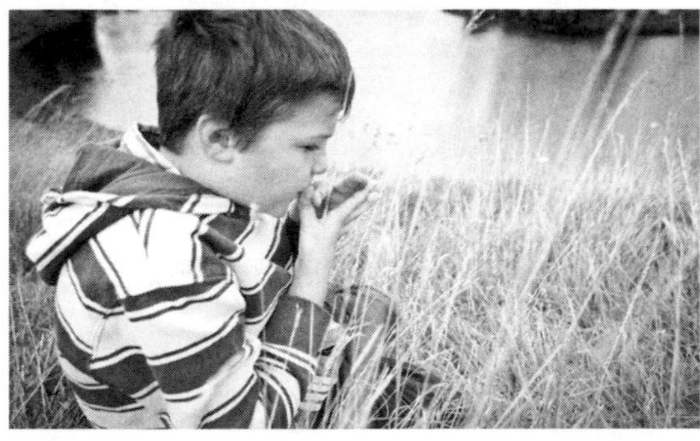

Teach Your Kid How to Play a Blade of Grass

First master it yourself. Pick a blade of grass that's 3 or 4 inches long and about a quarter inch wide. Put your palms together and your thumbs side-by-side, holding the grass blade between them in the middle of the gap between your thumbs. The blade should be taut. Now purse your lips, press them over the gap, and blow gently. The grass will vibrate, creating a loud, squeaky sound. Experiment with changing the pitch by moving the tips of your thumbs forward and back.

RULE # 4 **If you want to be a good father, be a good husband first.**

Know the Parts of an *Over-and-Under Shotgun*

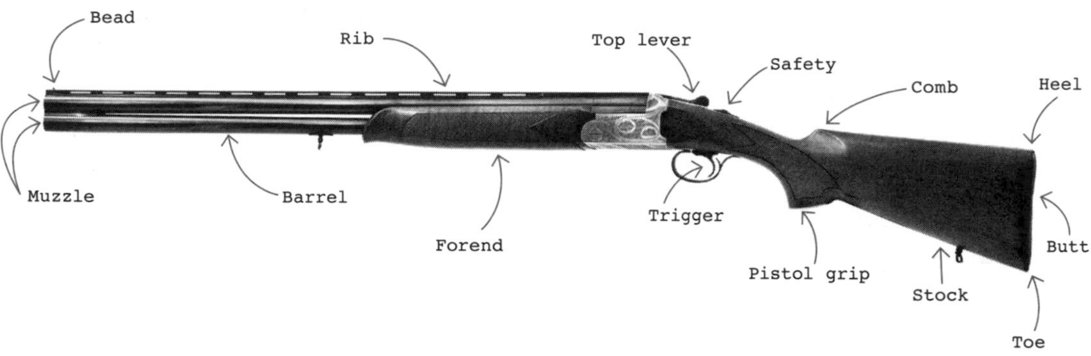

HOW TO OCCUPY A TODDLER FOR 2 HOURS

It's your sister's kid or your buddy's. You offered. So here's how to be a babysitting hero.

1. Break the Ice

Ask him about his favorite books or characters. Have him explain the character. You'll be as entertained as he will. The focus should always be on the child, so resist the urge to match his interests with your own superhero obsessions.

2. Head Outside

Be silly and imaginative. Go searching for leprechauns or fairies. (Remember that toddlers have poor balance, so watch the tyke carefully.) Or take a bowl of water and a paintbrush and "paint" on the sidewalk. The kid will love seeing the art evaporate in the sun before doing it again. This is good for at least 15 or 20 minutes.

3. Act Out a Bit

After you've worn the kid out, grab a picture book; reading is a great brain-building experience. But spice things up by using props. A story about a knight comes to life when you re-create the scene by making a castle out of couch cushions, chairs, and sheets.

RULE # 5

Women love to dance.

RULE # 6

Learn to dance.

How to Keep a Beer Bottle from Sticking to a Coaster

Sprinkle some salt on the coaster, and the bottle won't pick up the mat when you pick up the bottle. Marylanders use Old Bay.

How to Keep Your Edge (on Any Knife)

Use a natural Hard Arkansas Sharpening Stone. Put a liberal amount of honing oil on it. Turn the blade of the knife toward you and bring the knife across the stone in a circular motion, about a half-moon. Reverse it to sharpen the other side. The angle is the most important part, and you learn the right one by feel. Too flat and you'll wear down the side of the blade. Too much and you'll dull the edge. Wipe off the metal slurry and inspect the burr—that's the edge where the metal has folded over the apex or V of the blade. If you have burr from the knife's tip to heel, it's time to turn the blade over and sharpen the other side. Then work each side evenly until you have a razor's edge.

PARALLEL PARK—ANYWHERE

Russ Swift, owner of Russ Swift Precision Driving, set a record for parallel parking in the tightest space. Use his tips to score a personal best for speed and accuracy.

1. First, assess the spot. Pull up nearly alongside the space so your car's rear bumper lines up with the back car's front bumper. If you see 4 feet to spare ahead of you, then you can make it. Pull beside the front car, leaving about 18 inches between the doors; stop when your back bumper is about 2 feet ahead of the other car's back end.
2. For a spot on the right side of the street, look over your right shoulder; back up straight until your rear bumper clears the other car's rear bumper. Crank the wheel to the curb. Left side? Look over your left shoulder.
3. After your front bumper clears the car in front, straighten out your vehicle, ideally 3 inches from the curb. Now hop out of the car and execute a celebratory fist pump.

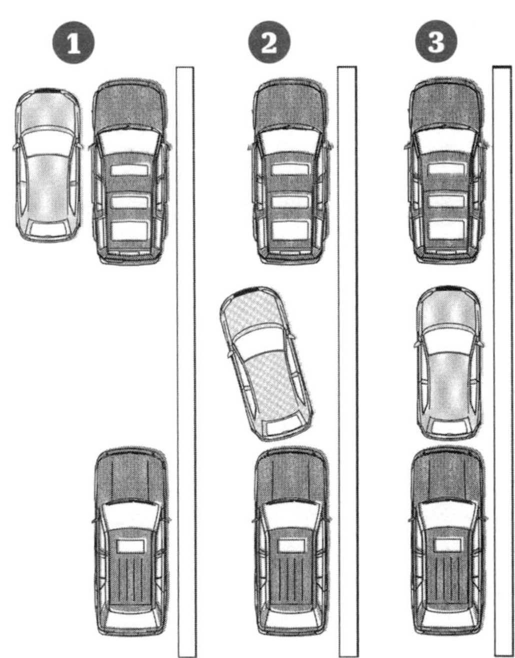

Slide a Beer Down the Bar

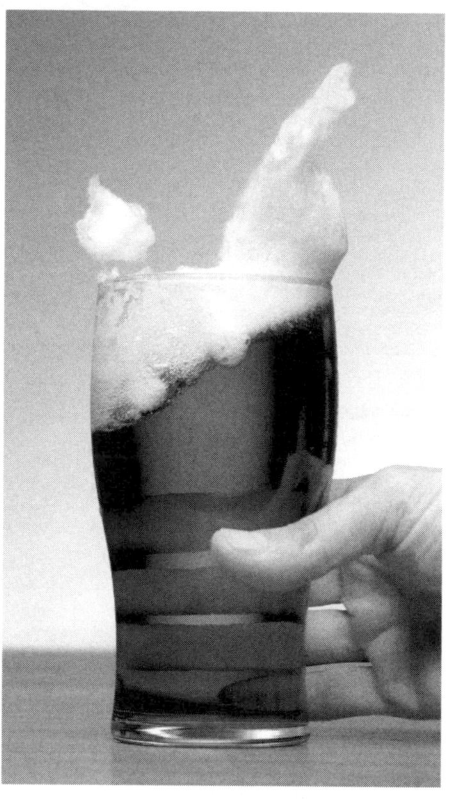

1. Prepare the Platform

If you're out at a pub, check the bar surface. A heavily lacquered wooden bar with a slippery sheen—and without pits or chips—works best. If it's your own basement bar, slick up the surface by hitting it with glass cleaner or wood polish.

2. Use a Bottom-Heavy Glass

You want a 16-ounce pint glass. Its solid base gives the glass a low center of gravity—essential for preventing a tip-over. Don't try this with a goblet, pilsner glass, or any other slender or top-heavy glassware.

3. Don't Fill It Too High

The glass should be about three-quarters full; that amount of liquid will weigh down the bottom half of the glass to give it more support as it travels. Any more could cause toppling. (Practice with water, lest you spill perfectly good beer.)

4. Send It Flying

Stand parallel to the bar, arm's length away. Wrap your hand around the bottom third of the glass. In a smooth, sweeping motion, gently push the glass toward your pal with little or no spin to keep the flight path on point. Now watch it slide . . .

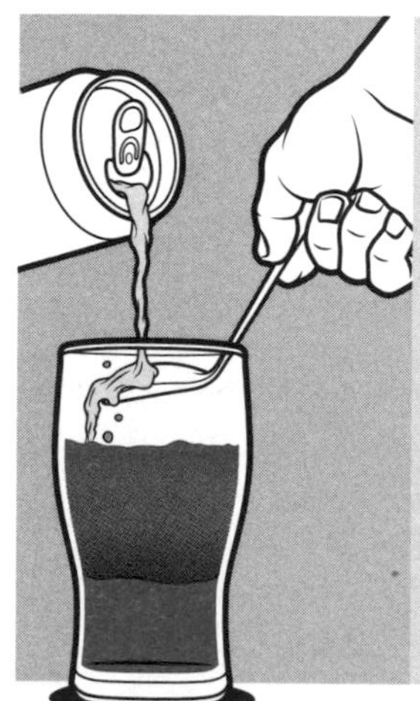

How to Pour a Black & Tan

There's a craft to pouring a black & tan that separates into two layers, and a large spoon and the right glass are key, says Adam Wells, bartender at Brendan Behan Pub in Boston. Start with a 20-ounce Guinness pub glass—its curve and big size make fitting the spoon in easier. Fill it halfway with Bass Pale Ale. Bend an old spoon 90 degrees, convex side up, and hold the spoon above the pale ale you just poured. Open a tall widget can of Guinness and pour it slowly and evenly on the spoon, pulling up as you go. If your two beers are the same temperature, they'll separate perfectly into two layers and you'll taste both in every sip.

Know Two Unbeatable Touch-Football Plays

When the boys from across the tracks challenge your buddies to touch or tackle, scribble these two plays in the dirt. They work for five- or six-man teams.

Lineman on the left takes four steps and cuts right. Guy to the right of the center goes 15 yards straight and curls over the middle. The halfback closest to the QB runs a post to the left corner of the field while the far halfback goes long, straight up the field. If the center can hold off the defender long enough, someone should be open for the pass.

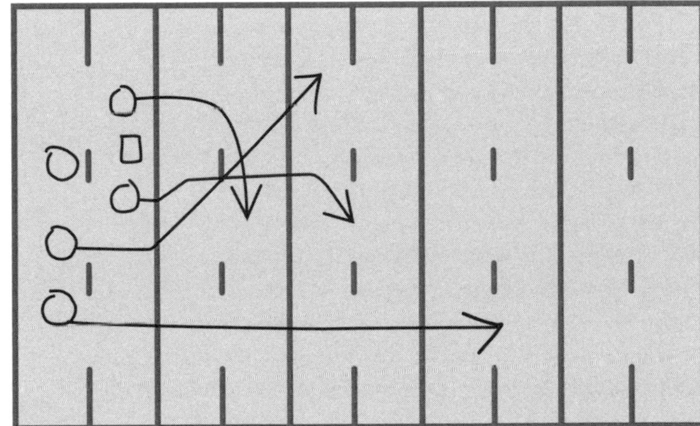

This one's called Lefty's Deceiver, and it has to happen quickly. As soon as the QB takes the snap, he pitches it to the halfback to his left, who runs right. Meanwhile, the player on the far right of the line runs a down-and-out. The halfback hits him with a bullet, or if he's covered, runs it upfield.

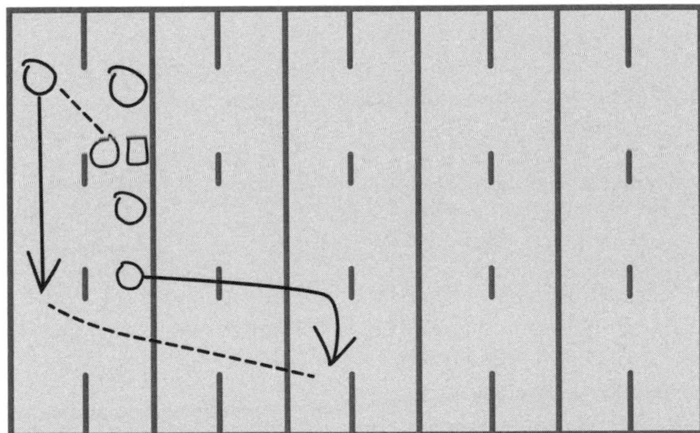

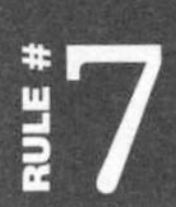

* The team that makes the fewest mistakes will win.

* Play for and make the breaks, and when one comes your way—SCORE.

The first two of Gen. Robert Neyland's "Seven Maxims of Football," which are recited by the University of Tennessee Vols football team before every game.

Own a *Signature Drink*

A beer works for almost any occasion, but when you're celebrating something special or your buddy's buying, it's nice to have a go-to classic cocktail, one with fewer than five ingredients. Care to try ours, the Sazerac?

This classic rye cocktail was originally a cognac drink invented in the 1830s by New Orleans native Antoine Peychaud, an apothecary owner best known for his bitters recipe, which to this day is a staple in most bartenders' arsenals.

Creating a Sazerac is simple . . . but not necessarily easy. Its preparation is a ritual for many devotees, and there are many ways to make it. Some recipes call for simple syrup; others use sugar cubes. Rye is the most common base spirit, but bourbon or cognac is fine if that's your preference. It's okay to use Herbsaint (an anise-flavored liqueur) instead of absinthe. But if you want to call your cocktail a Sazerac, there are a few rules you must abide by:

1. Never shake your Sazerac. Always stir.
2. Do not drop the lemon-peel twist into the drink. Hang it on the rim. (It is the drinker's choice to drop it in.)
3. Do not serve it with ice. Stir it with ice and strain it into a chilled glass.

The drink itself is a sophisticated, civilized affair. The absinthe rinse gives the cocktail a good dose of its herbal scent and more than a hint of its strong flavor. The bitters balances out the sugar, making it a well-rounded, complex-tasting cocktail that's reminiscent of a Manhattan but is still in a league of its own.

Our Sazerac recipe is courtesy of Marvin Allen, head barkeep at the Carousel Bar in the Hotel Monteleone in New Orleans. So you can bet this is indeed the real deal. Adieu!

The Sazerac

WHAT YOU'LL NEED:

2 ounces rye (such as Sazerac, or bourbon or cognac)

¼ ounce absinthe (such as Lucid)

4 or 5 drops Peychaud's bitters

½ teaspoon simple syrup

HOW TO MAKE IT:

Fill an 8-ounce rocks glass with a few ice cubes and add the absinthe, twirling to coat the glass. Set aside. In a Boston shaker add the Sazerac, Peychaud's bitters, and simple syrup. Stir (don't shake) until well chilled. Empty the rocks from the glass; it should have a thin coating of the absinthe. Strain the chilled contents of the shaker into the reserved absinthe-coated glass. Garnish with a lemon twist. Sit back and enjoy a taste of New Orleans history.

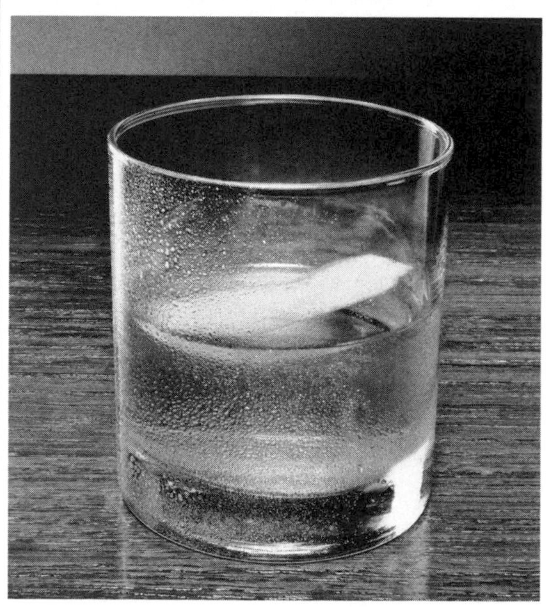

Avoid the Bait and Switch

Buy seafood from a fishmonger. DNA tests show that many fish sold in grocery stores and restaurants are mislabeled. To prevent getting hooked by the bait and switch, catch your seafood at a reputable local fishmonger. And download the Monterey Bay Aquarium Seafood Watch app (free for iPhone or Android) to locate restaurants that offer responsibly sourced seafood.

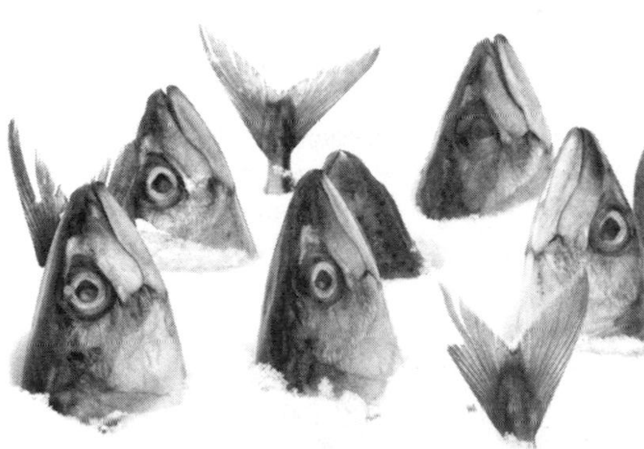

RULE # 8

Leave some food on your plate. The average china plate has enlarged 23 percent in the past century, which means we've been misjudging portion sizes since World War I.

How to Survive a Date in a Room Full of Women

Whether it's a first date, the thirtieth, or even if you've been married for 10 years, it comes down to this simple rule: Stay focused on her and never let your attention become distracted by the shape of another woman. Tip: When you're at a restaurant, always sit with your back to the room. Let *her* face out toward the crowd. That way, you'll avoid eyeing other women—that old moth-attracted-to-a-flame reflex that however innocent can annoy her to no end. Eliminate the threat of this ruining your date. Doing so will make it easier to give her your complete and rapt attention. Or you could just have your eyeballs removed.

Make a Dinner Toast

You will be called upon to do this on many occasions in life, so have a system at the ready because "I'm so drunk" is a bad start. Use this plan from Gary Schmidt, a past president of Toastmasters International.

Start

Don't stand up; that's for formal occasions. Just wait for a natural break in conversation before the meal is served. Then lift your glass and say, "I'd like to make a toast."

Talk

Think of a single word that summarizes the topic of your speech, something like "congratulate," "remember," or "honor." Keep it in mind as you talk to stay focused; you never want to be the guy who gives a long, meandering speech.

Stop

A toast can be a couple of sentences or last a minute or two, tops. After that, you're boring your audience.

Let the saw do the work.

50 TOOLS FOR EVERY TASK

With the following selection of basic hand tools in your garage (and the right know-how) you can build or fix almost any that needs building or fixing around your house. **Hint:** You can build this inventory of great tools at a fraction of the retail cost by hunting Saturday morning yard sales.

Adjustable Wrench
Allen Wrench
Angle Sash "Cut-In" Paintbrush
Ax or Splitting Maul
Bow Rake
Bow Saw
Center Punch
Circular Saw
Combination Square
Coping Saw
Cordless Drill
Drill bits
Duct Tape
Dust Mask
Earmuffs with 23 to 33 noise reduction rating (NNR)
Electrician's Pliers
Extension Cord (10-gauge contractor's quality)
Extension Ladder
Flashlight
Gooseneck Crowbar
Hacksaw
Hammer
Hand Saw
Laser Level
Level
Locking Pliers
Metal File
Metal Snips
Nail Set
Needle Nose Pliers
Pipe Snake
Pipe Wrench
Pocketknife or Multi-Tool
Pry Bar
Putty Knife
Orbital Sander
Reciprocating Saw
Rope (50 feet)
Round Nose Shovel
Safety Glasses
Screwdriver Set
Sledgehammer
Socket Wrench Set
Stud Finder
Square Nose Shovel
Tape Rule
Tongue-and-Groove Pliers
Wheel Barrow
Wood Chisel
Utility Knife

Fell a Tree

If you do this right, the tree won't fall on your house or bind your chain saw. First, figure out which way you want the tree to fall, ideally toward an open space, and not on your neighbor's aboveground pool.

Got it? Now make a horizontal cut about knee high to waist high on the side of the trunk where you want the tree to fall (1). Stop about two-thirds of the way through the trunk and pull out your saw. Next, cut a 60-degree angle down to the first cut until the wedge falls out (2). That notch should face the direction of the fall. Important safety note: Make sure you have a place to run away from the fall in back of the tree. It should be clear of other trees and brush. Now, get ready for the final cut. Start the back cut horizontally and slightly above the V notch (3). As soon as the tree starts to lean, pull out the saw and follow your escape route, yelling *TIMBER!,* and hopefully not, *Oh shit!*

2
3
60°
1

RULE # 10

Anything that comes in a shell is a bad thing to order on a first date: crabs, lobsters, snails, tacos, peanuts, gunpowder.

Change Your Spark Plugs

Save up to $150 by doing this yourself, says Cenek Picka of the Advanced Technology Institute. Check your owner's manual to see which plugs you need and when to change them. Replace them one at a time to ensure proper firing order.

Blast Away the Crud

With your engine completely cool, use compressed air to blow away dirt or debris around each spark plug. This reduces the risk of particles falling into the combustion chamber and causing major engine damage.

Clear Your Path

If your car has an older engine, the spark plug wires may be covered by rubber boots. The best way to remove the boots is with a boot puller, like the one from SummitRacing ($9, summitracing.com). Or you can remove a boot by twisting and pulling up on it. Never pull on the wires themselves.

If your car has a newer engine, coils are attached to the plugs. Pull back on the tab of each coil's harness, and then grab the coil and slowly pull up. You'll hear a pop of the vacuum seal breaking, and the coil should slide out. Don't use tools—they may snap the coil.

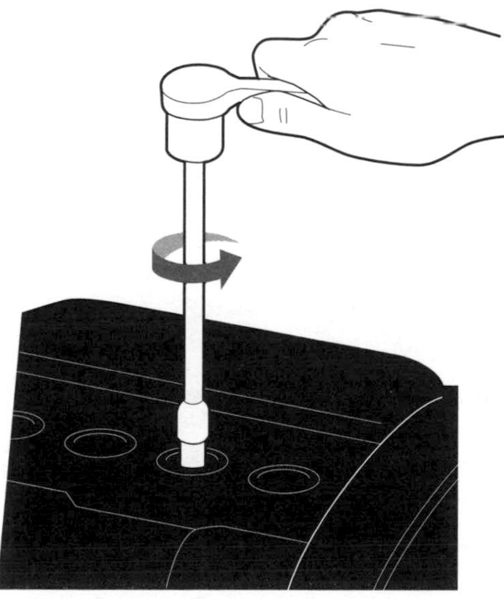

Remove the Plugs

Use a ratchet wrench, spark-plug socket, and extension to unscrew the plug. If the plug won't budge, it could be jammed. Put everything back together and take your car to the shop. You could damage the plug threads if you force it.

Set the Spark Plug's Gap

The space, or gap, between the two electrodes must be set for your engine. Use a gapping gauge to adjust the gap according to the figure in your owner's manual. The gap is correct when you pass the gauge between the electrodes and feel slight resistance.

Make the Swap

Apply a small amount of anti-seize lubricant, such as Permatex ($10, walmart.com) to the threads of the spark plug to prevent corrosion, and use the socket and extension to carefully insert the plug. Be careful not to bump the electrode. To avoid cross-threading, give the plug a twist in the opposite direction so the threads align and then hand tighten. Finish tightening with a torque wrench per your owner's manual. Reconnect the boots or coils.

RULE # 11 **Let the club do the work.**

Diagnose a "Check Engine" Light

When the little amber engine icon on your panel lights up, it's usually for a noncritical reason. (If the oil icon illuminates or your temperature gauge spikes, that's another story: Stop driving and have your car towed to a mechanic.) When you have to "check engine," you're most likely dealing with one of the three things below.

Culprit 1: A Loose Gas Cap

Your car detects air leaking from the fuel tank, something that can affect emissions. If the light comes on and there's no obvious engine trouble, check the cap, making sure you hear three clicks when you tighten it. (It may take several engine starts to make the light go away.)

Culprit 2: "Lean" Condition

This can result from too much air entering your engine. With the car running, check for hissing sounds in the vacuum hoses that enter the top of your engine. Once you pinpoint the leak, make sure the hose is properly seated on the port, or use oil-resistant tape to seal it.

Culprit 3: Old Spark Plugs

If the car's past 100,000 miles and the spark plugs or plug wires haven't been replaced, it might be time.

Run Your Own Diagnostic

Having your service tech read the engine code off your car's computer, which will ID the problem that triggered the light, could cost you about $75. For about the same price, you can buy your own OBD-II scanner. It'll tell you what the problem is and give you a shot at fixing it yourself. (It will also switch the light off.) We like the Actron PocketScan Code Reader ($85, actron.com).

3 WORDS TO LIVE BY

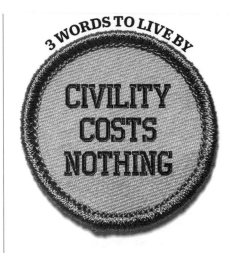

How to Instantly Earn the Respect of Anyone

Shake hands. Make your grip firm and confident, and pump no more than three times. Look the other person in the eye and smile.

Stand 3 to 4 feet away. This is the normal interacting distance. Closer and you'll make the other person uncomfortable. Farther away and you'll appear detached and disinterested,

Square off. Face the other person directly instead of standing slighting to the side. This suggests you're giving him or her your full attention.

Gesture. Occasionally extend your arms with the palms facing upward. This says you're being honest and have nothing threatening to hide.

Reach out and touch. If it's appropriate, punctuate or end the conversation with a pat on the shoulder or a touch on the arm. This connotes friendliness and warmth, especially if you're of a higher status. Be careful patting women, though. In fact, it's better not to touch them at all.

Calm an Angry Buddy

HOTHEADED COMEDIAN LEWIS BLACK TELLS YOU HOW TO KEEP YOUR FRIEND'S TEMPER IN CHECK.

1. Take It Outside
Dealing with someone who's about to blow his top is like walking a dog with a full bladder: You have to keep him moving to empty all of the contents. If your pal is fuming over a fumble by his team, coax him out of the house and into the yard, or from the bar to the sidewalk.

2. Make Him Yell
Telling him to calm down will only fire him up more. Angry men don't want to be told they're angry. So challenge him to yell louder. A few hearty primal screams can help stop his steaming. Better to have a few short bursts of rage than a whole day of frustrated stewing.

3. Buy Him a Drink
To help lend closure to the situation, invite him back inside with a round. But make it a scotch, not a beer. The better the booze, the slower he'll sip and the calmer he'll become. Before you know it, he'll have forgotten why he flew off the handle in the first place.

Pull Off the Two-Finger Whistle

PERFECT FOR SPORTS GAMES, CALLING YOUR FRIEND ACROSS THE STREET, OR HAILING YOUR HORSE

Step 1

Open your mouth and draw your lower lip tautly inward to cover the top of your lower teeth.

Step 2

Flatten your tongue and move it forward so that it hovers above the inside edge of your bottom lip.

Step 3

Touch the tips of your pinkie fingers together to form a 90-degree angle.

Step 4

Nails upward, insert the inverted V formed by your fingertips under the tip of your tongue. Roll the tip of your tongue upward and back slightly; it should curve up toward the front of the roof of your mouth, without touching.

Step 5

Take a deep breath and blow across the tip of your tongue. The harder you blow, the louder your whistle and the more people will look at you.

Source: Fred Newman, the author of MouthSounds *and the sound-effects man on* A Prairie Home Companion

RULE # 12

Pizza is generally a nutritious meal that derives 25 to 30 percent of its calories from fat—if you avoid meat toppings.

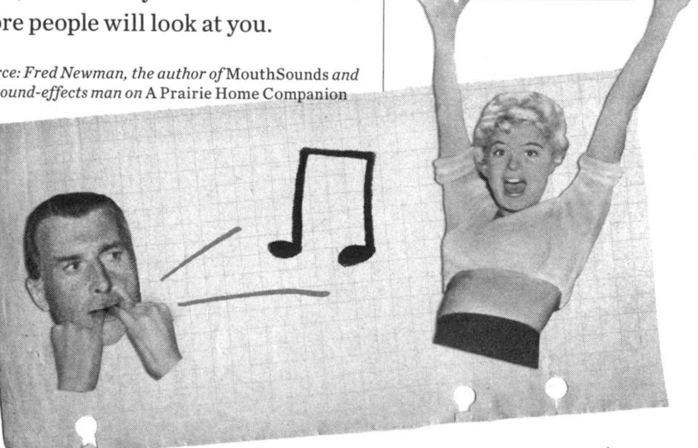

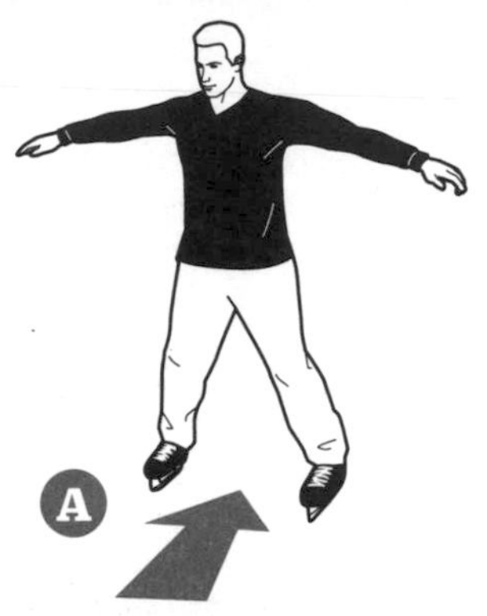

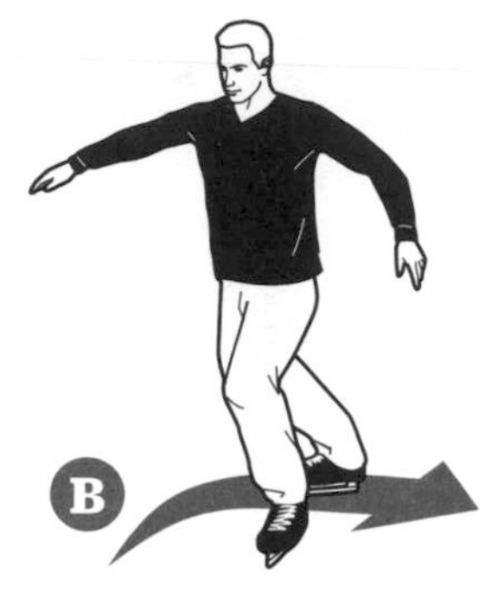

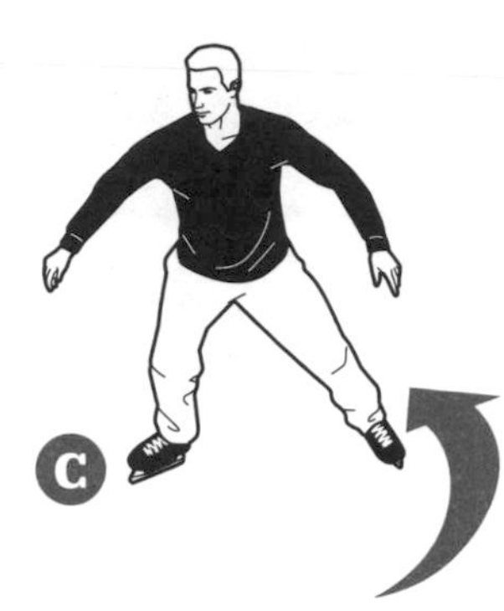

Ice-Skate Backward

Play better D during pickup hockey—or just impress your girl on a winter date.

Step 1: Stand Strong

Come to a stop. With your feet shoulder width apart, hold your arms out for balance (A). Bend your knees, which will help your hips provide push-off power.

Step 2: Build Momentum

Alternating your feet, start making slow, smooth cuts backward into the ice and slightly out to the side, turning your skates no more than 15 to 20 degrees from the path you want to travel. Squeeze your thighs together to bring your skates inward. Repeat.

Step 3: Stop—Or Spin

To slow and stop, put pressure on the inside edge of either boot and slowly drag it against the ice perpendicular to the direction you're moving (B). To turn around, bend your knees and rotate your shoulders against your hips. Then snap around by reversing that motion as you straighten your knees (C).

Source: Ryan Bradley, 2011 men's U.S. figure skating champion

---

RULE # 13

To avoid smashing your thumb with a hammer, use a comb instead of your fingers to hold a nail in place.

Launch a SNOT ROCKET

GROSS? YES. BUT FAR LESS NASTY THAN USING YOUR SLEEVE WHILE RUNNING.

STEP 1: Test the Launch

If you try this without enough buildup, you risk an epic fail. Lightly inhale through each nostril. Can't breathe comfortably? You're ready to blow.

STEP 2: Test Aim and Fire

In one swift motion, seal the opposite nostril tightly with the pad of your finger, rotate your hips and shoulders toward the direction of fire, inhale through and then close your mouth, and finally exhale in one swift blast through your nose. Now breathe easy.

Source: Zachary Soler, MD, of the Medical University of South Carolina; Donald Buraglio, blogger at runningandrambling.com

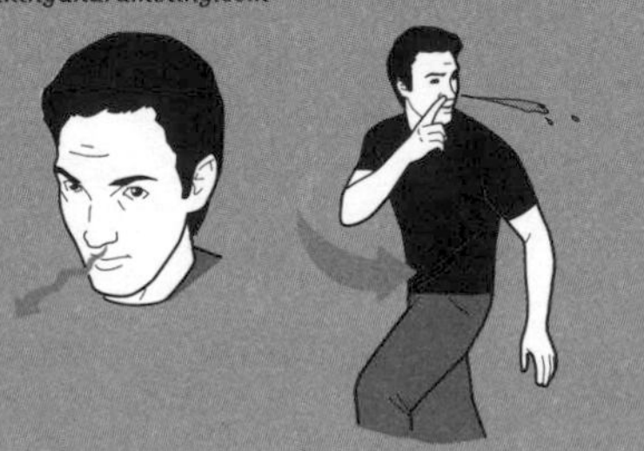

Throw a Wicked Curveball

Leave batters befuddled with this classic breaking ball, with tips from Austin Faught, former Division I All-American pitcher and current head coach at the University of Pitching.

Command the Mound

As in golf, your stance should be perpendicular to the path your ball will travel in order for you to derive the most power. Stand on the mound, feet shoulder width apart, and point your toes toward third or first base, depending on your stance. Align your front hip with home plate.

Grip It to Rip It

Rest the middle and index fingers of your throwing hand along the relatively straight part of the seams of the ball. Put your thumb on the ball's other side, pointed up toward the tip of your middle finger. Tuck your ring finger and pinkie beside the ball for support and spin.

Adjust Your Eyes

Most rookies aim too high. This can cause the ball to travel upward first, which fails to trick the guy at bat. Instead, drive the pitch toward the catcher's mask. That way the ball flies straight until the last second, when it breaks into the bottom portion of the strike zone.

Prime the Pitch

Wind up as normal, but at the release point your throwing elbow needs to be above your throwing shoulder, and that shoulder above your glove-side shoulder. Flat shoulders cause sidespin, which counteracts the topspin of your curve and can result in a sloppy pitch.

Throw the Hook

As you bring the ball over your shoulder, maintain your grip until the ball is pointed toward the catcher's mask. Release it with your pitching hand's palm facing inward, snapping your wrist as you release. Both feet should land with toes toward home—and the poor batter.

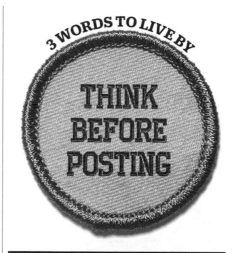

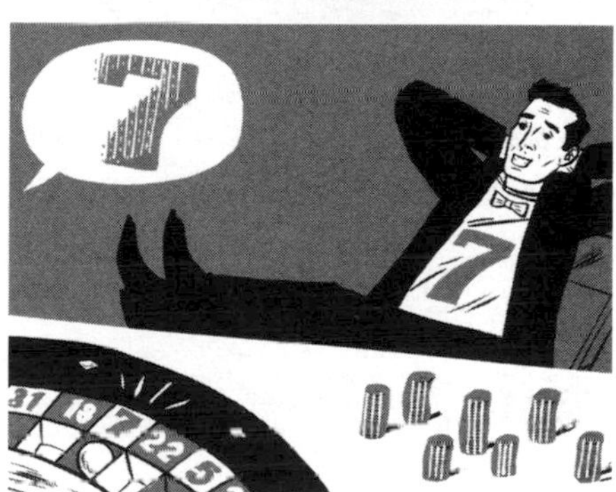

3 WORDS TO LIVE BY
THINK
BEFORE
POSTING

Blow $100 in a Casino

Why prolong your misery by losing on penny-ante games? Go out like a high roller: Hit the roulette table and put it all on one number, says Robert Hannum, PhD, a professor of risk analysis and gaming at University of Denver. "You'll win the straight-up bet on a single number in roulette once every 38 times," he says. So the odds offer a 35-to-1 payout of $3,500. To stretch out your play, bet in $20 hits for a 12.5 percent chance of pocketing at least $700.

Build a Wine Library

You don't have to install a cellar to have all the bottles you need on hand. Patrick Cappiello, wine director at Pearl & Ash in New York City, suggests the perfect vino stash—for everyday sipping, weekends, and special occasions.

GO-TO PICKS	WHITES	REDS
EVERYDAY		
$14 TO $20		
Anything from France's Loire Valley. "These wines are always a great value and extremely food-friendly," says Cappiello.	Sauvignon blanc (light, crisp); chenin blanc (rich, mineral)	Cabernet franc (full, leathery)
WEEKENDS		
$25 TO $40		
California wines, especially those that are lower in alcohol, which are meant to be sipped slowly and enjoyed.	Any chardonnay from Santa Barbara (bright, citrusy)	Syrah from the north coast (spicy, floral)
CELEBRATIONS		
$50+		
Wines from Burgundy and Bordeaux, "some of the most magical and ageworthy wines on the planet," Cappiello says.	Chardonnay from Chablis (intense, full-bodied)	Bordeaux (dense, potent); cabernet sauvignon blends (ageworthy)
AGE WELL		
Not all wines improve with the years. If you're looking for bottles to store, select high-acid, tannic wines with some sweetness. A bordeaux, burgundy, or rioja is a good choice, as is a dessert wine such as port, madeira, or ice wine, says Matthew Kaner, wine guru at Bar Covell in Los Feliz, California.		

Pour a Glass of Champagne

Don't commit sparklicide. A study in the *Journal of Agricultural and Food Chemistry* found that this is the best way to preserve bubbles and taste.

1. Chill the bottle to 39°F. (Just check your fridge thermometer.) That's the temperature at which champagne retains the most bubbles.
2. Hold the flute at a 45-degree angle, resting the flute's bottom edge on a table for support, so the champagne can slide in gently. Don't pour it directly into an upright glass; this destroys twice as many bubbles as pouring at an angle does.
3. For a smooth pour with minimal bubble loss, touch the bottle to the glass.

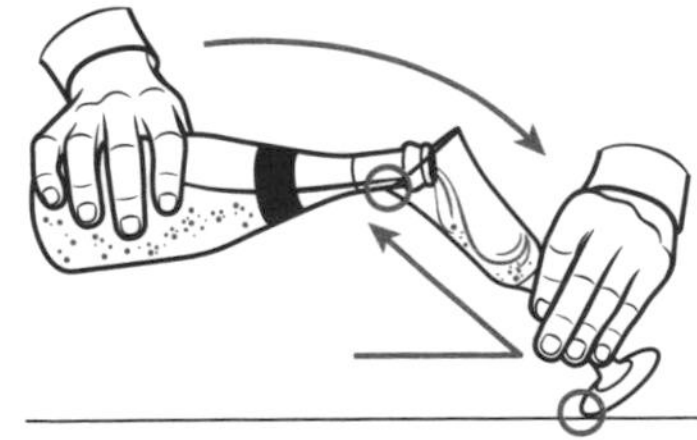

FEEL COMFORTABLE AT ANY PARTY

Become the guy with conversational firepower—the one everyone wants to hang out with. The key, says Tony Reali, host and conversation starter of ESPN's *Around the Horn*, and Leil Lowndes, communications consultant and author of *How to Create Chemistry with Anyone*, is to move from the general to the unexpected.

QUESTION 1

How do you know the host?

Yes, it may be a run-of-the-mill question, but you need to establish a basic connection with the person if you're ever going to divulge a few personal details as icebreakers. What's key here is your demeanor. Reali likes to open with a silly "I know we just met, but can I give you a hug?" You can achieve similar results (without awkwardness) by deploying some self-deprecating humor ("The host and I met as beauty pageant contestants").

QUESTION 2

What's the best live sports event/ burger/movie you've ever seen/ eaten/watched?

Good, open-ended questions provide people with opportunities to share anecdotes about their experiences. Be a good listener, but also be prepared for when your new acquaintance turns the question back on you. (That's the logical outcome of this type of inquiry.) Just don't act too eager to jump in with your own amusing story. No one likes the guy who is just waiting for his turn to talk.

QUESTION 3

What's your favorite curse?

This is a great Rorschach test to spring after you've established a good rapport—you can actually learn a lot about someone from their answer. (Is their preferred word based on its sound, or its meaning?) Plus, people love talking about cursing.

QUESTION 4

Was there one event or circumstance in your life that changed you as a person?

If your goal is to be memorable, this will do the trick. Asking how someone has changed can lead him or her to talk about both hardship and success. It also focuses the chat on the person as an individual. Use your judgment and ask accordingly.

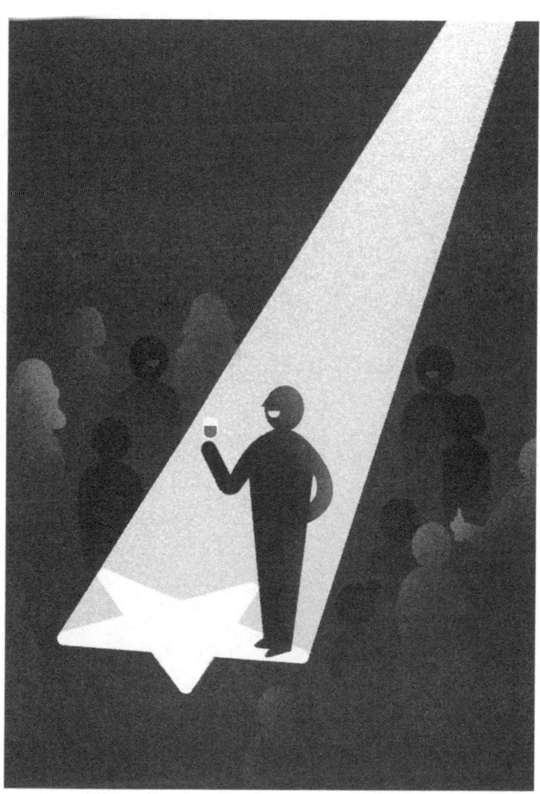

How to Ride a Horse

Hop into the saddle and stay there with an equine assist from Kent Desormeaux, a professional jockey and three-time Kentucky Derby champion.

Don't Horse Around

Greet your steed the wrong way and it could lash out. If you're allowed to pick your horse, go with a larger one—big horses tend to be friendlier. Step toward it from the side so it can see you, and pet it while talking quietly to form a bond. Then hop on from the left—that's the side it was trained to be mounted from.

Speak Equine

Trainers teach horses to respond to certain stimuli. To start the horse walking, squeeze your ankles together and make kissing noises. To stop, pull back on the reins with a "whoa." To turn, pull the reins in the direction you want to go, holding them about a foot away from your body. Be firm to earn respect.

Avoid Saddle Ass

To prevent the throbbing pain radiating from your groin after a ride, do what the pros call "posting." Instead of allowing the trotting motion to toss you up and down, stand in the stirrups slightly, bending your knees to act as shock absorbers as the horse increases its speed or steps over uneven ground.

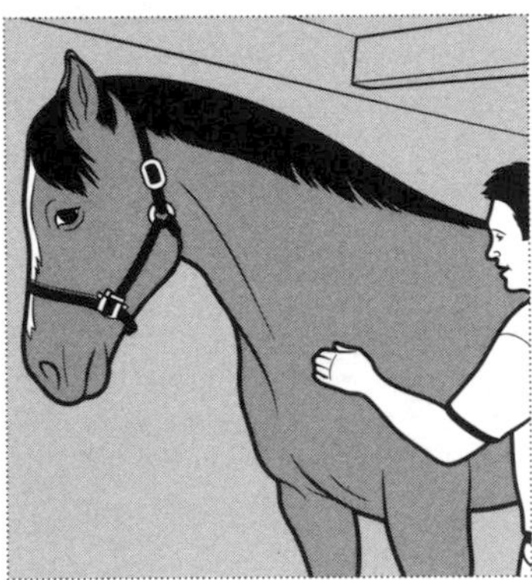

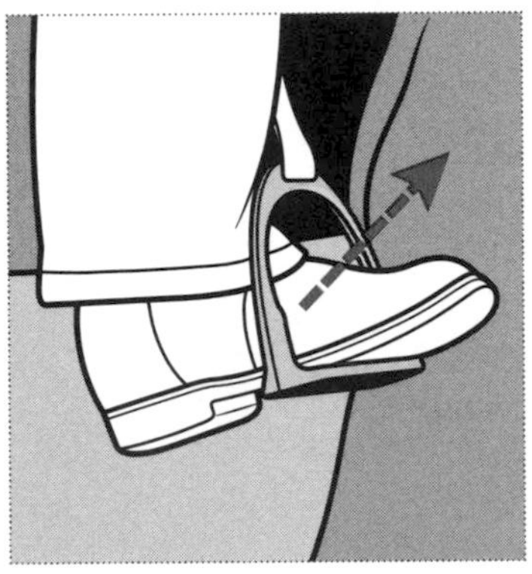

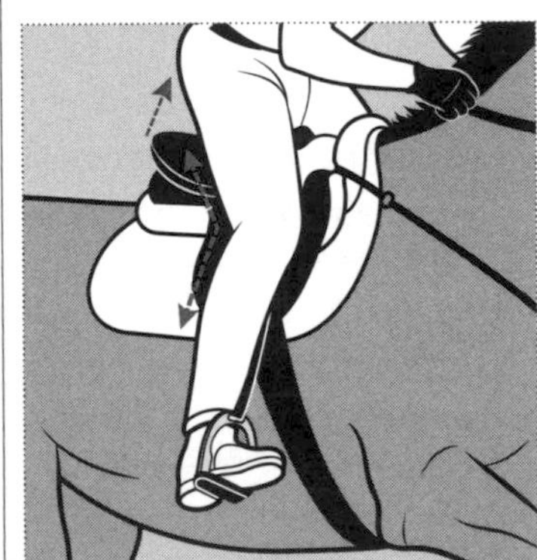

How to Ride a Bike

You think you've got this one down? Well, you're pedaling wrong if you're pumping your legs up and down the same way you did when you were racing after the Good Humor man. To cycle faster with less effort, learn to pedal in circles. Push down from the top of the stroke until the crank arms are horizontal. Now pretend you're scraping mud off the bottom of your shoes from this point until the next time the crank arms are horizontal, and continue to exert force by pulling across the bottom of the stroke. Finish by pulling up on the pedal to the top of the stroke (using pedals with toe straps or a clipless pedal system to anchor your feet).

RULE # 14

Do one high-intensity workout every other week. Researchers in Norway studying soccer players found that one HIIT workout every other week is just as beneficial as doing them weekly.

HOW TO COACH A KID

LOSE THE BOBBY KNIGHT ACT AND DEVELOP A STYLE THAT WILL KEEP KIDS ENGAGED AND HAVING FUN.

Level the Playing Field

Sit your tyke down and ask if you can "join the team." You'll probably get an emphatic "yes." The point is to let the little guy (or gal) know you're both on the same side.

Be Consistent

When critiquing play, always lead by citing something commendable ("Great job dribbling upfield!") before giving feedback ("Now try to keep your head up"). Then finish with another positive, encouraging comment ("You'll get it, keep working hard!").

Look Beyond Your Kid

If you're not a coach, hang out with other parents. Their comments (like "That was a sweet pass" or "They're crowding the ball") can help you lose the tunnel vision for your child and see the whole team.

Stoke Inspiration

If you see your lad's motivation dragging, whip up a game at home to focus on skills while still having fun. For kicking strength, tack up a target on a brick wall and see if he can nail it with the ball. For ball control, offer him ice cream for stringing together five juggles.

Discipline Privately

No kid responds well to public scolding, so if yours is acting out or not being a team player, pull him aside; then you can switch to parent mode. Explain why it's important that he accept the consequences for his actions just like any other teammate does. Don't make a scene. If he's not receptive, say you'll finish the talk at home with mom—but try to avoid mixing at-home disciplinary tactics with on-the-field ones.

Sources: Jimmy Nielsen, former goalkeeper for Sporting Kansas City; Larry Lauer, PhD, of the Institute for the Study of Youth Sports at Michigan State University

Remember a Phone Number

STEP 1 Repeat

Ask the person to slowly repeat the number. This gives your brain time to split the digits into manageable chunks and begin making connections with numbers that are already stored in your memory.

STEP 2 Divide

Don't think about the individual digits, because your mind needs more substance to help you remember long-term. Group them into two-, three-, or four-digit chunks; doing this reduces the number of items you have to remember.

STEP 3 Associate

Link the digits to numbers you already know. Try sports jerseys (for 2399, think Jordan chilling with Gretzky) or years in history (for 7644, the American Revolution and D-Day). For a 314 area code, think pi. Or 256 is you at age 25 holding a 6-iron.

STEP 4 Speak

Repeat the number back to the person.

STEP 5 Visualize

"Dial" the number on an imaginary keypad. You may be able to remember the motor sequence better than you remember the individual numbers.

Source: Alan Castel, PhD, an assistant professor of psychology at UCLA's memory and cognitive aging lab

Deliver a Moving Eulogy

Stephen D. Boyd, PhD, is a minister and professional speaker who has given 175 eulogies. Here are his tips for speaking eloquently about someone who's passed on.

1. When You Sit Down to Write It

Don't give the bio—that's covered in the obit. First, establish your connection to the person, and then move on to an anecdote that reveals something about the person's character. Talk about a time when the person went out of his way to help you when you didn't expect it, for example. Don't be afraid to be lighthearted. At funerals, people are desperate for a chance to laugh. But keep this in mind: You want them to remember your talk as moving, not funny. Keep it to about 3 minutes.

2. The Day Before the Funeral

Print your eulogy in a large font, double-spacing the lines. Use only the top two-thirds of the page, to keep from having to glance too far down and preventing the audience from seeing your face. Practice reading your comments at least five times aloud, preferably in front of a few friends to see how people react.

3. Before the Ceremony

Find as many familiar faces among the attendees as you can so you feel anchored. Speak with the memorial's leader about having someone else read your eulogy if you can't finish it.

4. During the Eulogy

Keep a bottle of water by the lectern in case you lose your composure. Take a sip, pause, and focus on your breathing. Make eye contact; if that's too hard, fake it by looking at the back wall or at strangers, who are less likely to trigger emotions.

Write a Memorable Thank-You Note

Class Up Your Paper

Correspondence cards are more businesslike than average folded cards, and they offer just as much blank space. For special occasions, splurge on personalized Crane & Co. Navy Blue Bordered Ecruwhite Correspondence Cards ($115 for 25, crane.com).

Write As You Speak

Avoid language that sounds formulaic. Instead of "Dear John," just say "Hello John." Instead of "Yours truly," just write "Regards" or "All my best" followed by your name.

Be Legible

Type out a draft to compose your thoughts. When you're ready, use a ruler as a guide just beneath your pen to keep lines straight. If your print is sloppy, switch to cursive. The change should slow you down, improving your penmanship.

Keep It Neat

Smudges will make your note look like an afterthought. Avoid fountain pens on glossy paper because they may streak. For card stock, use a fine-point. We like the Sheaffer Agio ($50, sheaffer.com).

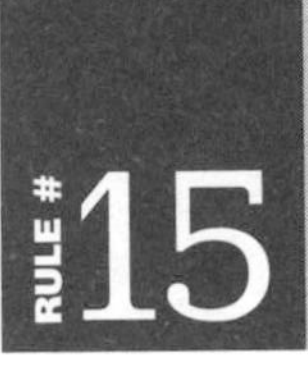

Avoid long jokes that keep going and going like the Energizer Bunny. They drive women away. A joke should have at the most two parts, the second part sort of funny.

Give a Proper Holiday Tip

YOU CAN'T JUST ASK "HOW MUCH?" SO WE POLLED 30 SERVICE WORKERS TO FIND OUT HOW MUCH THEY'RE TYPICALLY GIFTED.

Your Personal Trainer

The tip: An amount equal to the cost of one session

How to deliver it: To make the transaction easy, just tell your trainer to take a session off your current prepaid package.

Your Barber

The tip: The cost of a haircut

How to deliver it: Make sure to hand the tip to your barber before you're in his chair. He may miss the cash on the counter as he preps for his next client.

Your Dog Walker

The tip: A week's pay

How to deliver it: Include a note so there's no confusion about where the extra money came from. And yes, lots of people have Fido "sign" the card.

Your Mail Carrier

The tip: A job-well-done note

How to deliver it: Mail carriers aren't allowed to accept cash tips. A letter of praise to their supervisor often means more.

Your Bartender

The tip: An extra $20

How to deliver it: Add it to your regular tip and say, "Happy holidays." If your bartender is hosting your annual Christmas party, throw in another $100.

Your Newspaper Carrier

The tip: $20

How to deliver it: If your carrier doesn't send a card first, leave a message with the paper's customer service line saying that you're leaving a card near where the carrier drops the paper.

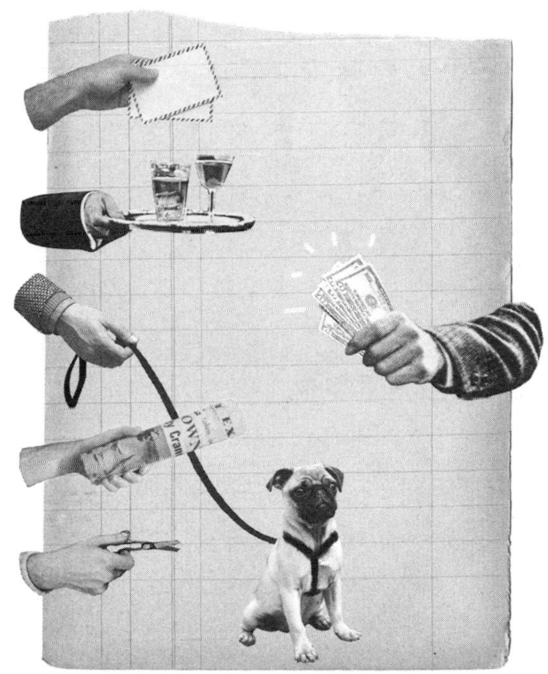

Don't Become Chum, Chum

Of shark-attack victims, 93 percent are male. September is peak chomping season as more divers and surfers hit the water in tasty, seal-colored wetsuits. To learn how to survive a shark attack, swim over to page 47.

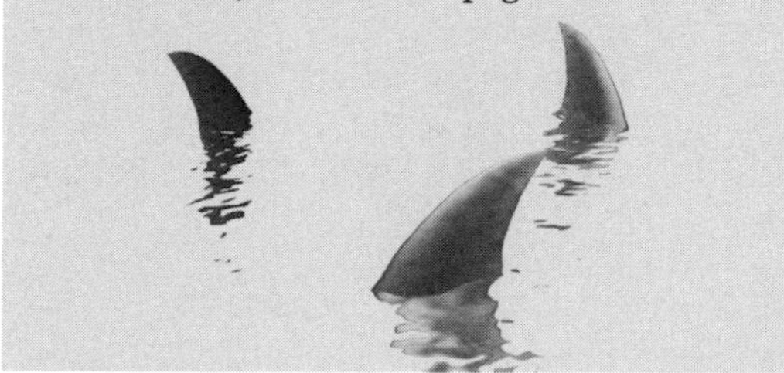

HOW TO TIE THE TRUCKER'S HITCH

NEED TO TIE A CHRISTMAS TREE, CANOE, OR LUGGAGE TO THE ROOF RACKS OF YOUR CAR?

A trucker's hitch will give you a 3-to-1 mechanical advantage when cinching the load down tight. Once you've tied one end of your rope to the roof rack and tossed the rope over your load, you're ready to secure it with the hitch.

Step 1. Tie a slippery half-hitch or slipknot. Do this by forming a loop in the rope about halfway between your load and the rack, cleat, or hook (a). Next, push a "bight" or bend in the rope through the loop as shown (b). Grasp the loop in one hand and the standing ends of the rope in the other and pull the knot tight. The loop you created forms a pulley.

Step 2. Grab the running end of the rope and push it under the roof rack, cleat, or other fixed point and then through the back of the "pulley" or loop in the slippery hitch you just tied (c).

Step 3. Pull down on the end of the rope to cinch your load down taut. Now, keeping tension on the running end of the rope with one hand, pinch the rope where it goes through the "pulley" loop with your other hand so it won't slip loose and finish with one or two half hitches (d). This beats the hell out of a bungee cord.

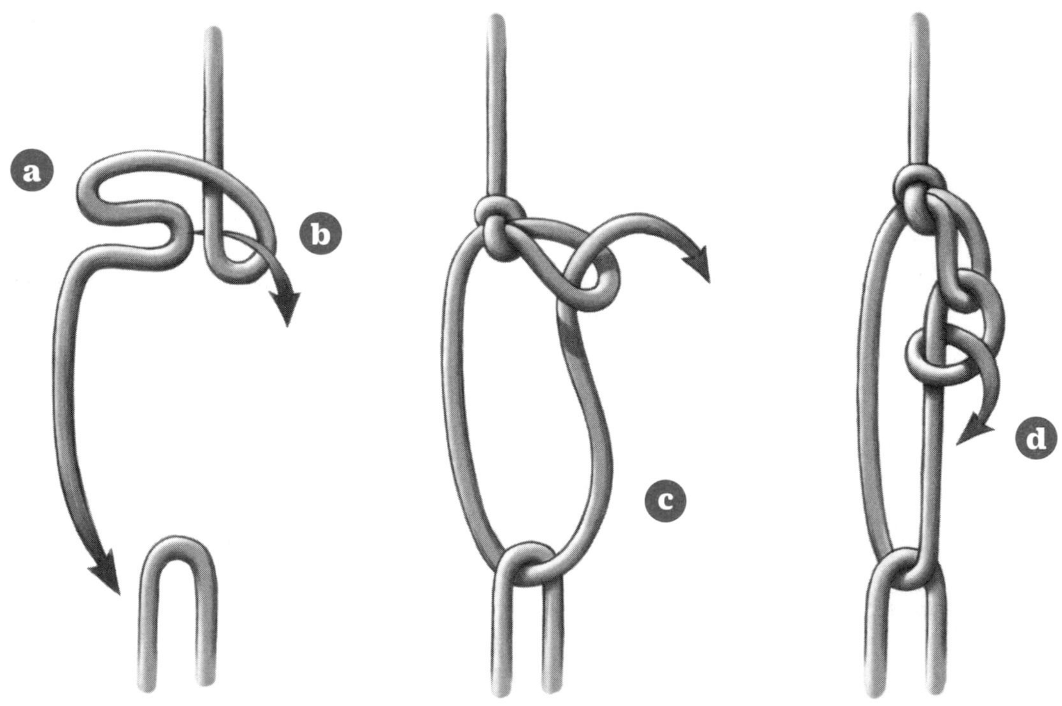

Kick In a Door

Save the day (and your shoulder) with breakthrough tips from police officer Bob Charpinsky, training director for the New York Tactical Officers Association.

A. Assess the Obstacles

Kicking down a door may be your only option if someone needs help immediately. If the person is on the other side of the door, alert him or her to stand back before you go into action-hero mode. You can probably kick down a door that swings away from you. If it swings toward you, find another way to enter. Deadbolts make the job harder.

B. Set Your Stance

Stand a bit less than a leg's length from the door, keeping your shoulders square and your feet about shoulder width apart. You want to kick as close as you can to the knob or lock, which is usually the weakest part of the door.

C. Go Van Damme on It

Raise the knee of your dominant leg above your waist. In one swift move, kick, leading with your heel. As soon as your entire foot makes contact, transfer your momentum to push your body weight through the door, knee bent. Your upper body should lean forward slightly for maximum force.

D. Kick and Kick Again

The door may require multiple blows. If it or the frame begins to crack, good. The casing may also move, causing the doorknob to twist. See these signs? Keep kicking the same spot. If after a few kicks the door won't budge, call 911 if you haven't already.

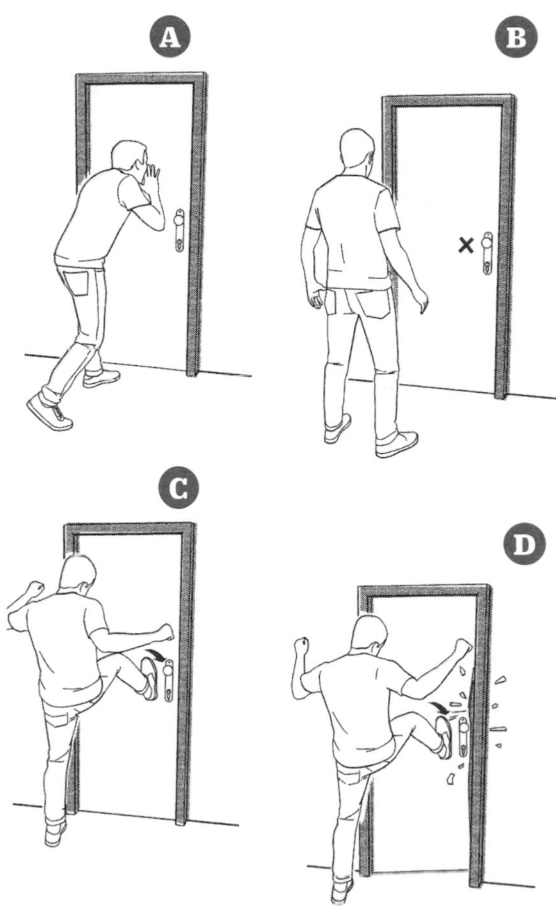
A
B
C
D

RULE #16 Your cereal won't go mushy if you pour the milk just until the cereal starts to rise.

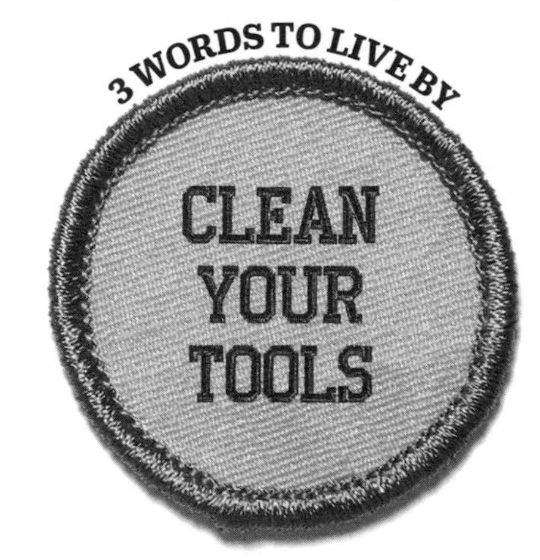
3 WORDS TO LIVE BY
CLEAN
YOUR
TOOLS

How to Escape the *Hound from Hell*

You're out for a run. You hear barking and scratchy paw steps of an angry dog behind you. Horror movies from the 1980s spring to mind as you picture your vital organs being torn out by vicious canine teeth.

The basics:

Animals are not humane.
If you panic, they panic.
If they panic, they bite.

The details:

Nearly two million people are bitten by dogs annually. To make sure you don't join them, the best strategy is to overcome your urge to outrun the animal (you won't). But most of the time a dog is lots of bark and no bite.

Humor him. Stand still, turn, and face the dog. Play it cool, don't stare in a threatening way, and don't make any quick movements. Talk in a quiet voice: "Hi, there, Brutus, go home now, nice doggy." Show him you're not a threat. He'll probably circle you, maybe urinate on your khakis, then leave you alone. After the dog has calmed down, back away slowly, keeping your eye on the animal.

Throw the dog a bone. Got a snack in your pocket? Share it. The old saying is true: Dogs are less likely to bite the hand that feeds them.

Mad dog options. If the dog doesn't calm down, intimidate him. Face him down. Make yourself as big as you can be, scream, and stare him right in the eye. While you're putting on this show, take off your jacket and wrap it around your fist. If the dog lunges, feed him your padded hand. Back away until you can get to safety, then sacrifice the garment.

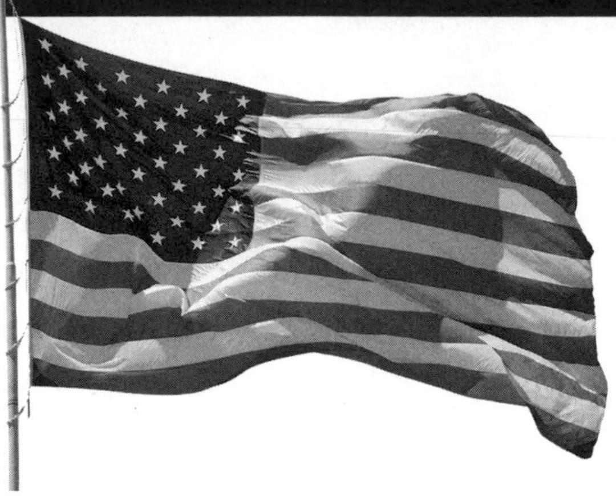

How to Display Old Glory Correctly

- When shown with other flags, the US flag should be taller or extend out farther, and it should hang above any other flag on the same pole.
- In a row of flags, it should be farthest to its own right.
- When hung horizontally or vertically from a wall, the union should be at the top and to the left of anyone looking at it. When displayed in a window, it should be displayed in the same way.
- When hung over the street, the field of stars should be to the east on a north-south street or north on an east-west street.
- If a flag is tattered, it should be "retired" by burning. Or take it to a local VFW, where the members will handle it properly.

How to Choose a Doctor

Find a doctor who is roughly your age give or take five years. If your physician is facing the same health issues you're facing, it'll help him anticipate what tests and treatment you need.

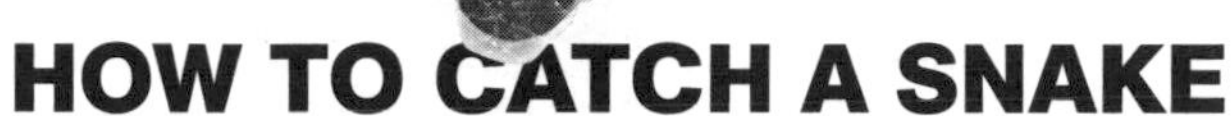

HOW TO CATCH A SNAKE

If you come across a snake, it's best to leave it be. But if you find one in your shed or garden and want to relocate it, grab a long stick or broom handle and follow along.

Make its acquaintance. First, try to ID the snake to make sure it's not venomous. You don't want your first snake snatch to end in a trip to the ER.

Shift its attention. Point one end of the stick in front of the snake's head to give it something other than you to focus on.

Choose heads or tails. If it's a small garter snake or similar nonpoisonous serpent, you can quickly but gently grab it behind its head. It'll probably wrap its tail around your arm. Cool. For larger snakes and those you can't ID, grab the tail and lift up but leave the front quarter to half of the snake's body on the ground facing away from you. Extend your arm and keep your legs away.

Carry a big stick. Now, still holding the stick, slip the free end of the stick under the front half of the snake and lift. This will make it easy to control the business end of the snake. It's also less likely to freak a big snake out than grabbing its neck.

Assist with relocation. Carry the snake out of your yard and into a field or woods and release it with its head facing the direction you'd like it to slither—away from you. Want to help it move further away? Slip it into a pillowcase that you can tie shut for a short car ride across the tracks.

Soap up. Wash your hands with soap and hot water after touching the snake. Reptiles can carry bacteria that can make you very sick.

RULE # 18 Be outspoken when you know a lot about a subject, but keep your mouth shut when you don't.

Degrease with Oil

Soap and water suck at cleaning motor oil and oil-based paints from your hands, so turn to your kitchen cabinet. Vegetable oil helps remove them better than soap and water. Just dab a tablespoon or two on a paper towel, rub to break up the grime, and finish with soap and water.

RULE # 17

Get more protein without eating meat. How? Learn to use quinoa. Chilling the nutty grain after cooking restores firmness. Then drizzle on some olive oil and lemon juice. Mix in some vegetables along with olives or feta cheese for saltiness. Yum, and good for you, too.

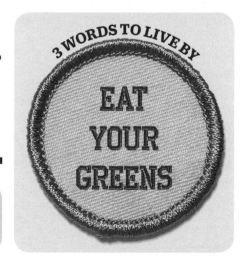

Flirt LIKE A PLAYER

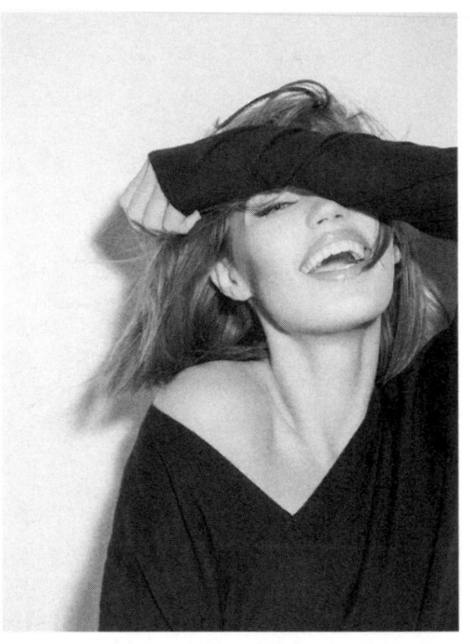

There are many paths to a woman's digits, but only one shortcut: humor. Now, you may be thinking, "But I try to be funny, and it never works!" Therein lies your problem: Humor is tough to pull off, especially if you try for laughs. Theresa DiDonato, PhD, an assistant professor of psychology at Loyola University Maryland, suggests building from something you have in common, such as a hot topic in the news or an event you both just witnessed. But if you just saw the waitress spill a tray of drinks, don't turn it into a line. That sends the wrong message about your personality. DiDonato's research shows that the best flirtation strategy is affiliative humor—warm, low-key, playful joking—rather than mean-spirited quips. In fact, in that tray-spilling scenario the best thing you can do is help the waitress clean up. Your consideration will catch a woman's eye and make her more open to your attempts to converse. Oh, and bet on self-deprecating humor. Women like a guy who can laugh at himself.

Make a Pit Stop

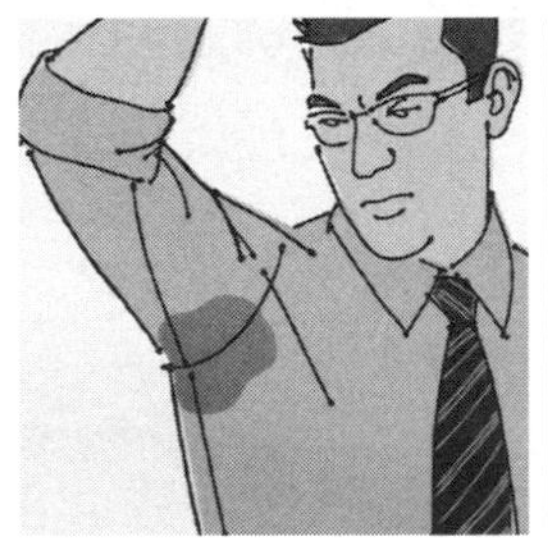

Three ways to fight embarrassing underarm sweat stains:

1. Try an over-the-counter antiperspirant like Gillette Clinical Strength. Apply before bed and it will settle into underarm pores over night.
2. Insert Garment Guard Disposable Underarm Shields into your armpits to block sweat from reaching clothing.
3. Ask your doctor for a prescription antiperspirant like Drysol, which contains a high amount of aluminum chloride, which plugs sweat glands, thereby preventing sweat from reaching the skin. Apply before bed.

Build Brand "YOU"

Want to boost your earning potential?

Develop your personal brand. It describes the qualities that differentiate you and what you can deliver. Find it at the intersection of your passions, values, and job strengths, says personal branding guru William Arruda, founder of Reach. Then write a creed that hits those three areas for your résumé and LinkedIn profile.

RULE # 19 **Max out your 401(k) contribution. You won't see the cash until retirement, but it gives you two things you need to become wealthy: compounded gains and annual tax deductions.**

Say Howdy (Almost) Anywhere

Arabia	Al salaam
China	Ni hao
Czech Republic	Nazdar
Finland	Paivaa (PIE-vah)
France	Bonjour
Germany	Guten tag
Greece	Yassas (YAH-sas)
Hungary	Szia (SEE-ya)
Ireland	Dia Dhuit
Israel	Shalom (shah-lohm)
Italy	Buon giorno
Japan	Konichiwa
Korea	Annyong ha shimnikka
Norway	God dag
Poland	Czesc
Portugal	Bom dia
Russia	Zdravstvuite
Spain	Hola
Turkey	Merhaba
Philadelphia	Yo (y-OH)

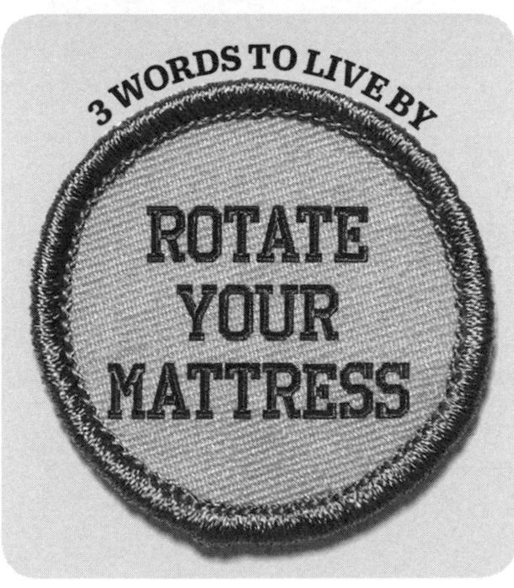

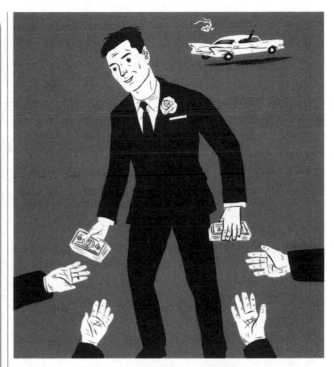

3 WORDS TO LIVE BY
ROTATE

MATTRESS

How to Be a Better Best Man

As the groom's go-to guy, you should do more than just party hard and deliver a killer toast. Anja Winikka of TheKnot.com offers these tips for handling your responsibilities with style:

Make a grand gesture. If your wedding party has the bank, buy one big gift. Look for an item the couple might need that they didn't register for, like a TV or a high-end grill.

Direct traffic. For 24 hours, you're the event mastermind. Memorize the timing and location of events. Point guests to the reception, parking, or men's room.

Volunteer as trip advisor. Take on whatever the groom can't leave to kayak.com. Help negotiate a group hotel rate for out-of-town guests and coordinate airport pickups. Your job is to make this whole getting-married business easier for your buddy.

Dole out the dough. For one day in his life your pal shouldn't worry about money. That's where you come in. "Help the groom with any day-of payments," Winikka says. "This includes tips for vendors like the caterer, the florist, the musicians, even the altar servers."

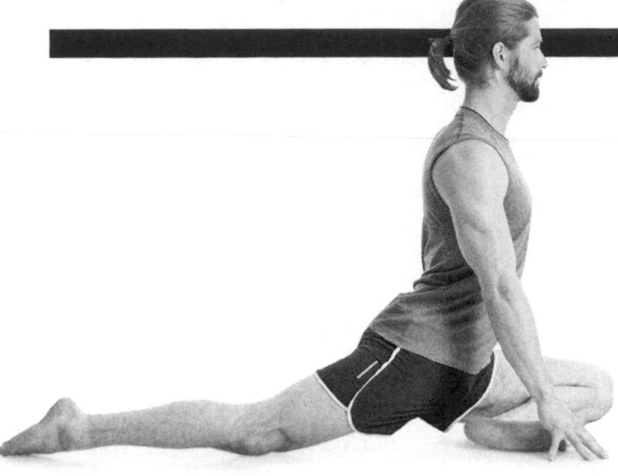

How to Fix a PAIN IN THE ASS

When your butt muscles tighten, they pinch your sciatic nerve, causing a pain in your ass, technically called piriformis syndrome. If you run or cycle, you are especially prone because the focus on forward motion tends to weaken hip muscles. Fix it by foam rolling your muscles and relaxing them with yoga's pigeon pose, shown above.

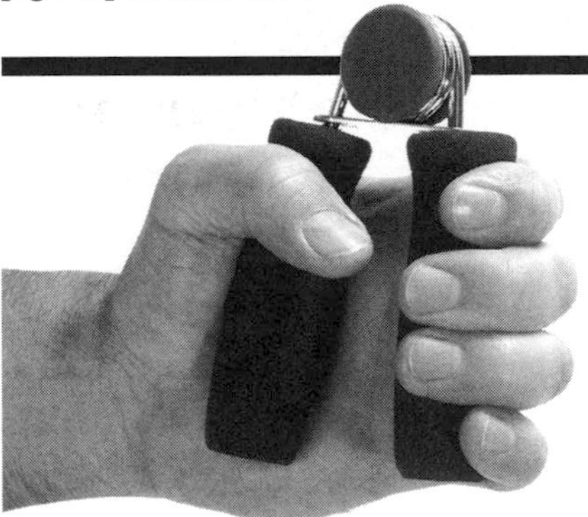

Master the Power Handshake

It's not about a crushing grip or turning the other guy's hand under yours. Just be sure to reach out first so your arm has more extension than his. When he takes your hand, his elbow will be bent inward, toward his body; that's a sign that he's claiming less personal space. Match his grip strength and give three or four pumps. That's how you subtly dominate the interaction.

7 SIMPLE WAYS TO LOSE WEIGHT

1. Drink diluted fruit juice. Natural fruit juices contain lots of calories. Cut them in half by diluting them with water.
2. Stop eating when you've eaten 80 percent of your normal amount, and wait 20 minutes. You'll feel satisfied because it takes 20 minutes for your stomach to signal your brain that you're full.
3. Eat breakfast. A survey of more than 2,000 people who lost significant weight and kept it off for at least 5 years found that 78 percent ate breakfast 7 days a week.
4. Cut 100 calories a day. That's roughly the amount of calories in a handful of chips or a light beer. Eliminating one of these a day would be the equivalent of 700 calories a week and could lead to nearly 10 pounds of weight loss in a year.
5. Eat your largest meal at breakfast or lunch. And lighten up at dinner. This gives you hours of activity to burn off the calories. If you consume a lot of calories late in the day, you're more likely to store these calories as fat.
6. Walk for 30 minutes daily. That's all you need to do to move from couch spud to moderately fit, a change that will provide significant health benefits.
7. Strength train to build muscle. After age 30 your muscle mass starts to shrink by about 1 percent per year. That's why older folks get fat. Muscle is more metabolically active tissue than fat. By building more you automatically burn more calories 24/7.

How to Survive a HEART ATTACK

The outcome of a myocardial infarction depends on how much heart muscle dies, so speed of treatment is often critical. Knowing heart attack warning signs is key: chest tightness or heaviness; extreme fatigue; pain in shoulders, neck, jaw or arms; shortness of breath; sweating; lightheadedness; or nausea. If something feels amiss, don't delay, do this:

- **Call 911 or another emergency medical number.** Don't drive yourself to the emergency room. Wait for EMTs, who can begin treatment en route and alert the ER docs of your vitals.
- **Take an aspirin.** Chew it to speed the blood-thinning medicine more quickly into your bloodstream.
- **Be assertive in the emergency room.** Your life could be at stake.

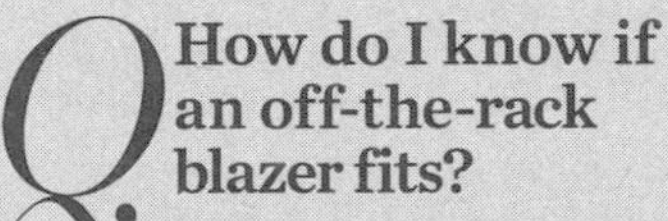

Q
How do I know if an off-the-rack blazer fits?

A. It should be snug in the shoulders. Everything can be tailored, but if the shoulders are off, you'll spend twice as much on alterations.

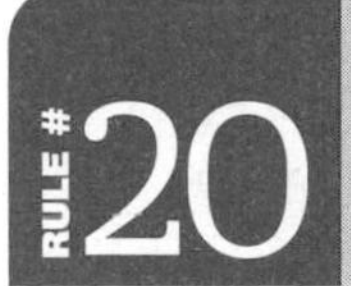

Looking down at one's penis makes it look smaller than it really is.

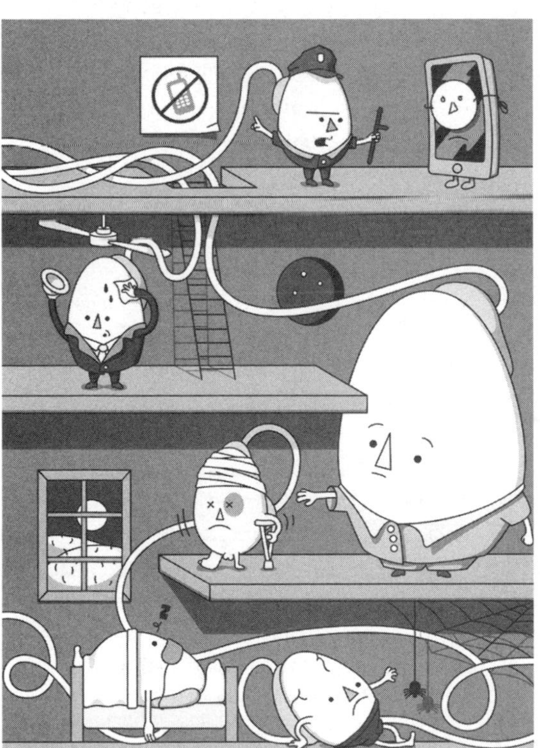

Your Balls: An Owner's Manual

4 FACTS YOU SHOULD KNOW ABOUT YOUR BOYS

Keep 'Em Cool

A laptop on your lap raises your balls' temp, which may harm sperm quality.

Eyeball Their Size

Bigger balls may indicate increased heart trouble risk, according to a report in *Journal of Sexual Medicine.* In the study, older men with a testicular volume of 20 milliliters or more risk heart problems due to blood vessel damage, which may increase testes size.

Hold the Phone

Numerous studies have linked cell phone exposure to decreased sperm count and quality. So keep your phone in your back pocket instead of in the front one, says *Men's Health* urology advisor Larry Lipshultz, MD.

Hit the Sack

Less sleep means more stress hormones flooding your body, which can reduce sperm production.

HOW TO SAVE FOR ANYTHING

You've got financial goals, big and small. And now you have a foolproof plan.

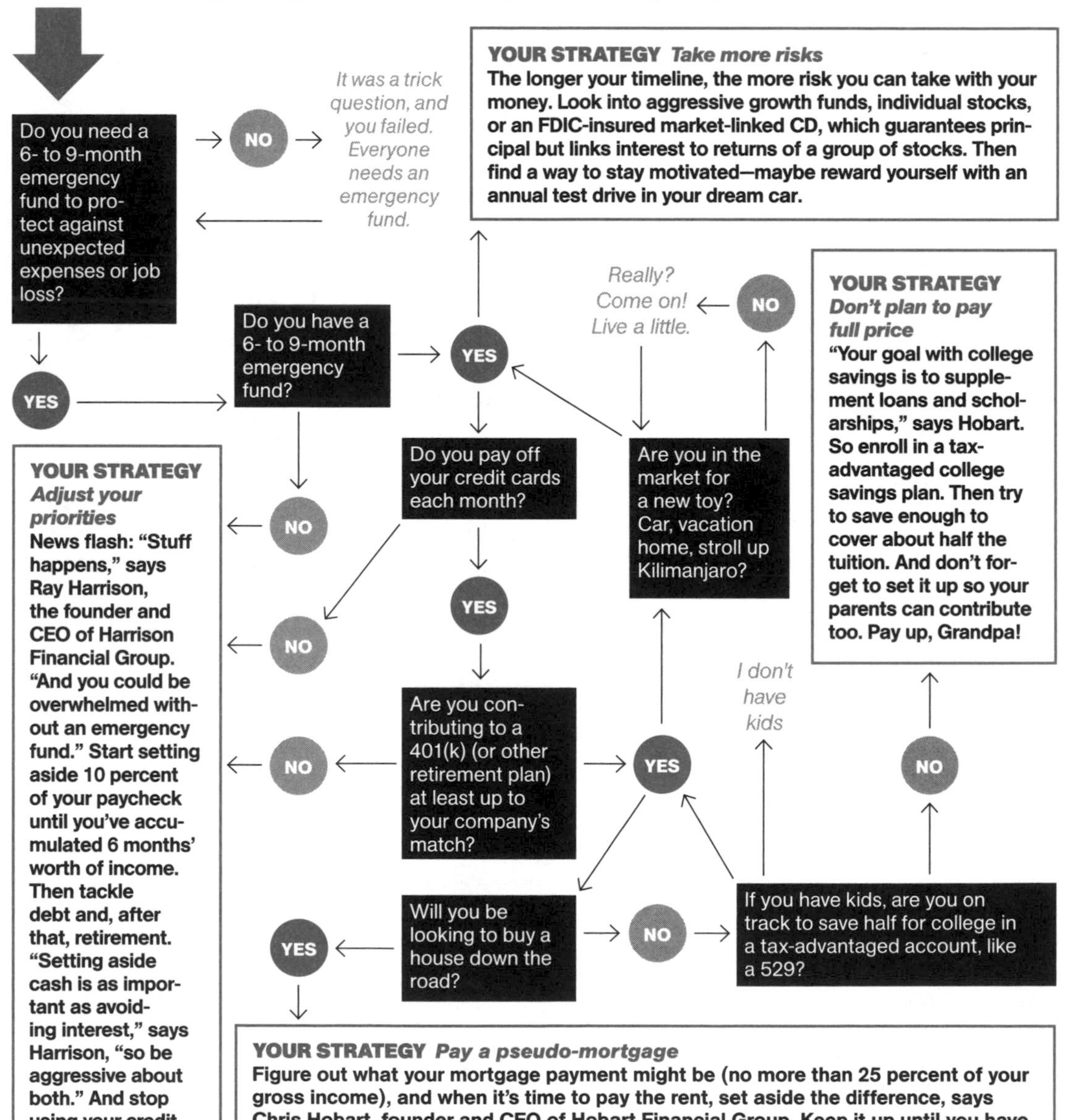

Do you need a 6- to 9-month emergency fund to protect against unexpected expenses or job loss?
NO
It was a trick question, and you failed. Everyone needs an emergency fund.
YES
Do you have a 6- to 9-month emergency fund?
NO
YES
YOUR STRATEGY Take more risks
The longer your timeline, the more risk you can take with your money. Look into aggressive growth funds, individual stocks, or an FDIC-insured market-linked CD, which guarantees principal but links interest to returns of a group of stocks. Then find a way to stay motivated—maybe reward yourself with an annual test drive in your dream car.
Do you pay off your credit cards each month?
NO
YES
Are you contributing to a 401(k) (or other retirement plan) at least up to your company's match?
NO
YES
Are you in the market for a new toy? Car, vacation home, stroll up Kilimanjaro?
NO
Really? Come on! Live a little.
YOUR STRATEGY
Adjust your priorities
News flash: "Stuff happens," says Ray Harrison, the founder and CEO of Harrison Financial Group. "And you could be overwhelmed without an emergency fund." Start setting aside 10 percent of your paycheck until you've accumulated 6 months' worth of income. Then tackle debt and, after that, retirement. "Setting aside cash is as important as avoiding interest," says Harrison, "so be aggressive about both." And stop using your credit card!
Will you be looking to buy a house down the road?
YES
NO
If you have kids, are you on track to save half for college in a tax-advantaged account, like a 529?
I don't have kids
NO
YOUR STRATEGY
Don't plan to pay full price
"Your goal with college savings is to supplement loans and scholarships," says Hobart. So enroll in a tax-advantaged college savings plan. Then try to save enough to cover about half the tuition. And don't forget to set it up so your parents can contribute too. Pay up, Grandpa!
YOUR STRATEGY Pay a pseudo-mortgage
Figure out what your mortgage payment might be (no more than 25 percent of your gross income), and when it's time to pay the rent, set aside the difference, says Chris Hobart, founder and CEO of Hobart Financial Group. Keep it up until you have saved a down payment of at least 10 percent.

How to Land On Your Feet

Sometimes life just doesn't go your way. For example: Some day you may need to jump out of a window to escape sure incineration or the unexpected return of her boyfriend/husband. There are wrong ways and right ways to land back on your feet:

- If you must jump from a two-story window or (God forbid) higher, hang from the window ledge to start your fall as close to the ground as possible. Look for an awning, bushes, a vat of female mud wrestlers, anything to cushion the fall.
- Try to land on the balls of your feet. As your body contacts the ground, allow your knees to bend slightly and use your hands to break the fall as much as possible. Immediately start forward into a shoulder roll.
- Falls off of barstools and sidewalk curbs are far more likely to occur than planned window jumps so be ready for these six-inch falls that can land you in the ER. Land on the balls of both feet at the same time. Bend at your knees and waist to absorb some of the shock and extend each arm in front of you for balance.

RULE #21

Never eat out of the original container. How many times have you dipped your hand into the chip bag only to find yourself staring at the bottom 15 minutes later?

Make Simulated Snot

HOMEGROWN SLIME WILL OCCUPY 6- TO 17-YEAR-OLDS FOR HOURS.

YOU'LL NEED:

- ½ *cup white craft glue*
- ¼ *cup water*
- 6–10 *drops of food coloring (we recommend snot green, but blue, red, or orange are cool, too)*
- ½ *cup liquid clothing starch*
- *Large bowl*
- *Plastic mixing spoon*

DO THIS:

1. Pour the glue and water into the bowl and mix well.
2. Add your food coloring.
3. Mix in the liquid starch. Stir well until you get a blobby, slimy bowl of slime.
4. Knead it with your fingers.
5. Store it in a zipper-lock plastic bag so it won't dry out.

THICKEN THINNING HAIR

You can make your thinning hair look thick and strong throughout by using a light gel and blow-drying it while fluffing it with a round brush.

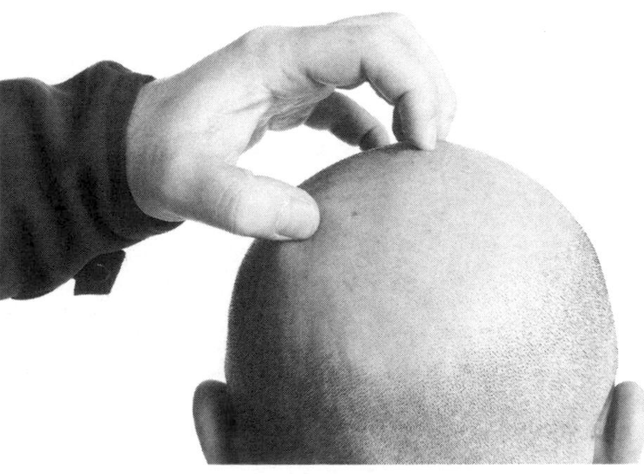

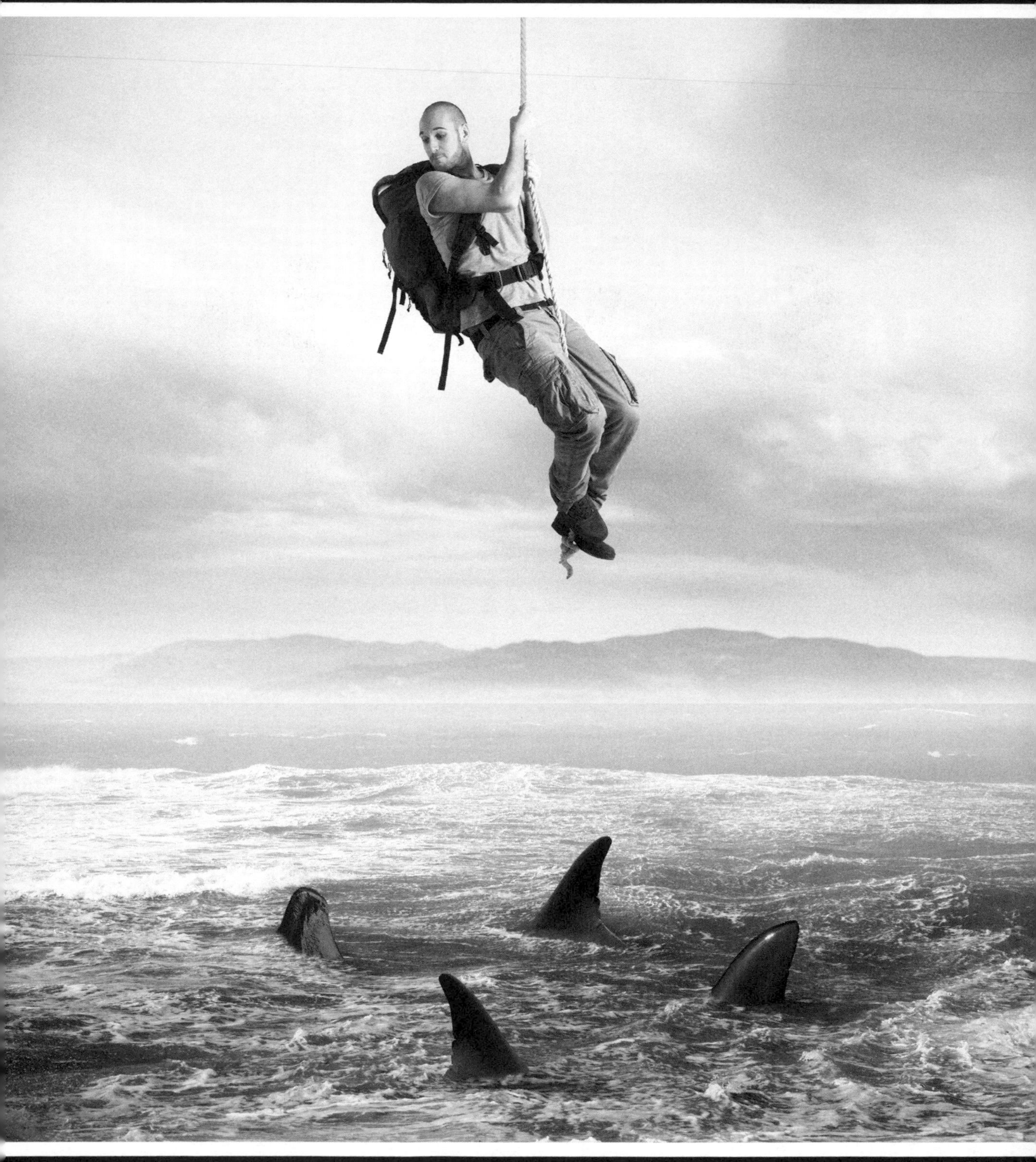

Survive in the Wild

Skills You Learned in Boy Scouts and Forgot as Soon as You Noticed Girls

Some years ago, at Delaware Water Gap National Recreation Area, a car with New York license plates pulled up at a campsite at 9:30 at night. In it were four guys from Queens in their early twenties, and it was pretty clear they weren't experienced campers. From the trunk of the car, they pulled a cooler of beer, an ax, and a brand-new tent still in the Dick's Sporting Goods bag. While three guys busied themselves with beer drinking and tent construction, trying to follow the paper instructions by flashlight, the fourth set out to build the campfire. He carried two bundles of firewood wrapped in plastic and dumped the wood in the fire ring. Next, he siphoned gasoline from the car's tank into an empty iced tea jug. He poured the gasoline onto the wood, then tossed his cigarette on it.

Nothing happened.

He bent down, sparked his cigarette lighter, and the gasoline ignited—*poof*—no more eyebrows!

The great outdoors presents many dangers but even more opportunities for looking stupid. The following pages offer a crash course in outdoor wisdom and skills so you won't look stupid.

Build the Perfect
CAMPFIRE

An impressive fire requires plenty of air to fuel the flames. At your next campout, structure your fire-pit fuel this way for a long-burning blaze.

Step 1: Safeguard the Site

Remove flammable objects from an area about 8 feet in diameter and place several containers of water nearby.

Step 2: Build a Cabin

Three logs **(a)** form the base of the fire. Stack two more layers of two logs each, placed perpendicular to the layer below **(b)**. For a longer-lasting fire, make five layers. Fill the "cabin" with kindling and tinder **(c)**. Then, atop the final layer, make a roof with sticks **(d)**.

Step 3: Build a Tepee on Top

Make a mound of dryer lint (the best fire starter) **(e)** or a store-bought fire starter (second best) and then small twigs, or tinder **(f)**. The more tinder, the quicker the fire ignites. Never use leaves, needles, or cones—they absorb more heat than they produce and can shoot out sparks.

Carefully lean many sticks together in a small tepee structure surrounding the mound **(g)**. Leave an opening facing the prevailing breeze. Use thinner sticks for the foundation, and then thicker ones.

Step 4: The Fire

Ignite the kindling inside the tepee and let it burn. The tepee will eventually collapse and fall into the log cabin. To put the fire out, drown the embers with water. Stir. Repeat. Don't leave until you can feel the ground with your hand to confirm that it's cool.

Source: Mike Cooney, Boy Scouts of America, senior district executive, eastern Maine

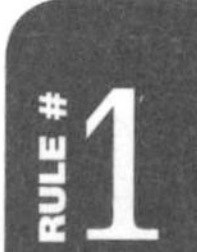

Strips of white birch bark make an excellent fire starter and will burn even when wet.

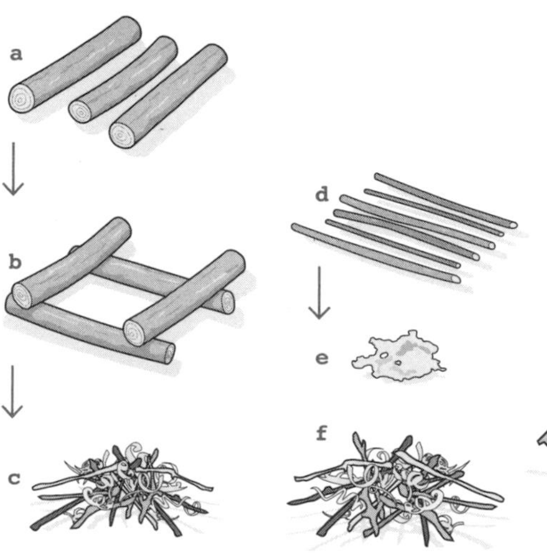

g

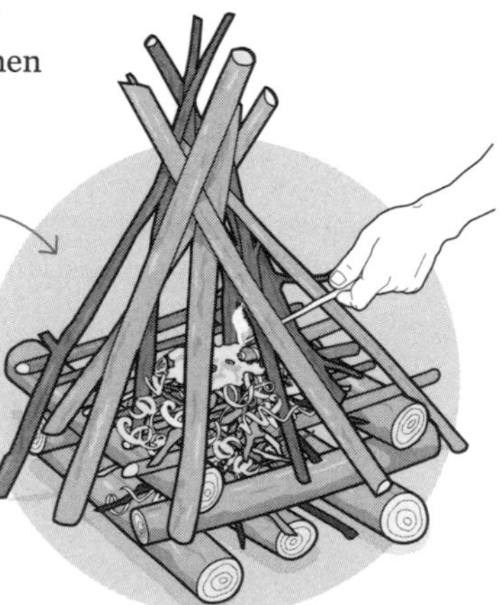

Start a Fire With a Flashlight

Out of matches? No Bic? If you have a fresh flashlight battery and very fine steel wool, you can start a fire. Roll the wool between your hands into a cigarette shape. Then pull the ends apart gently so there is only a fine mesh of steel wool in the center. Now touch one end to the battery's positive end and the other to the negative end. The current will make the wool in the center spark and burn. Touch some dry tinder with it and blow to get a flame.

How to Make Trail Mix

A bag of GORP (**G**ood **O**l' **R**aisins and **P**eanuts plus) not only energizes the body, it lifts the spirit during a long, hard slog up a steep and rocky trail. Here are the base ingredients for a tasty trail mix. Feel free to get creative.

2 cups popcorn
3 tablespoons raw almond slivers
3 tablespoons peanuts
⅓ cup raisins
⅓ cup dried cranberries
Cinnamon to taste

Combine all ingredients.

Makes 4 servings

Per serving: 150 calories, 6 g fat, 4 g protein, 3 g fiber

1. Complex carbs equal energy; fiber fills you up.
2. Monounsaturated fats provide long-lasting energy.
3. Peanuts contribute protein, healthy fats, and L-arginine, an amino acid that helps control blood flow.
4. Raisins' iron content boosts oxygen delivery.
5. Cranberries house antioxidants and have antibacterial properties.
6. Cinnamon flavors the mix without relying on the salt many prepackaged mixes contain.

RULE # 2

Never build a campfire ring with river rocks. If they have been in water for a long time, they are cold and more porous. When heated, they can expand and blow apart like grenades, shooting shrapnel around your campsite.

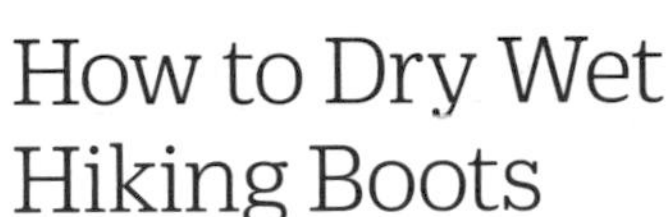

How to Dry Wet Hiking Boots

Never put them close to a campfire to dry them. The heat can crack the leather or melt rubber soles or synthetic uppers. Instead, stuff the boots with small fire-warmed rocks placed inside socks.

RULE # 3

Change your scenery. Block out a week for a camping trip. Sleeping outdoors naturally syncs your circadian clock to the sunrise and sunset, according to a study in *Current Biology.*

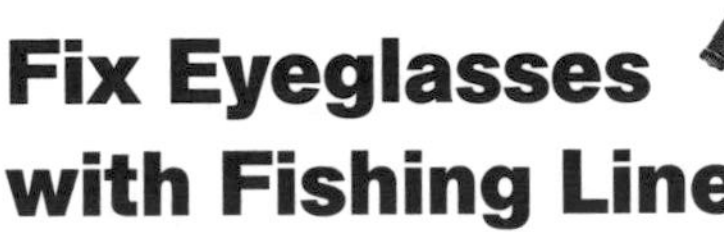

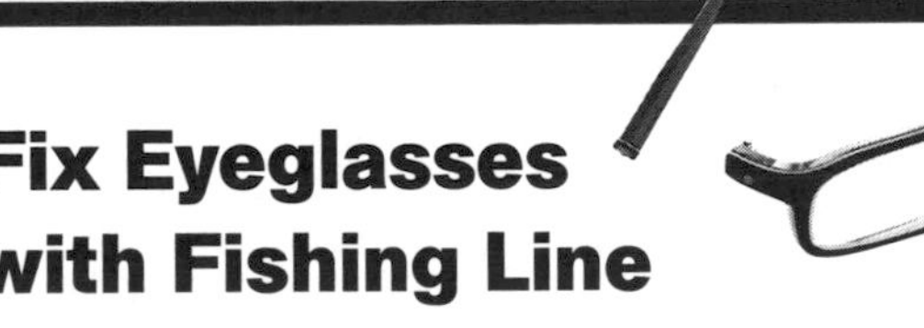

Fix Eyeglasses with Fishing Line

If you lose the little screw that holds the temple of your eyeglasses to its frame, knot one end of monofilament, then slip the other end through the screw hole and tie it. Melt both knots with a match to form a rivet. Fixed! Just in time to see the bear that's been watching you fix your glasses.

Paddle Her Properly

WE CAN. CANOE?

There's no easier way to look like a doofus on the water than trying to paddle a canoe when you don't know how to make the vessel go straight. First thing to know is how to sit in a canoe: If you're paddling solo, sit in the stern, facing the bow, the front of the canoe. You'll know it by studying Anatomy of a Canoe on the next page. You can sit, but you'll get more stability and power by kneeling in front of the seat to lower your center of gravity. Ready to paddle? When paddling on the right, or starboard side, of the boat, your right hand should grasp the throat just above the blade; your left hand should be on top of the grip, never around the shaft, a common beginner mistake.

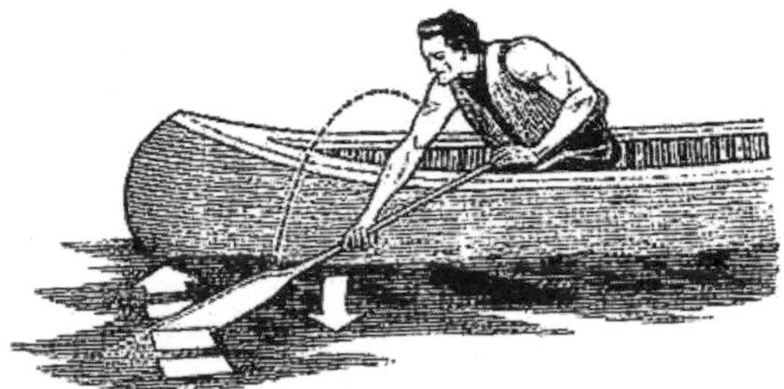

Cross Draw Stroke

This stroke is created for the bowman, or front paddler, to help steer the front of the canoe quickly, for example, to avoid a boulder just beneath the surface in a whitewater river. The cross draw is like the draw stroke but performed on the side opposite (or "off") from which you are paddling. For example, if you are paddling on the right side of the canoe and want to turn the bow to the left, don't change hand grips, but rather lift the paddle blade from the water, rotate your torso to bring the blade to the left side of the canoe, reach out as far as you can (as shown above), dip the paddle blade, and pull it to the hull. The bow will pivot left.

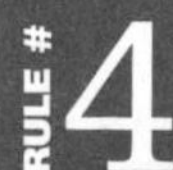

RULE #4

If you fall out of a raft or canoe in a whitewater river, never try to stand. Your foot can become wedged between rocks, and the force of the water will force your upper body (and head) underwater. Instead, see Rule #5.

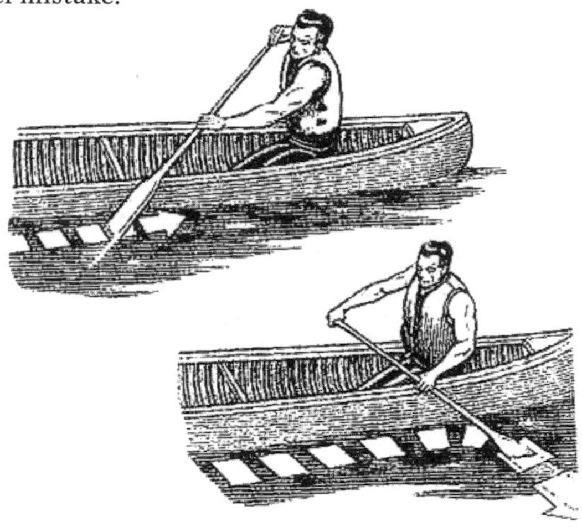

Forward Stroke (A)

The primary stroke for canoeists. Extend your arm nearest the blade straight and place the paddle in the water ahead of you. Pull back with that hand while pushing forward with the hand on the grip.

J-Stroke (B)

This stroke is used by the canoeist in the stern to keep the canoe tracking straight, since with each forward stroke, the canoe wants to turn to the opposite side. The J-stroke corrects this. Start a forward stroke as shown in drawing A. When your left hand reaches your hip, rotate your right wrist thumb down toward the water. That will turn the paddle blade into a rudder position underwater. Now simply pry the blade away from the canoe to bring the boat back on track.

By using both strokes properly, you won't have to switch sides with your paddles.

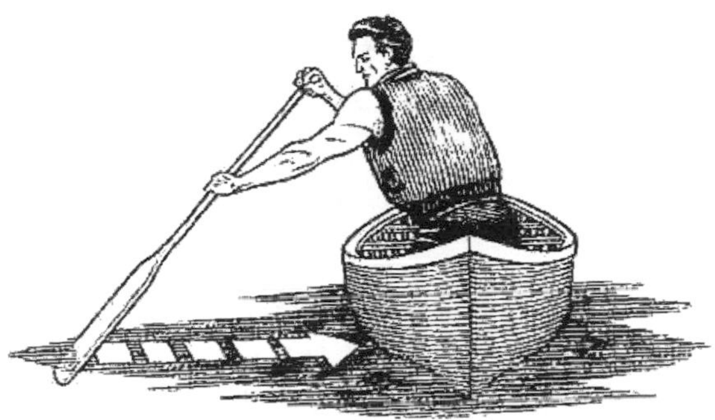

Draw Stroke

Used primarily by the bow paddler to turn quickly to avoid a rock in whitewater, this stroke is useful for pulling the boat up to a dock by either paddler. With the blade held parallel to the canoe, reach out to the side away from the boat, dip the paddle in the water and draw the blade back toward the side of the canoe.

RULE # 5

This goes along with Rule #4. After being dumped out of your boat in a whitewater river, float on your back facing downstream. Stay upstream of your canoe, kayak, or raft. A boat full of water can crush you if you get between it and a big rock. Keep your toes poking above the water's surface and use your feet to kick away from any boulders. Backstroke toward shore and away from any "strainers," or downed trees that are in the river. River water can go through these strainers, but you can't; you can be pinned against them and forced under. Stay away.

Anatomy of a Canoe

You know you paddle, not row, a canoe, right? Now learn its parts.

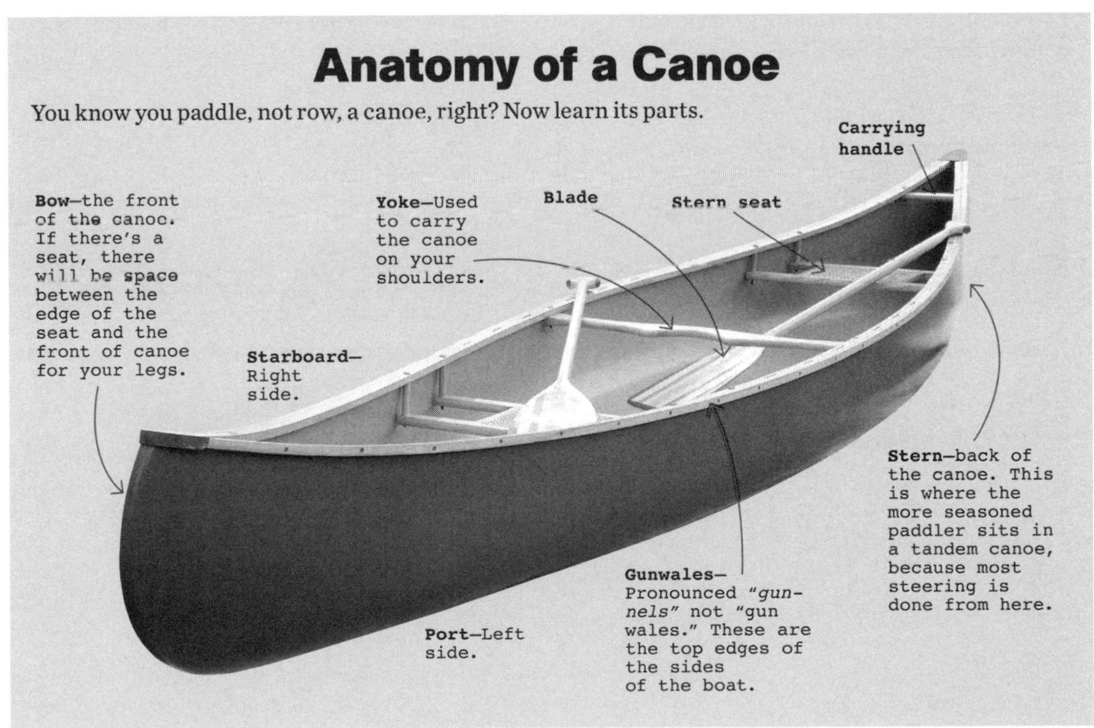

Carrying handle
Bow—the front of the canoe. If there's a seat, there will be space between the edge of the seat and the front of canoe for your legs.
Yoke—Used to carry the canoe on your shoulders.
Blade
Stern seat
Starboard—Right side.
Stern—back of the canoe. This is where the more seasoned paddler sits in a tandem canoe, because most steering is done from here.
Gunwales—Pronounced "gun-nels" not "gun wales." These are the top edges of the sides of the boat.
Port—Left side.

Estimate a Jump from a Cliff

You want to end summer with a splash, but that cliff looked a lot smaller from a mile away. Before you leap into the abyss, you should know exactly how far you're about to plunge. Because this could be legendary.

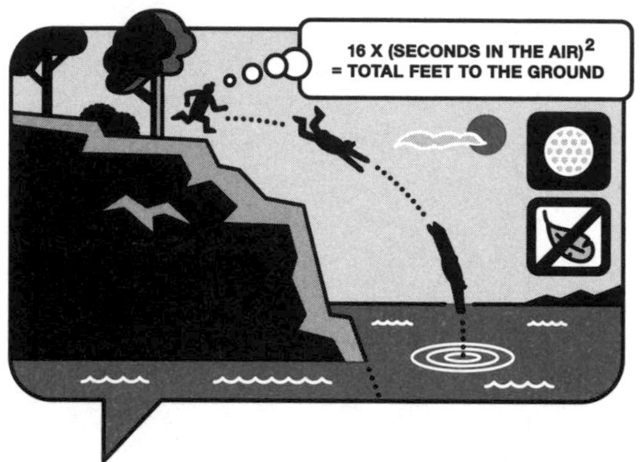

Here's how: Pick up a rock, toss it straight out over the edge, and count the seconds until it hits bottom. Then let Newton's second equation of motion run the numbers. Simply put, gravity exerts the same pull on all objects regardless of weight. That means just about anything dense and solid, whether it's a rock, a baseball, or a human body, will generally fall at the same rate.

As things plummet, they also pick up speed. In other words, during a 2-second fall, you'll drop 16 feet the first second and 48 the next. While there are other ways to gauge distance, counting hang time has another perk: You can grade other people's dubious claims from any angle or even by looking at their iPhone videos. And it's worth betting that your buddy is exaggerating when he brags that he's free-fallen from some crazy height. A *Men's Health* review of 20 YouTube videos in which people boasted they'd jumped 100 feet (total hang time: $2^1/_2$ seconds) revealed that 75 percent of those tall tales fell short.

Make your off-the-cliff calculations even easier by downloading the Cliff Height Timer app. It's a stopwatch that does the math for you.

Now you can Geronimo in with confidence. No jump should be a leap of faith—not when science can help you calculate a reliable personal record.

Assumptions: This math is most accurate for heights up to 200 feet. After that, air resistance on any object becomes a bigger factor.

Safety note: Never jump or dive into water that you don't know for sure is plenty deep and free of hazards. Scout the water first.

Source: Mark Rober, a former NASA engineer who hosts his own science and creativity channel on YouTube.

16 × (SECONDS IN THE AIR)^2 = TOTAL FEET TO THE GROUND

Flip Flapjacks

To turn a pancake over in the air with a flourish, sweep the frying pan forward, up, and around in a smooth, looping-the-loop motion.

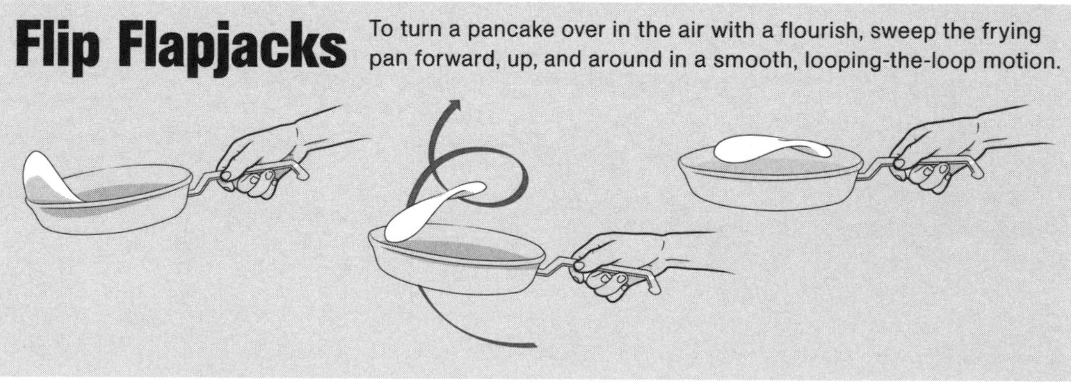

Know Your Knots

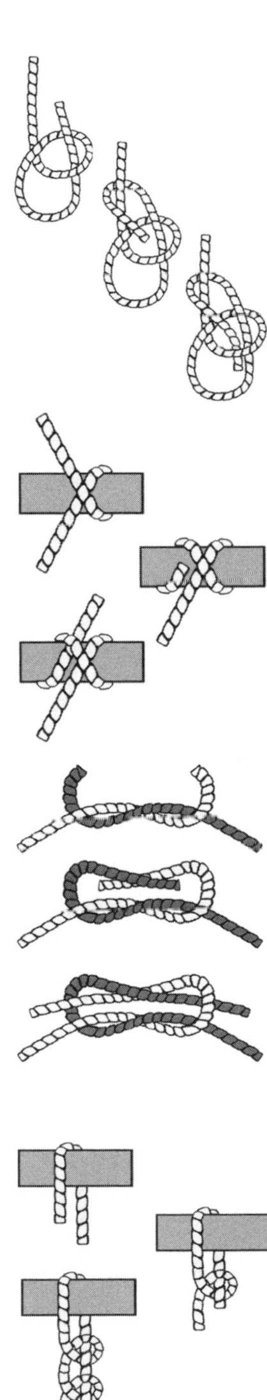

Bowline—forms a secure loop.

Form an eye hole in the rope with the standing part of the rope extending underneath. Take the end of the rope and form a large loop below the eye, then snake the end up through the eye. Turn the free end of the rope around the standing part ("the rabbit runs around the tree") and back down into the eye ("and jumps back in his hole"). Pull the standing part to tighten.

Clove Hitch—Ties up to a post fast and releases easily.

Turn the rope's end around a post and run it underneath the standing part. Take a second turn around the post in the same direction and poke the working end through the eye of the second turn. Pull tight.

Square Knot—Often called a reef knot because it was used to tie up a reef (sail).

Used to tie two ropes together so they can easily be untied. Cross the left end of a rope over the right end of the other rope. Tuck the left end under the right. Then tuck the working end that lies on the right side of the knot over and under the working end on the left side of the knot. Remember: "Left over right and under; right over left and under." Pull to tighten.

Two Half Hitches—A simple knot to tie a rope to a tree or boat.

Form a clockwise loop around the object with the working end of the rope over top of the standing rope. Tie an overhand knot by bringing the working end through the loop. That's one half hitch. Repeat with a second overhand knot.

Carry a Big Stick

Choose the right hiking stick with these tips from Simon Fryer, a guide with the Colorado Mountain School. (Speaking softly, optional.)

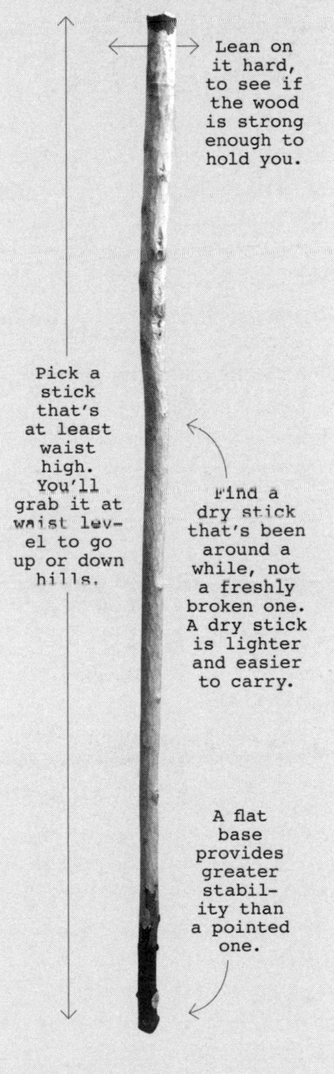

Lean on it hard, to see if the wood is strong enough to hold you.
Pick a stick that's at least waist high. You'll grab it at waist level to go up or down hills.
Find a dry stick that's been around a while, not a freshly broken one. A dry stick is lighter and easier to carry.
A flat base provides greater stability than a pointed one.

Pilot a Kayak through Rough Waters

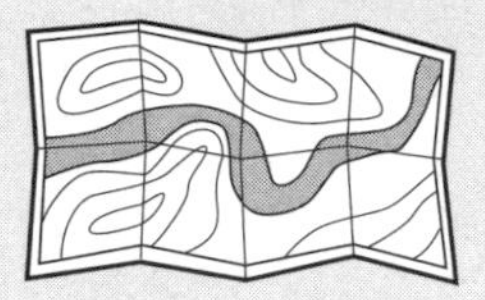

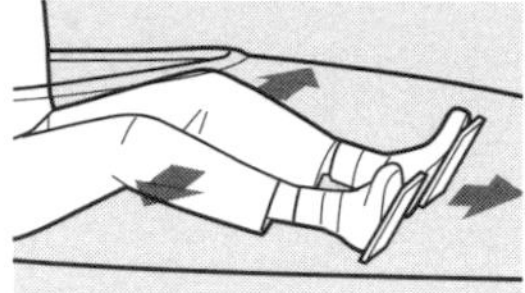

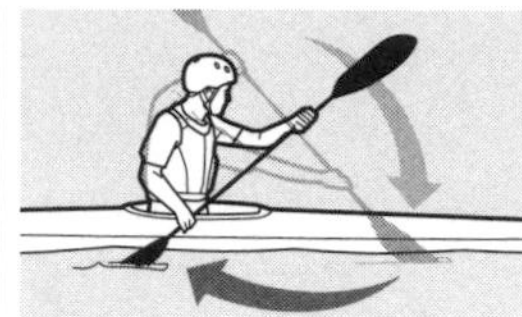

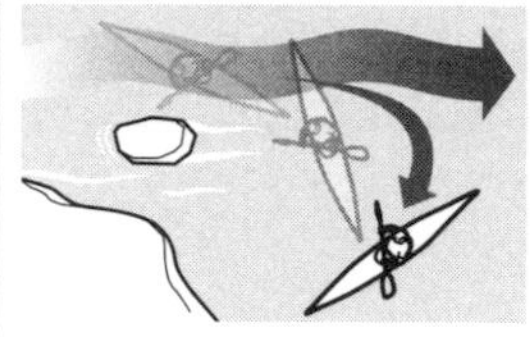

Map Your Route

Survey the water before shoving off. Make a mental note of calm-water chutes and hazards such as large rocks and branches of fallen trees (known as "strainers.")

Also try to pick out eddies. These counter-current pools gather behind obstructions and can help you control your speed and offer slow-water places to rest.

Take the Helm

As you enter the kayak, slide your legs all the way to the front, placing the balls of your feet on the foot pegs. Your legs should bow, with your knees bracing the craft's top inner wall.

Plant your butt in the seat and your hips in the hip pads. You should feel as if you're wearing the kayak, your posture strong and body slightly forward for power. Secure your spray skirt over the lip of the cockpit to keep water out.

Paddle Properly

Don't rely only on your biceps for power. Instead, paddle from your torso. Hold the paddle with your hands shoulder width apart, striving for a 90-degree elbow angle.

Reach with the paddle as far forward as possible and pull until it passes your knee. The first 30 percent of the stroke applies the most forward momentum.

Bob and Weave

To catch an eddy, position your kayak so you enter at an angle. Otherwise the eddy's flow may tip your ride.

If the eddy is to your left, bank the boat by lifting your right knee while pushing down with your left butt cheek (or vice versa), and enter it using a hard forward stroke. Use this method to connect the dots on your way to calmer water.

Stay Warm, Like a Scarecrow

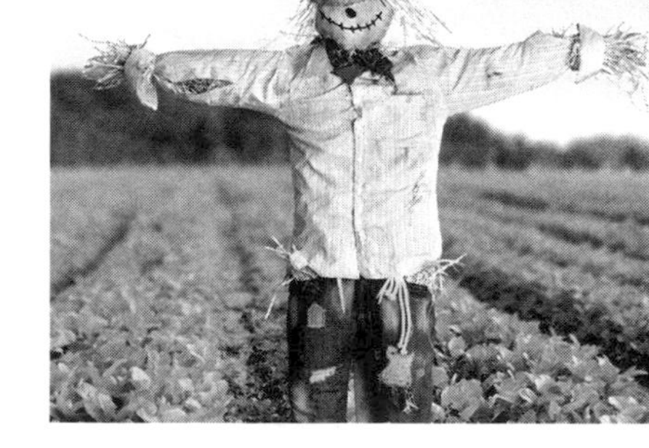

If you're caught in a storm, keep hypothermia at bay with the scarecrow technique. Take your shoelaces and tie your pants cuffs around your ankles. Then stuff your pants and shirt with dry leaves or pine needles as insulation. If trapped in your car during a snowstorm, do the same thing using the stuffing from inside the seat cushions.

Survive with a SPEAR

Avoid panic in a survival situation. Focus on taking action, using a "SPEAR":

Stop

Plan

Execute

Assess & Reevaluate

Avoid a Bee Sting
(WITHOUT LOOKING LIKE A MORON)

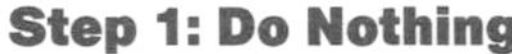

Step 1: Do Nothing

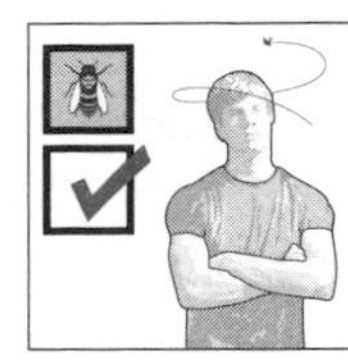

Most bees don't attack. A circling bee is usually curious about why you're near their home or about your smell; its scent glands may be agitated by a grooming product you're wearing. Stand still. Fast movements make you an aggressor.

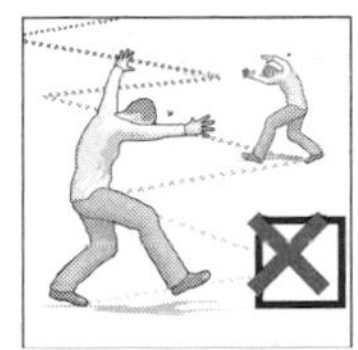

Step 2: Retreat!

If the bee aims for your face, if it brings friends, or if it's around for longer than a minute, you might be in its territory. Time to go:

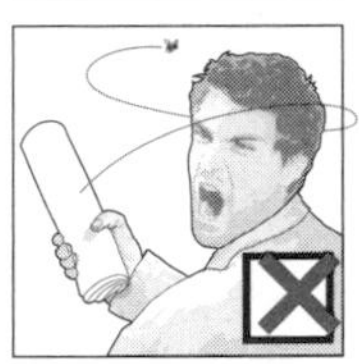

- Jog in a straight line for a few seconds to gain distance quickly. Bees give up the chase if you're too far away.
- Don't zigzag. The bee can follow your scent, and zigzagging makes for a lot of running but not a lot of distance.
- It doesn't know what your rolled-up magazine is. All you're doing is pissing it off at close range.
- Forget about jumping into a lake. Bees are happy to follow your scent to the water and sting your face when you resurface.

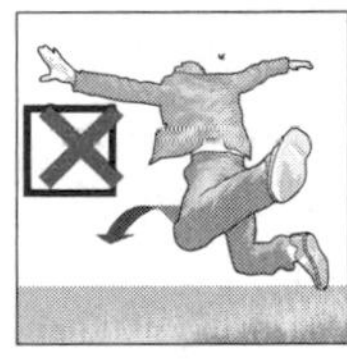

Source: Paul Jackson, chief inspector of Texas A&M University's honeybee identification lab

Primary Stingers

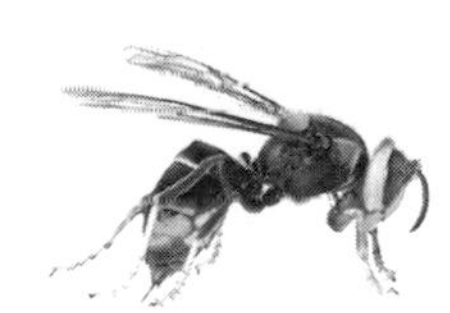

Hornet
Sleek; usually nests in trees; can sting multiple times

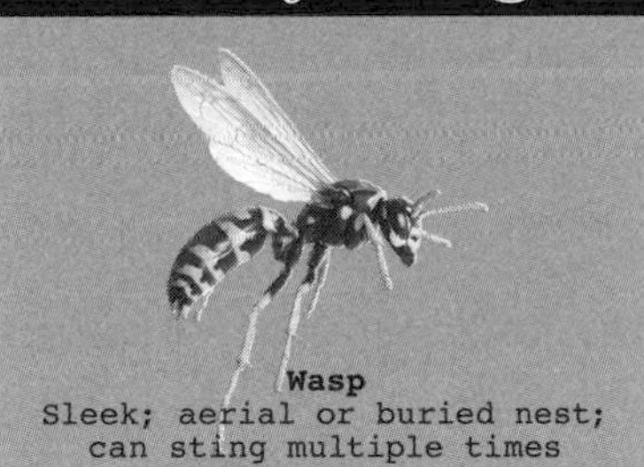

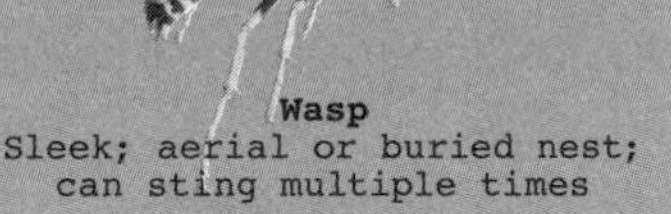

Wasp
Sleek; aerial or buried nest; can sting multiple times

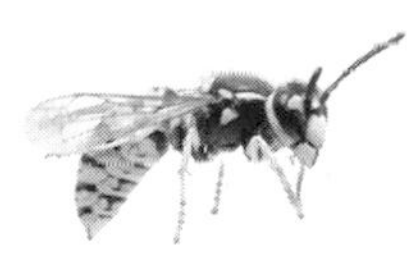

Yellow jacket
Distinctive black-and-yellow-banded wasp; aerial or buried nest; can sting multiple times

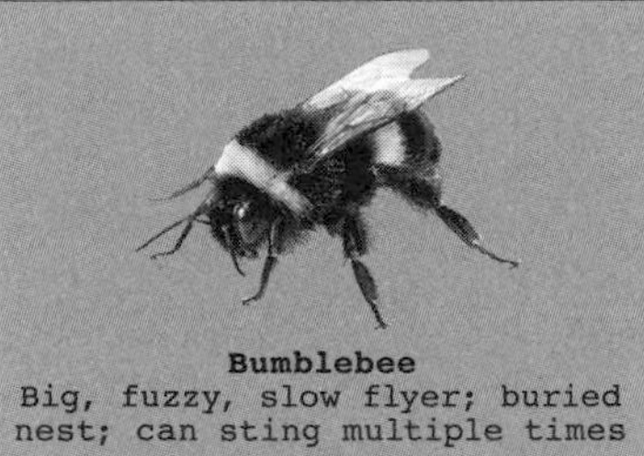

Bumblebee
Big, fuzzy, slow flyer; buried nest; can sting multiple times

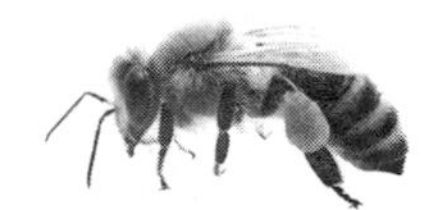

Honeybee
Relatively small; nests in trees and wood; stings once, then dies

Sting First-Aid

If a honeybee stings you, try to extract the stinger ASAP or venom will seep into your skin. Don't pinch the stinger (the venom sac may burst). Instead, scrape it out with a credit card or your fingernail. Apply ice to reduce swelling. Take an antihistamine such as Benadryl to help stop itching. Also, try applying a paste of baking soda and water.

RULE # 6

To estimate how long a hike will take, figure a half hour for each mile and a half hour for every 1,000 foot increase in altitude.

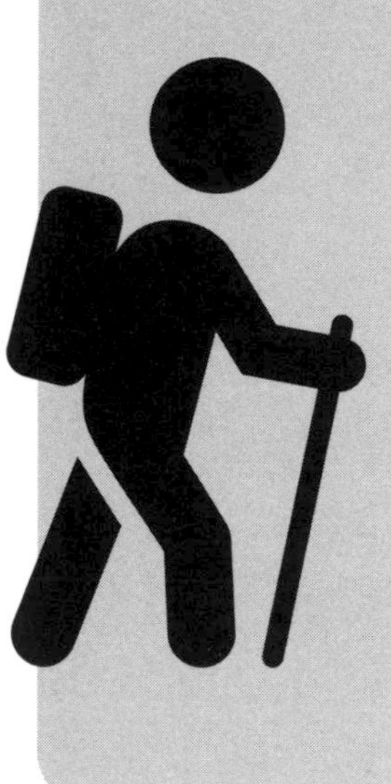

Find North without a Compass

With a stick. Press a stick into the ground and angle it directly at the sun so it doesn't cast a shadow. After a while, the sun will create a shadow of the stick that will point toward the east. Drawing a perpendicular line across the shadow will give you north and south.

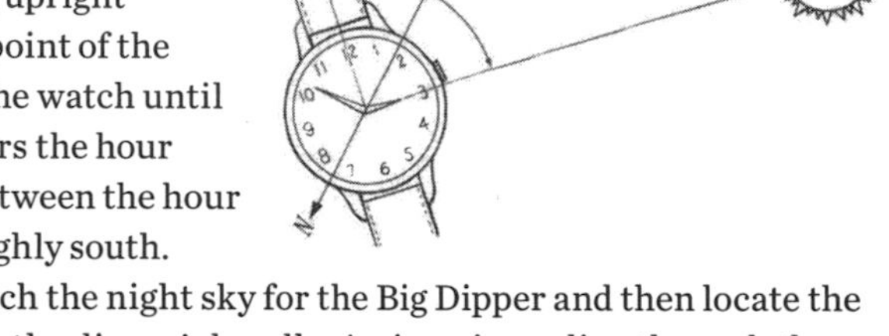

With a watch. Holding an analog watch flat, place a twig upright against the dial at the point of the hour hand. Now turn the watch until the twig's shadow covers the hour hand. A line halfway between the hour hand and 12 points roughly south.

By the North Star. Search the night sky for the Big Dipper and then locate the two stars farthest from the dipper's handle. An imaginary line through them points almost straight at Polaris, the North Star. Polaris is also the last star in the handle of the Little Dipper.

Guesstimate Wind Speed

	MPH
Smoke rises straight up	0
Smoke drifts	1-3
Leaves on trees rustle	4-7
Small branches move	8-12
Larger branches move	13-18
Small trees sway and flags ripple	19-24
Larger trees sway; flags flap, making a beating sound	25-31
Whole trees sway and flags extend straight; it's hard to walk against the wind	32-38

Stay Warm in a Sleeping Bag

Common sense might lead you to believe that bundling up with every piece of warm clothing you have will keep you warm in your sleeping bag. But you would be better off stripping to the skin or wearing only long underwear. That will give your body heat a chance to warm the air inside your sleeping bag, which will keep you comfortable. In the morning, change out of whatever you slept in. Those clothes will be damp from perspiration and will chill you as soon as you step outside.

RULE # 7

A pee bottle in your sleeping bag will make you feel very intelligent on a cold or wet night in the tent.

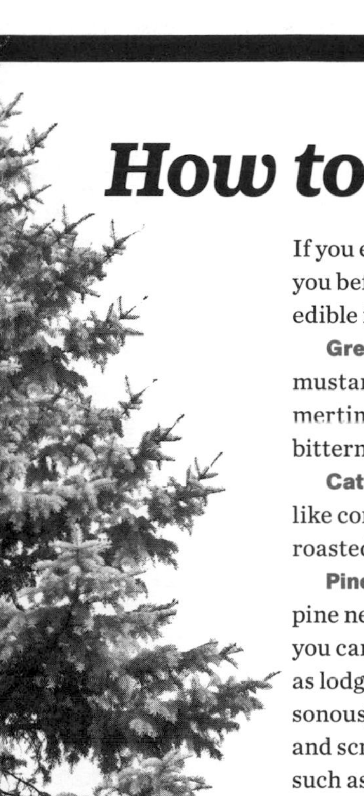

How to Eat a Pine Tree

If you ever get lost in the woods, rescuers will probably find you before the buzzards do. Still, it's wise to know what's edible in the wild.

Greens. Watercress, dandelion, young goldenrod, black mustard, or chicory leaves make a good salad. By summertime, some greens turn bitter. Boil them to cut the bitterness.

Cattail. Boil the young green pollen heads and eat them like corn on the cob. The thick root of this plant can be roasted.

Pine-needle tea. Chop a handful of green lodgepole pine needles and steep in hot water for a fragrant tea. Also, you can eat the inner white bark of certain pine trees, such as lodgepole and Scotch pine (but NOT yew, which is poisonous), raw or boiled. Strip the brown bark from the tree and scrape out the inner white pithy bark. Some pine trees, such as piñon pine nuts, can be eaten, too.

Caveat: Before you go gnawing on anything in the great outdoors, pick up a guidebook like the *Peterson Field Guide to Edible Wild Plants*. Getting sick is often worse than going hungry.

Make a Homemade Survival Kit

Toss this stuff in the trunk of your car for the time you break down 40 miles from the nearest Days Inn.

- 25 feet of nylon cord for stringing up a tent and a zillion other uses
- Two large, heavy-duty plastic bags. Can be cut to make a tent or a rain suit.
- A metallized space blanket for warmth
- A large candle and 20 waterproof wooden matches
- A small, sharp pocketknife
- Water purification tablets
- Some fishhooks and line
- Small flashlight with extra batteries
- Large bandanna. Use it as a sunhat, sweatband, sling, bandage, and for catching minnows.
- Chocolate bar and dried meat
- A collapsible cup
- A small first-aid kit

Cram it all in a 2-pound coffee can, which doubles as a cook pot. Put the plastic top on it and wrap 4 feet of duct tape around the can. You can use the tape to repair equipment and—in a pinch—people.

BEAR *Essentials*

- When hiking in bear country, yodel, talk loudly, or sing. Making human noises allows the animal to move away before you get there. You never want to surprise a bear.
- If a black bear enters your camp, bang on a pot to scare it away.
- If a black bear noses you awake at night, don't make sudden moves, but don't play dead, either. Talk to the bear in a calm, deep voice to let it know you aren't roadkill.
- Never run or climb trees—two things bears do better than humans. Instead, stand your ground and get big and loud. Clap your hands and yell. If in a group, gather together to appear bigger and show that you aren't afraid. Drop any food that might be attracting the bear.

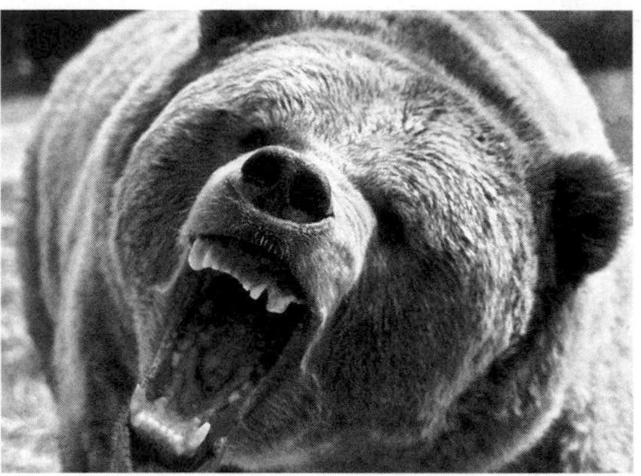

- If attacked by a brown bear, curl into a ball, holding your head and neck with your arms. Leave your backpack on for protection. Most brown bears will stop attacking when the threat is gone.

Conquer the Trail

Keep your feet happy with tips from long-distance hiker Justin Lichter and Georganna Morton of Mountain Crossings Outfitter.

Outfit your feet. Go with trail shoes—they lack the stiffness of boots and don't need to be broken in. If the top or side of your foot rubs during the hike, stop to relace, skipping the grommet closest to the hot spot to relieve the pressure.

Calibrate your stride. Rookie hikers tend to stomp. Instead, walk as if you were on the street—naturally. Over time, any unnatural motion in your stride can fatigue your joints.

How to Shit in the Woods

Find a secluded area that isn't within 200 yards of a water source right off the trail. Use a trowel to dig a hole 6 to 8 inches deep. "The best enzymes for decomposition are in the top layer of soil," says Kathleen Meyer, author of *How to Shit in the Woods.* No TP? Hunt for soft fallen leaves that haven't dried up or even a smooth stone.

Assume the position. Squat in a surfer's stance, butt below your knees, arms extended for balance. Done? Bury the leaves or stone along with your waste, or if you used toilet paper, seal it in a plastic bag and carry it out of the woods with you and flush it at home. Don't forget to wash your hands.

Source: Kathleen Meyer, author of How to Shit in the Woods.

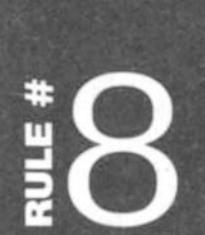

When lost in the wilderness, think: first shelter, then water, then food.

Swim with Sharks

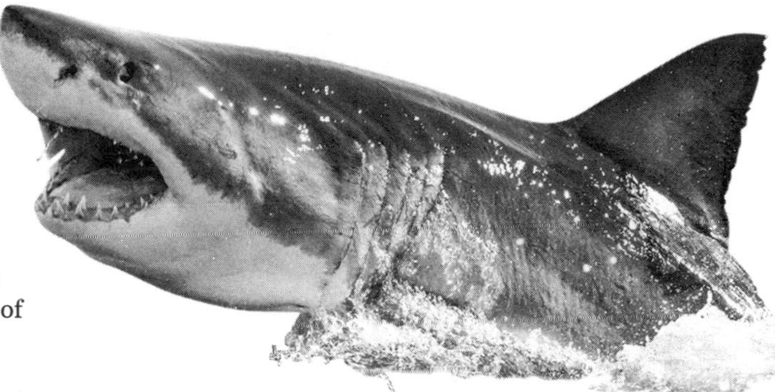

Your chances of being attacked by a shark are about 1 in 75 million. So the odds are better for you that Jennifer Lawrence will show up at your motel-room door with a bag of pretzels and a party hat. Of course, we don't have to tell you that you won't get very far trying to tell that to the fin in the water. So use this uncommon knowledge to get out of the water with your limbs.

The Basics:

1. Don't act like bait.
2. Punch an attacking shark in the nose.
3. Sharks are dumber than pit bulls. Meaner, too.

The Details:

1. **Don't panic or splash.** You'll look like a wounded seal—but swim away with slow, even strokes.
2. **Go deep.** If you are scuba diving, move to the bottom against a rock so you are protected from the rear. You might also scare the shark away by sending a stream of bubbles his way from your regulator.
3. **Duke it out.** If the shark attacks, poke it sharply in the snout, eye, or gills. Sharks, like many other animals, are sensitive around the schnoz, and a good punch in the nose makes you too much trouble for dinner.
4. **Dress down.** Don't wear brightly colored swim trunks or flashy silver chains.
5. **Don't tinkle.** How many times do we have to tell you? Don't pee in the water. No matter how scared you are. Sharks love that stuff.

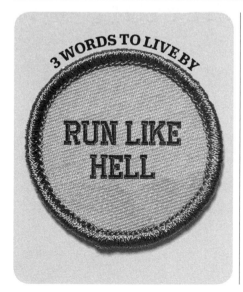

3 WORDS TO LIVE BY
RUN LIKE
HELL

How to Escape a Rip Current

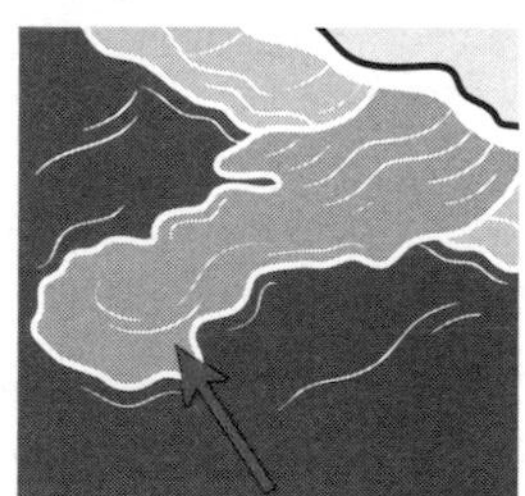

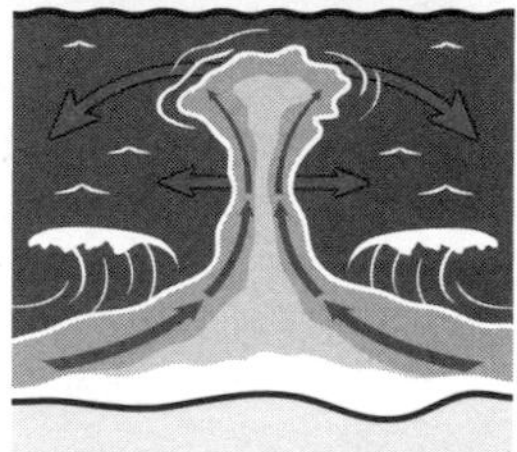

Your instinct will be to swim straight to shore, but the current is too strong. Instead, move parallel to the shoreline. Can't break the grip? Tread water and go with the flow. Eventually the current will carry you out of the rip current and you can swim to shore. You can avoid a rip current by spotting the clues: a channel of churning, choppy water; a change in water color; a break in the incoming wave pattern; or a line of seaweed or foam moving out to sea.

Catch More Fish

When you don't catch anything on your fishing trip, you've been skunked. And that stinks. Improve your odds of landing a lunker with these tips.

1. Before you set a line, ask a question. Visit a tackle shop near where you'll be fishing and ask which lures and baits are best and how to fish them.
2. Be sneaky. Fish frighten easily. Sneak up on them quietly. Don't bang your tackle box on the boat or talk loudly on shore. When approaching a good fishing spot, walk slowly and crouch down so the fish won't see you.
3. Think small. When finicky fish aren't biting your big nightcrawlers or minnows, try using smaller bait. Cut your worm or minnow in half and put a piece on your hook. Sometimes fish prefer smaller portions.
4. Think shade. On sunny days, bass like to hang out in the shade of half-sunken stumps and submerged logs. Cast your lure a few feet in front of the stump and then reel the lure through the shade.
5. Use lightweight line. It should be thin and invisible to fish. For bluegills, perch, and trout, use 4- to 6-pound test monofilament. For larger fish, use 6- to 12-pound test line.
6. Brook trout are easier to catch than a cold because they feed on food that floats by. Use a spinner lure and cast it perpendicular to the current. Aim for a part of the stream with eddies and small, standing waves and let the lure drive downstream while reeling in. No bite? Take two steps downstream and cast again.
7. Sunrise is one of the best times to fish. Get up early. Be casting at first light.
8. Pick a fish's favorite color. The best rubber worm colors are black for night fishing and purple for daytime fishing.

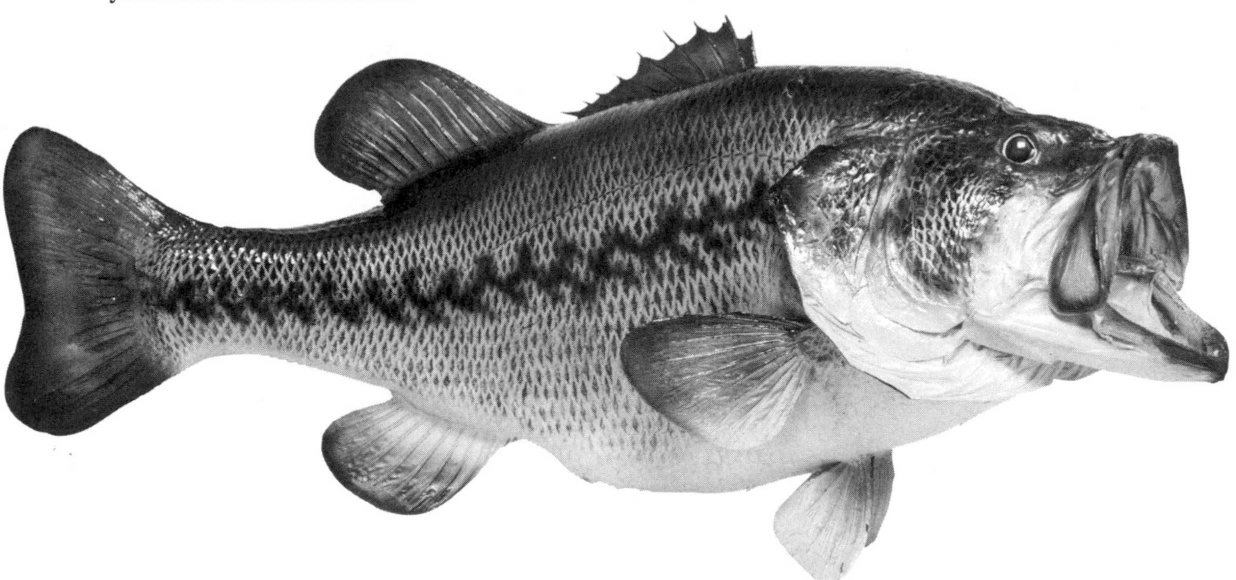

9. Go and stop and go. To make your spinner or rubber worm look more realistic, use a stop-and-go retrieve: Reel in five to seven turns, then stop for a few seconds and repeat this pattern.
10. Use homeboy minnows. When fishing with live baitfish, catch them in the same water you are going to fish. That way you won't introduce new diseases or fish species to a lake or river.
11. Play a double-header. Bring two rods. Bait one, cast, and let it sit propped up on a Y-shaped stick. Put an artificial lure on the other one, cast, and retrieve. You'll double your chances of catching.
12. Try crickets. Big bluegills love crickets. Buy about 50 live ones from a bait store. Use a number 10 long-shanked hook and run the hook through the cricket's back, just behind the head. Add two large split shots to the line to make the insect easy to cast, no bobber. Cast into water that's about 10 feet deep and has a weedy bottom. Let the split shots hit bottom, then raise your rod tip and start reeling in slower than slow.
13. Avoid hooks bigger than size 10. The fish will notice them. Size 12, which is smaller than 10, is perfect for trout.
14. To catch more fish, set the hook right. Many beginners yank the line too hard, pulling the hook right out of the fish's mouth. When your bobber goes under or you feel the "tap tap" on your rod, lift your rod tip with a quick jerk. That'll help the hook bite into the fish's jaw. Then keep your rod tip high as you reel it in.

HOW TO *Toss a Fish Back*

By returning your fish to the water, you improve your chances of catching more fish another day. How to do it right: Wet your hands before touching the fish. Handle it as little as possible when taking it off the hook. Hold it under the head and tail and gently place it back in the water, moving it forward so water passes through its mouth and gills until it swims away.

Master the Sidearm Cast

To avoid snagging your line in the trees with an overhand cast, try this side style instead, recommends Chris Lane, 2012 Bassmaster Classic champion.

Step 1. Stand with your feet shoulder width apart and your body squared with where you want the lure to land. This stance provides power from your hips; the result is a stronger cast.

Step 2. Hold the rod in front of your hip on your dominant side and keep it parallel to the ground. Swing it back around your hip, turning so your knee bends slightly.

Step 3. In one smooth motion, rotate your hips and the rod back toward your starting stance. Swing the rod forward, and when it passes your hip, flick your wrist toward where you want the lure to land. At the same moment let out your line.

How to Clean a Fish

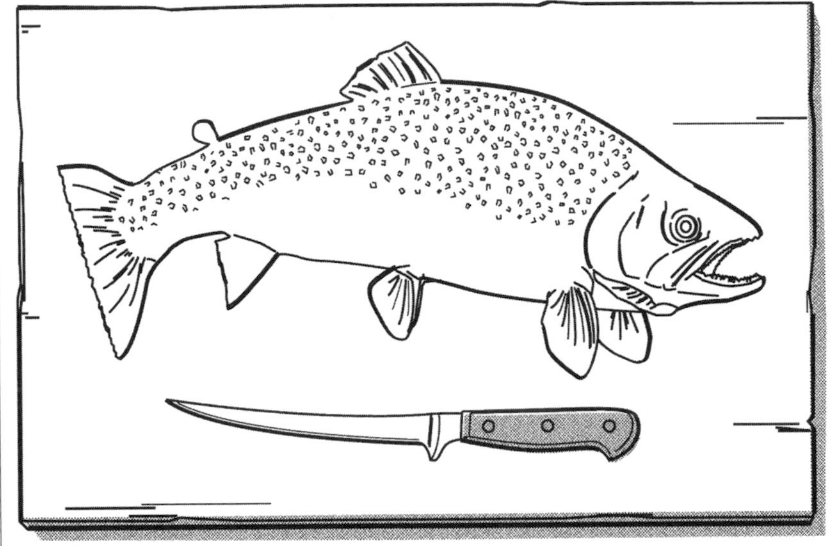

Strip the Scales

Grab a knife with your dominant hand. Flop the fish onto a cutting board and hold the head with your nondominant hand. Position the blade perpendicular to the fish. Using firm strokes, scrape from tail to head. (Scales will fly!) Flip it and repeat.

Slice It Open

Rinse the fish. Holding the fish the same way as before, insert the knife tip into the slit between the belly and rear fins. Work the blade toward the head until you reach the bone beneath the gills. In one motion, force the knife through to cut the bone.

Gut It!

Remove the knife, pinch the guts near the head, and pull them out. Yank out the bacteria-ridden gills too—that way the fish won't spoil quickly. Hold the gills between your thumb and forefinger and pull up and away from the body. For a large fish, use your knife for help.

Finish the Job

If you look inside the body cavity, you'll see a dark blood line running along the top. Don't leave it there, or you'll have bitter-tasting fish. Use the tip of your knife or your fingernail (a spoon works great) to scrape out the line. Then rinse the entire fish well under cold water. Pat your dinner dry. Now you're ready to cook.

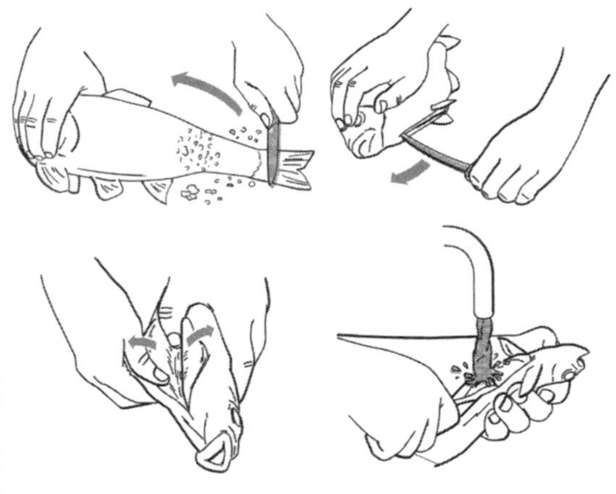

If you can see the fish, the fish can see you.

Best Fishing Lures

THESE WORK SO WELL, THEY SHOULD BE ILLEGAL

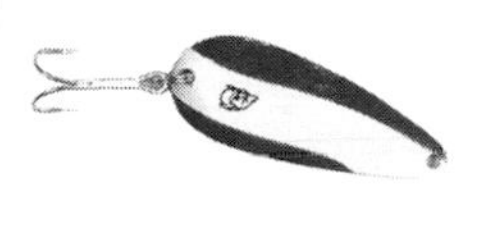

Dardevle. For bass and big trout. A good lure to use with the go-stop-go retrieve.

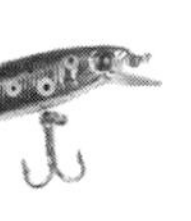

Rapala. This floating plug with treble hooks looks like a pike's favorite food: a minnow.

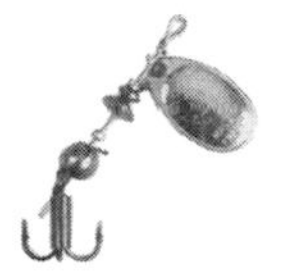

Mepps spinner. Great for small, rocky trout streams.

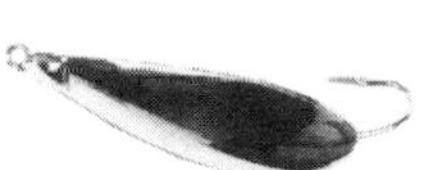

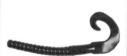

Johnson silver minnow. Toss this weedless lure into the weedbeds and watch the bass jump.

Black rubber worm. Choose a 7-inch size with a curly tail for extra action.

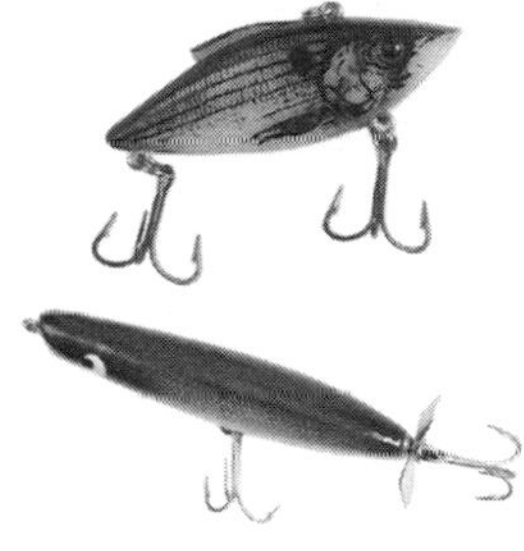

Rat-L-Trap. Looks like a wounded shad. Good for trout and pike.

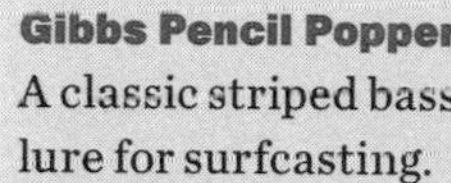

Gibbs Pencil Popper. A classic striped bass lure for surfcasting.

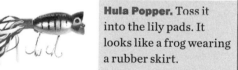

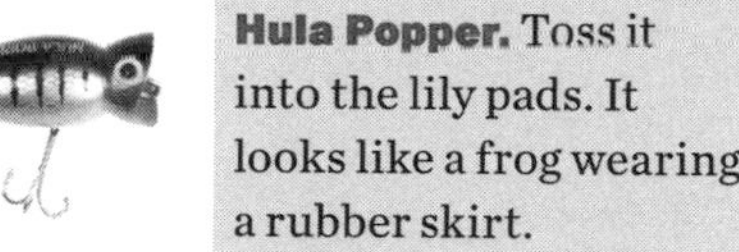

Roostertail. One of the best rainbow trout spinners ever made.

Hula Popper. Toss it into the lily pads. It looks like a frog wearing a rubber skirt.

Jitterbug. The *glub-glub* sound it makes as you reel it in rings the dinner bell for bass.

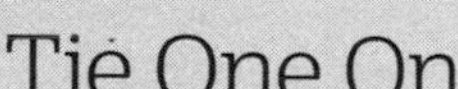

Tie One On

The "improved clinch knot" is simple and can be used for hooks and lures.

- Thread the line through the eye of the hook, leaving 3 inches. Twist the excess five to seven times around the standing line.
- Hold the coils and thread the end through the first loop above the eye, and then through the large loop you just created.
- Pull on the standing line and the excess simultaneously. Use your fingernails to slide the knot tight against the hook's eye.

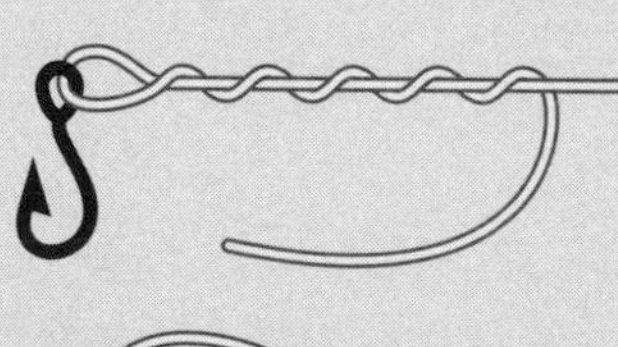

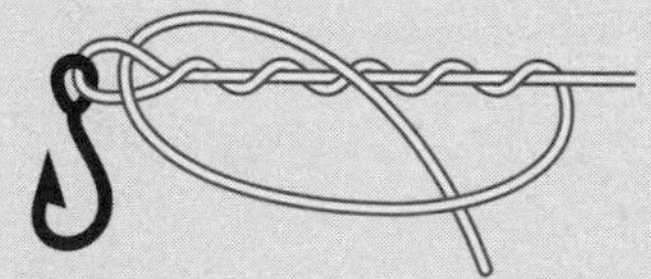

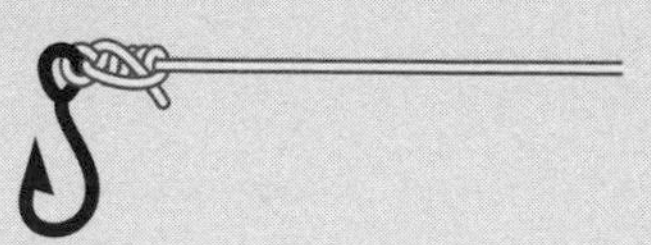

A Fish Finder

Do you know a brownie from a crappie? Try this match-the-catch quiz. Write the letter of the fish picture on the line next to its name. Answer key is on page 58.

Freshwater

___ Largemouth bass
___ Smallmouth bass
___ Bluegill
___ Pickerel
___ Rainbow trout
___ Brown trout
___ Brook trout
___ Crappie
___ Channel catfish
___ Walleye
___ Perch
___ Muskellunge
___ Northern pike

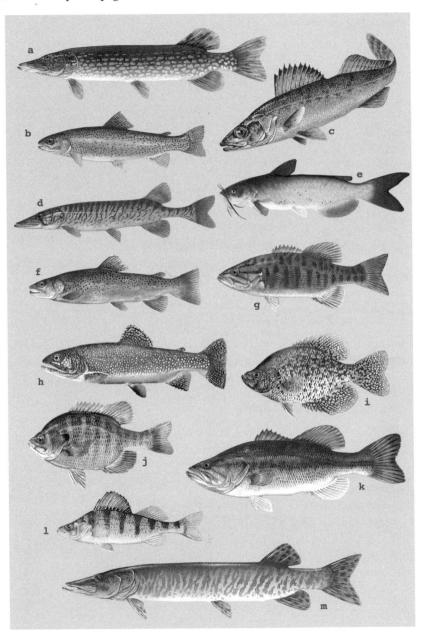

Saltwater

____ Bluefish
____ Striped bass
____ Tarpon
____ Billfish
____ Sea bass
____ Tuna
____ Weakfish
____ Pompano or jack
____ Red drum

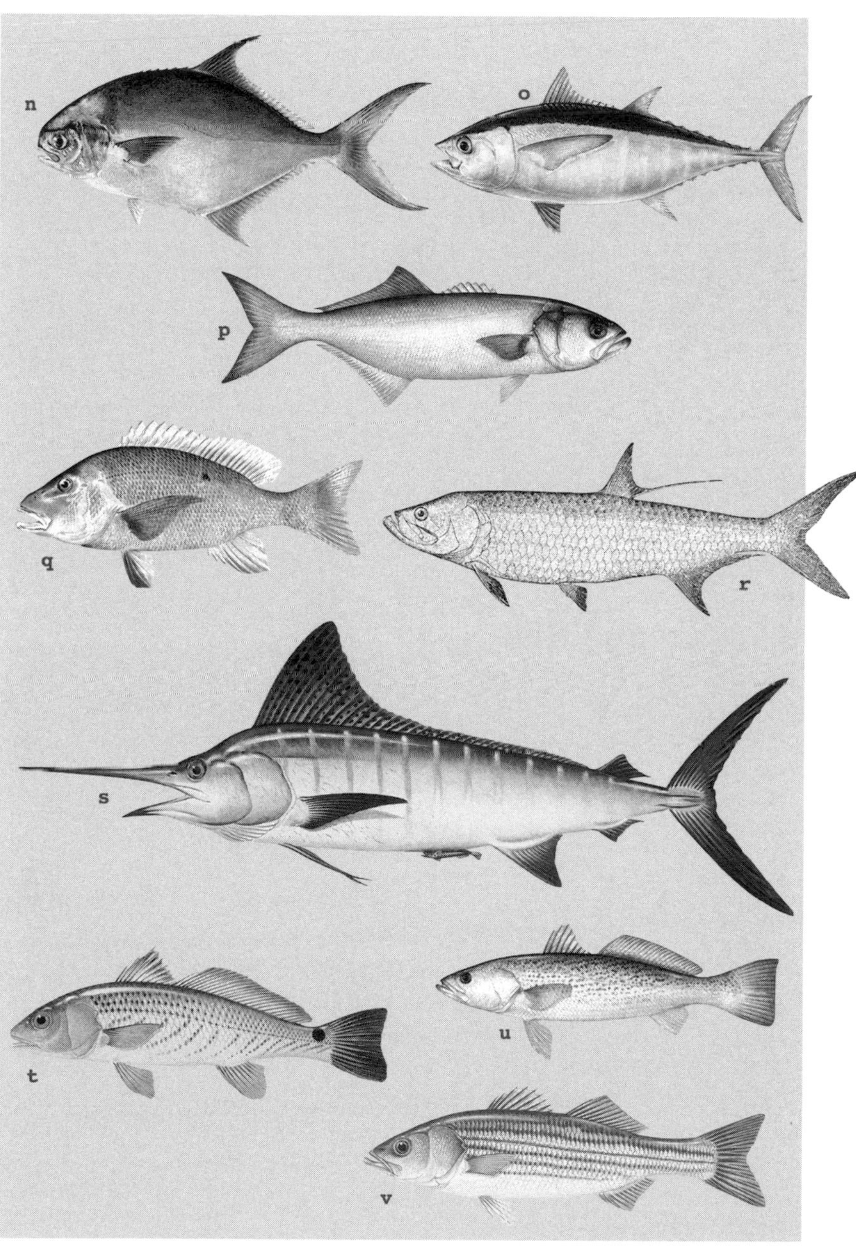

Keep Sweat Out of Your Eyes

During a hike or trail run, you can divert the sweat from stinging your eyes by rubbing lip balm over your eyebrows.

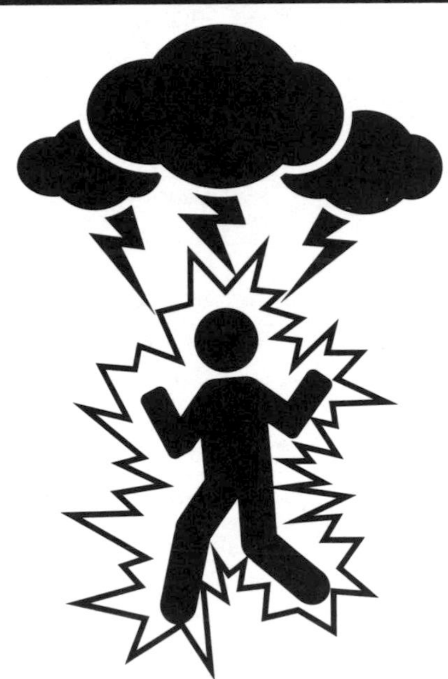

Don't Get *Fried by Lightning*

If you are caught in a lightning storm, get low, but don't lie on the ground. Instead put your feet together so they touch, squat down, grab your legs, and rest on the balls of your feet. If a bolt strikes the ground, the current may bump over the balls of your feet and reenter the ground without traveling into your body. If there's a space between your feet, the current may travel up one leg and into your body. If you're with a group of people, spread out away from each other and have everyone squat as described above.

Scale a Big Boulder

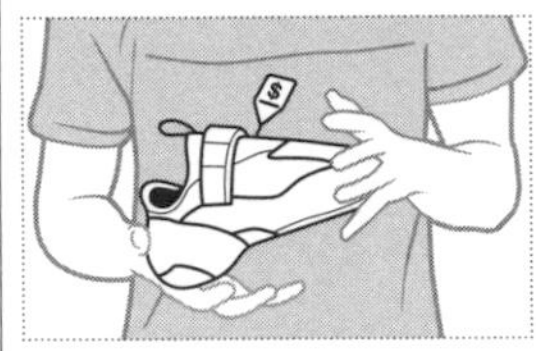

Assemble Your Gear

You don't need ropes and harnesses for bouldering. Just find a large, thick crash pad, like the Metolius Sketch Pad ($115, metoliusclimbing.com), and thin, sturdy climbing shoes, such as the Five Ten Blacks (fiveten.com, $160). You'll also want a basic chalk bag, like evolv's Roundtangular bag ($19, rei.com).

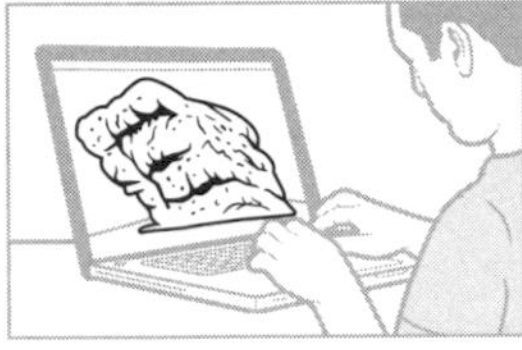

Scope Out Your Rock

Hit up rockclimbing.com to find great boulders near you, or scout your own. Your wall should be 10 to 16 feet high with a flat area for your crash pad and handholds or cracks you can follow, says Chris Potts, co-owner of the Seattle Bouldering Project. Chalk marks from previous climbers signal preapproval.

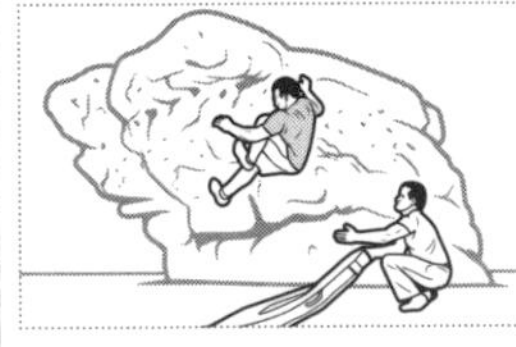

Plan Your Route

Set up a challenge—reaching the top, traversing a face, or going all the way around the boulder, says Patrick Odenbeck of montanabouldering.com. Have your buddy spot you, moving the crash pad as you move. His goal shouldn't be to catch you but instead to prevent you from falling on your back or neck.

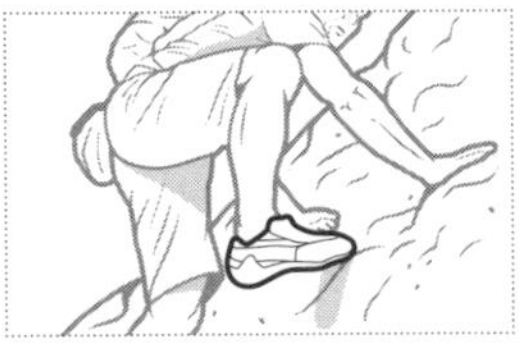

Keep Your Momentum

Rookies tend to stand on the middle of their feet when climbing, placing their feet parallel to the boulder, which saps power from their legs. Instead, stand on your toes. This helps you engage your calves, aiding balance and letting you power up the rock, says Potts. Your legs should absorb most of your weight.

How to Use Your Pants as a **LIFE JACKET**

You're in the middle of a lake, and the boat sinks, and you're not wearing a life preserver. Do this: Make one out of your trousers. While treading water, slip off your pants and tie the legs together at the cuffs, tightening the knot with your teeth. Grab the belt or waist of the pants and throw the pants over your head to catch air inside. Or, hold the waist in one hand under water to inflate them by cupping air in your other hand, pushing it underwater, and releasing it into the pants. (You can even blow air into the pants to inflate.) When inflated, hold the waist closed and lean the back of your neck across the crotch to keep your head above water. Reinflate as needed.

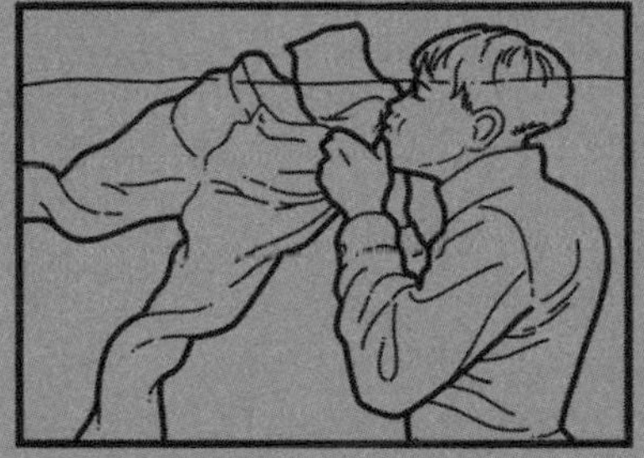

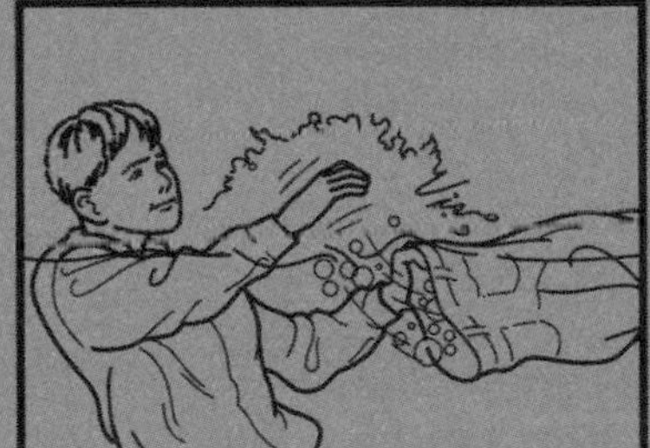

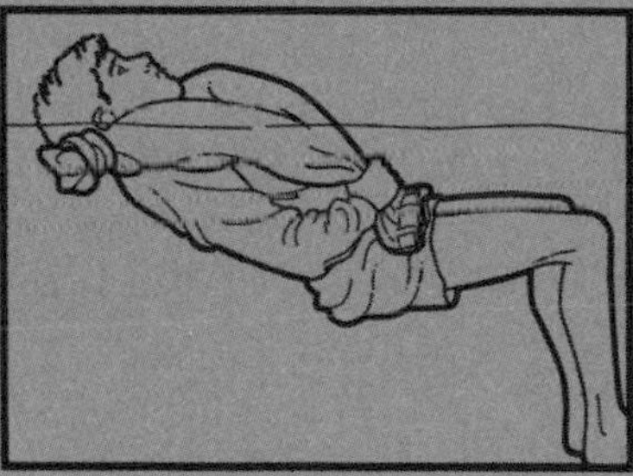

Illustrations of life jacket and arm splint courtesy of The Boy Scouts of America.

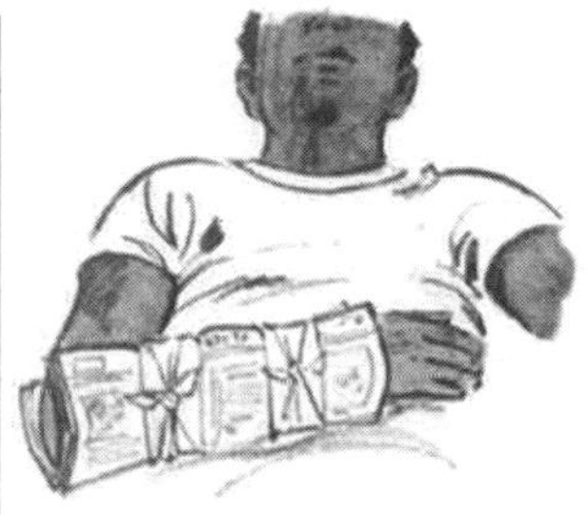

Secure a Fractured Bone

WITH A COPY OF *MEN'S HEALTH*

Create a splint from your favorite magazine or rolled-up newspaper. Secure it in three places with tape, ensuring that the splint supports above and below the break.

RULE # 10

When cooking over an open fire, use flame for boiling, coals for broiling and frying.

Tighten a Loose Ax Head

Soak the head in a bucket of water for a few hours (only if the handle is made of wood, Einstein). The wood will swell and tighten the ax temporarily.

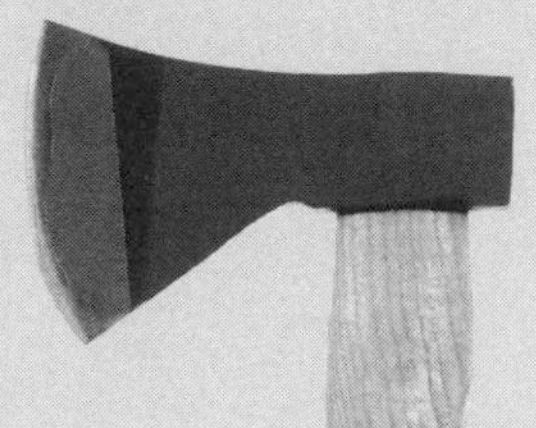

Learn How to Fly Fish in About 600 Words

"The equipment does the work," says Bob Sousa, PhD, author of *Learn to Fly Fish in 24 Hours.* "You are the conductor."

Rod

A good freshwater fly rod for a beginner is a 5-weight, between 8 and 9 feet in length. Shorter rods are good for the tight little streams of the east and longer rods for wide-open lakes and big rivers of the west.

Line

A 5-weight rod takes a 5-weight line, but if you are a new caster, fit it with a 6-weight, weight-forward fly line. It'll be a little heavier and therefore easier to cast. (Remember, unlike in any other style of fishing, the line, not the weight of the lure or a sinker, carries the bait to the fish.) If you're fishing water that's 5 feet deep or less, use a floating line; 5.5 to 15 feet deep, a sinking-tip line; over 15, use a full sinking line. To the line, tie a 9-foot tapered leader. Your leader will shorten as you change flies during the day. After losing 2 feet or so, tie on a "tippet," a thin piece of line, to bring the leader back to 9 feet in length.

Reel

Choose a reel with a good, functional drag. You'll lose fewer fish if you "reel fight" them versus bringing them in by retrieving line by hand. Line typically comes in 110-foot lengths. Since many fish can strip off 100 feet of line, you'll need to add what's called "backing," a Dacron line, to the reel. "I recommend winding the fly line on the reel *first,* then tie your backing onto the end of the fly line, and fill the reel to capacity," says Sousa. "That way you know how much backing you need." Then strip the line off the reel and reverse it so that you wind the backing onto the arbor first, followed by the fly line.

Flies

"Match what the fish are eating at that moment and you will catch a lot of fish," says Sousa. Or, if you can't figure out the hatch, try one of these six classic flies below. "If you put 1,000 fly fishers in a room and ask them to write down their 10 favorite flies, 95 percent of them will have these six on their list," says Sousa.

DRY

Adams

Black gnat parachute

Elk-hair caddis

WET

Wooly bugger

Bead-head golden-ribbed hare's mast nymph

Pheasant-tail nymph

How to Cast a Flyrod in Four Simple Steps

1 Make sure your thumb is on top of the rod handle.

2 Lift the rod up briskly, stopping abruptly when the rod tip reaches the 1 o'clock position.

3 Look behind you to watch the fly line float back. Wait for it to fully unfurl before starting the forward cast. This is crucial, and why beginners using a slightly heavier 6-weight line will find it easier. You want to feel the little tick in the rod when your line is fully extended behind you.

4 Bring the rod forward, stopping when the rod tip is at 10 o'clock and allowing the fly line carrying the leader to unfurl, and delicately present the fly onto the water. All you need to do is cast 30 feet to catch fish, says Bob Sousa, PhD, author of *Learn to Fly Fish in 24 Hours*.

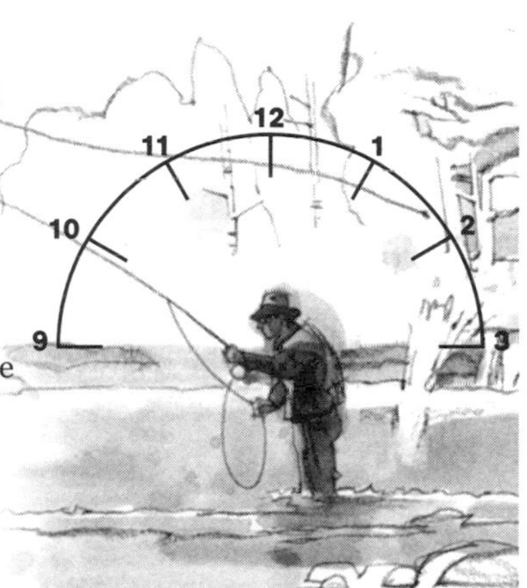

Weather a Storm

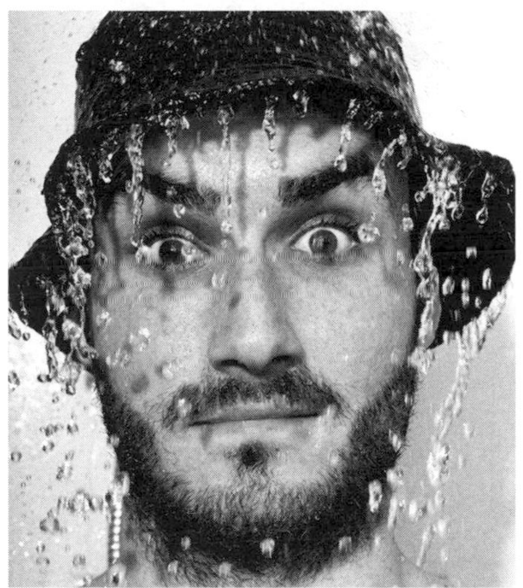

Hurricanes, tornadoes, blizzards, floods—disaster is never far from us, it seems. If nature's wrath descends on your town, survive with tips from Keith Stammer, director of emergency services in tornado-ravaged Joplin, Missouri.

Quick Tip: Is your home vulnerable to high winds? Pick the lowest, most central interior room, like a bathroom. If you're in a flood zone, go to the garage.

Cell Phone

Ahead of time, make sure your phone can receive wireless emergency alerts. (Ask your carrier.) Download Red Cross apps for weather, shelter, and first-aid information.

Social Media

If trouble looms, pick one person outside the region who can receive messages from you and relay them or post updates to social media. In many situations, text messages can be sent and received even if call service is out.

Radio

Buy a radio synced with NOAA, such as Midland's hand-cranked ER102 ($60, midlandusa.com).

Supplies

Pack work clothes, a hardhat, gloves, and boots. Store rope, duct tape, flashlights, a tarp for shelter, and On Duty's 4-in-1 Emergency Tool. It can turn off gas and water and pry doors open ($20, ondutynetwork.com).

Rations

You'll need 72 to 96 hours of food and approximately 1 gallon of water per person per day.

ID Key for "A Fish Finder" (pages 52-53)

Freshwater Fish
a. Northern pike
b. Brown trout
c. Walleye
d. Pickerel
e. Channel catfish
f. Rainbow trout
g. Smallmouth bass
h. Brook trout
i. Crappie
j. Bluegill
k. Largemouth bass
l. Perch
m. Muskellunge

Saltwater Fish
n. Pompano or jack
o. Tuna
p. Bluefish
q. Sea bass
r. Tarpon
s. Billfish
t. Red drum
u. Weakfish
v. Striped bass

Q What's the fastest way to adjust to high altitude when skiing or backpacking?

A. The rule of thumb for preventing the nausea and headache of altitude sickness is this: Once you're above 10,000 feet, limit the elevation increase of your sleeping environment to between 1,000 and 1,500 feet a day, says Andrew Luks, MD, an associate professor at the University of Washington's division of pulmonary and critical care medicine. Breaking your ascent into chunks will give your body time to acclimatize to the reduced oxygen supply. But if you're planning to summit a peak, you may need more than 3 days to acclimatize. Monitoring your ascent is critical because of the possibility of cerebral or pulmonary edema, a rare but potentially fatal swelling of the brain or lungs.

How to ID a Big Bird

LOOK! UP IN THE SKY! IT'S A, A . . . WHAT THE HELL IS THAT?

You see them gliding on the thermals above, silhouetted against the blue sky. And the (kid, girlfriend, wife, buddy, used car salesman) asks, "Golly, what in tarnation is that big bird flying in the sky?" If you know the telltale shapes of America's big raptors, you'll seem pretty damn smart.

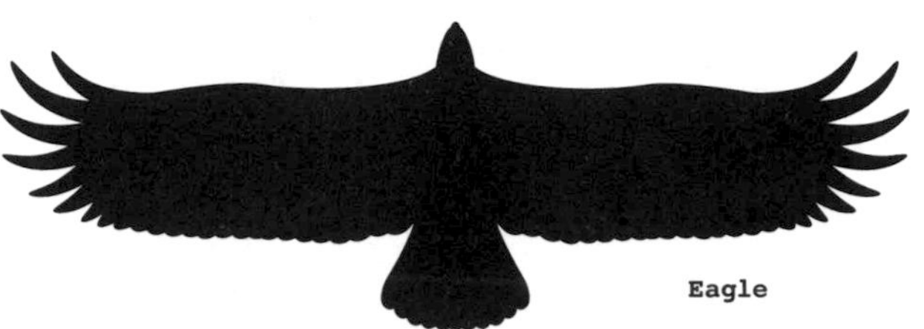

Eagle

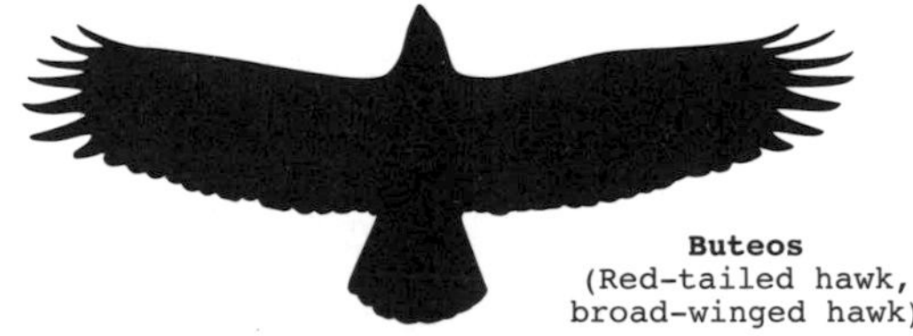

Buteos
(Red-tailed hawk, broad-winged hawk)

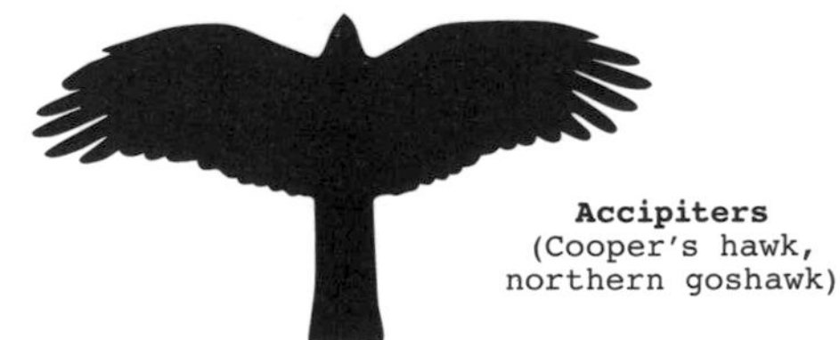

Accipiters
(Cooper's hawk, northern goshawk)

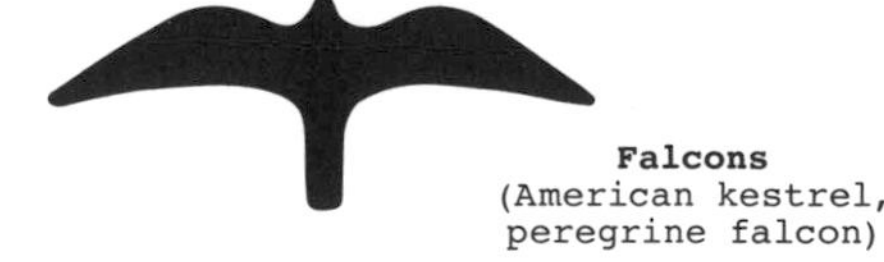

Falcons
(American kestrel, peregrine falcon)

Remove a Tick—Safely

Choose Your Weapon

If you don't have a tool like Pro-Tick Remedy or Ticked Off, tweezers work. Don't apply Vaseline, lotion, or alcohol-based substances, and never burn the tick. Any of these can make it spew blood into your skin. Yeah, gross.

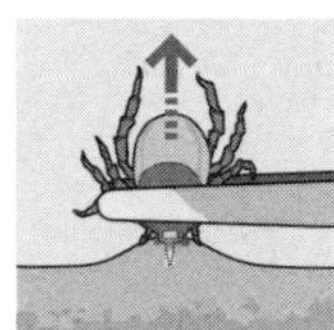

Be Gentle

Don't squeeze too hard; you want the tick intact. Stay away from its gut and aim for where its mouth is inserted into your skin. Then pull up straight. If the tick breaks, remove as much of it as you can and monitor the site closely.

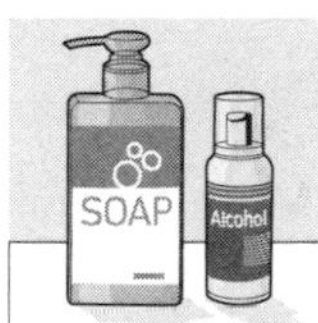

Wash

Use soap and warm water to thoroughly clean the bite area. Then disinfect it with alcohol or cover it with Neosporin. With a tick bite, you should expect a minor skin infection even if you're not infected with a tick-borne illness.

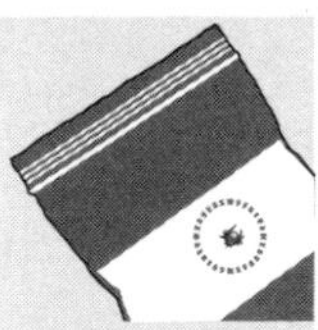

Store the Tick

Save the tick in a zipper-lock bag and store it at room temperature in case it needs to be tested in the future. Watch for joint pain or the bull's-eye rash that indicates Lyme disease.

Fix a Blister on the Trail

Pack the tools you need to treat your feet with help from Jeffrey Page, DPM, a hiker and director of the Arizona School of Podiatric Medicine at Midwestern University.

Prevent Infection

If the blister is ruptured, clean it before bandaging. Soap and water are best for flushing dirt and debris, or you can use an antiseptic towelette to wipe the blister and an inch around it. Apply an antibiotic ointment, such as Neosporin, and then bandage the area.

Pop with Care

If the blister is unbroken, pop it. Use an antiseptic wipe to sterilize a pin or pocketknife. Pierce the blister's edge, leaving the "roof" intact. Carefully press on the roof with another antiseptic wipe until the blister is drained.

Reduce Irritation

Apply a small piece of a hydrogel material and secure it with adhesive (2nd Skin makes both) or athletic tape. For added relief, surround the blister with strips of adhesive felt.

Speed Recovery

You don't have to let the blister "breathe." For faster healing, keep it slightly moist after the hike with antibiotic ointment and an adhesive bandage.

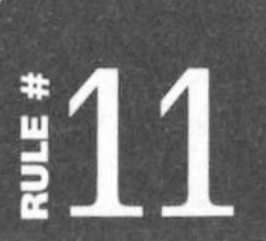

When choosing a spot to pitch your tent, look down, then look up. Down—will you be lying on rocks and roots? Up—look for "widow makers," large, dead branches that may fall on your tent (and you) in a windstorm.

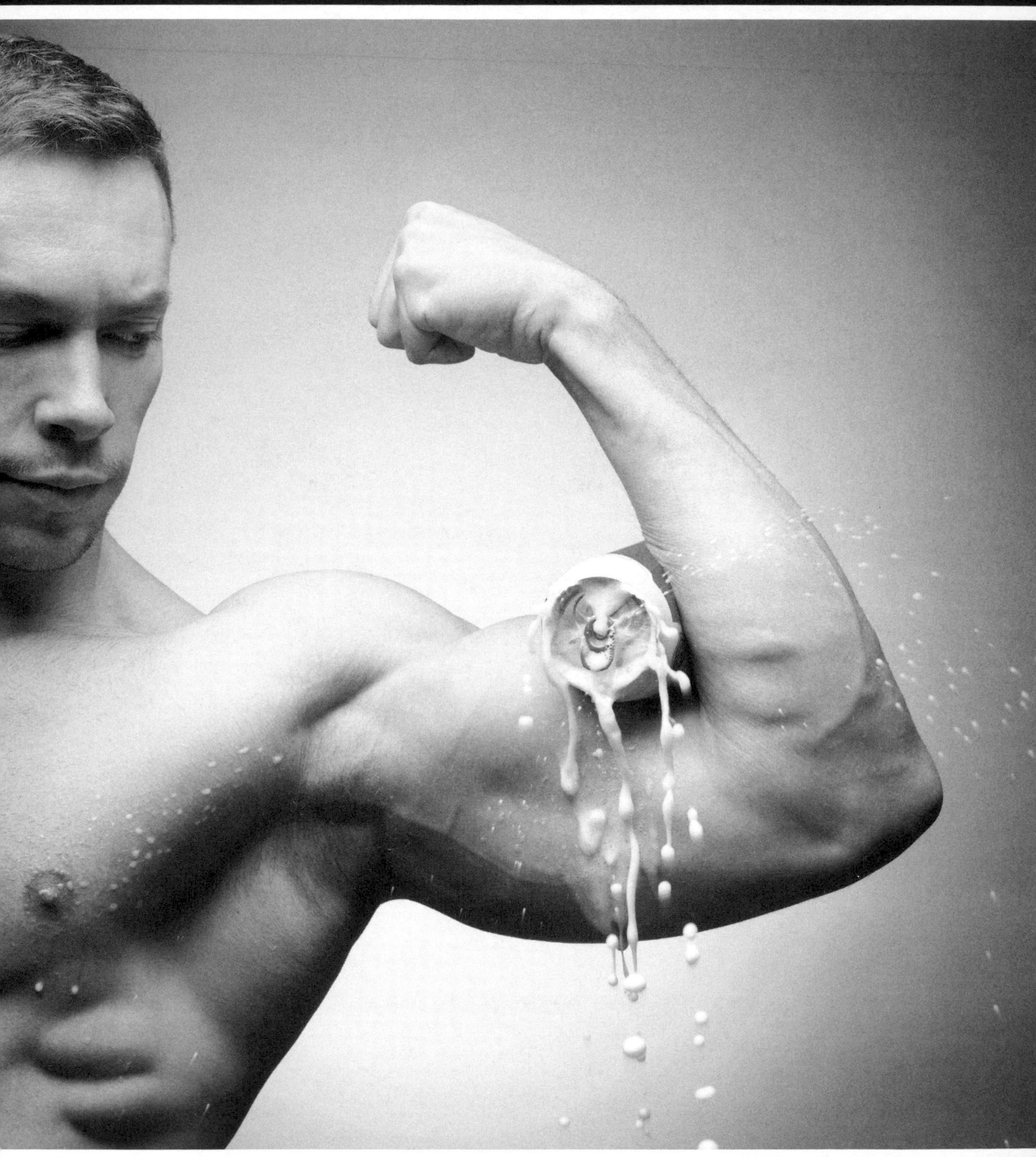

Muscle and Fitness

Dozens of Training Hints and Tips, Plus Wicked Quick Workouts That Will Burn Fat and Give You a Shredded Physique of Hard, Rippled Flesh

If you're in lousy shape, you're in luck. With a little effort you can quickly make significant strides toward improving your strength, aerobic endurance, and health. Results come big and fast when you're starting from being out of shape. It's when you have those last 5 stubborn pounds to lose or you're training for a triathlon that things start to really get tough. That's when you get into DOMS (delayed-onset muscle soreness), protein bars that taste like sawdust, and early-morning swims in frigid pools. But that's also when you've witnessed the results of exercise, and you love that feeling. Wherever you fall on the fitness spectrum, we have something useful for you in this chapter that'll help you become stronger, leaner, fitter, and quicker. We've even peppered in Amazing Feats of Fitness in case you really want to become sadistic about your body improvement project. Are you ready to sweat buckets? Turn the page and start with a simple circuit of body-weight exercises that'll kick off your total-body reboot.

Blast Fat Anywhere

Your body is all you need to get back in shape. Do the moves in the order shown, resting 15 to 30 seconds between exercises (or, if you're a gamer, jump rope for 1 minute in between). Complete three lung-busting circuits.

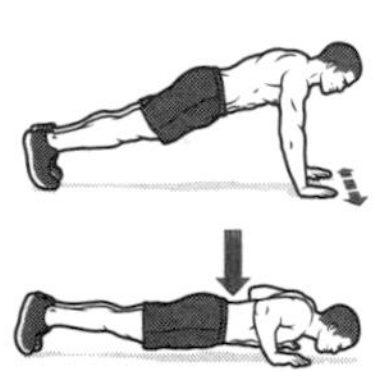

1. Pushup

Get down on all fours with your hands slightly beyond shoulder width. Put your feet together; straighten your arms and legs. Lower your body until your chest nearly touches the floor. Pause; push yourself back up. Do 20 reps.

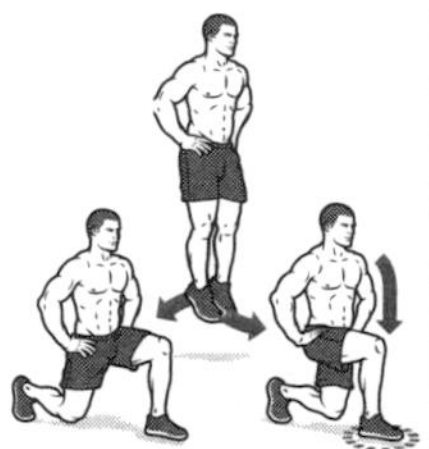

2. Split Jump

Assume a staggered stance with your left foot in front of your right. Lower your body into a lunge. Jump with enough force to propel both feet off the floor. Land with your right leg forward. Alternate legs each rep. Do 20 reps.

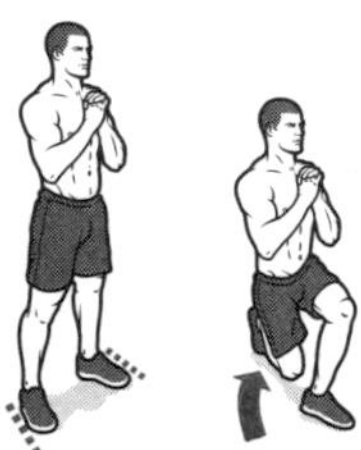

3. Drop Lunge

Stand tall with your hands clasped in front of your chest. Step back with your right foot, crossing it behind you as you sink into a lunge. Reset and repeat with your left leg. Continue alternating. Do 10 reps on each side (20 total).

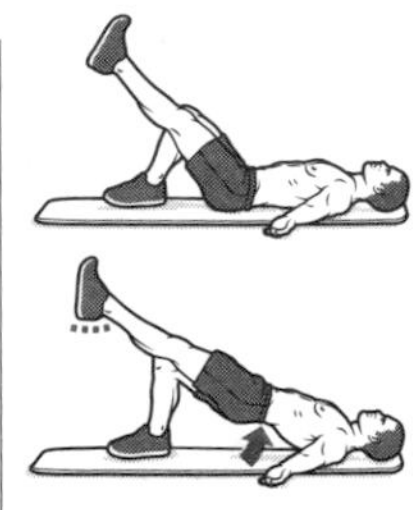

4. Glute Bridge

Lie faceup on the floor with your right knee bent and your left leg straight and in line with your right thigh. Push your hips up. Pause, and slowly lower your hips to the starting position. Do 10 reps, switch legs, and repeat (20 total).

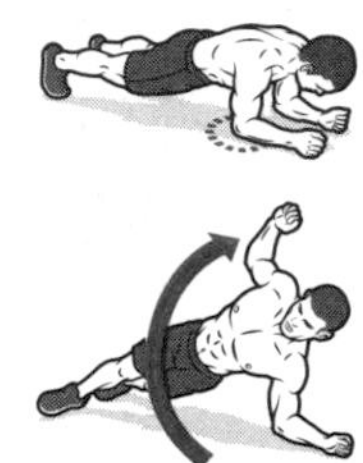

5. Rolling Plank

Assume a pushup position, but rest your weight on your forearms instead of your hands. Rotate your torso up and to the right. Repeat to your left. Continue alternating sides. Do 5 reps per side (10 total).

Q What's the best exercise to improve my tennis backhand?

A. Twisting medicine ball throws, because backhand power comes from core strength, not muscular arms, says Orlando tennis coach Brad Minns. "You must twist your body so your nondominant hand can lead when you strike the ball," he says. That means your hips, shoulders, arms, and core muscles must work together. The perpendicular medicine ball throw works them all as it mimics the shot. Practice with a partner or, if alone, don't release the medicine ball, but swing it from midtorso to over your shoulder as you twist your body.

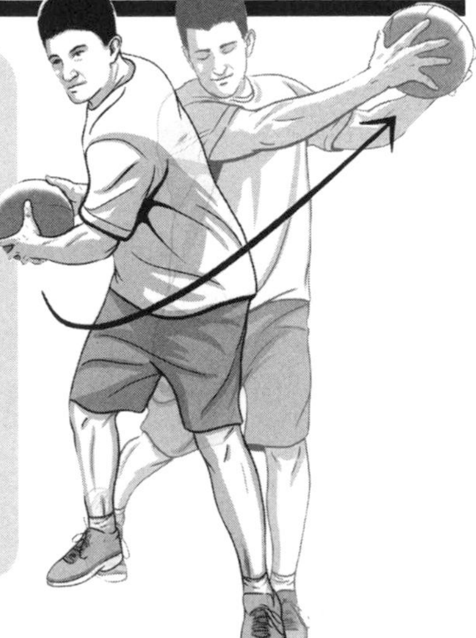

4 Mistakes That Can Make You Fat

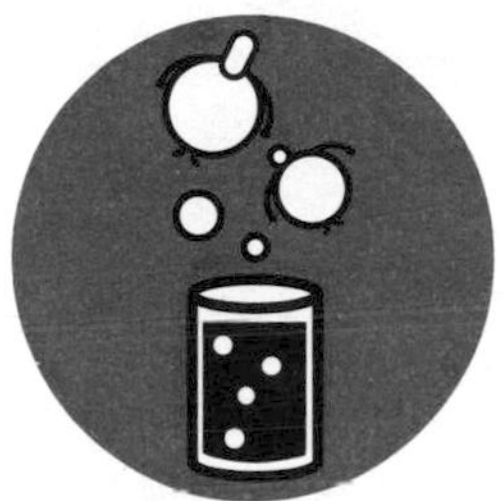

You Drink Diet Soda like It's Water

A University of North Carolina at Chapel Hill study found that when people swapped their favorite sugary soft drink for the diet variety, they ate more desserts and more bread than people who swapped their go-to beverage for water. Artificial sweeteners may increase your hunger for sweets, says study author Barry Popkin, PhD.

You Try Too Hard

Adopting a very rigid diet almost guarantees that your weight-loss efforts will be sabotaged by food cravings, suggests a new study in the journal *Appetite*. So cut yourself some slack. Flexible dieters have just as many cravings and give in to them just as often, says study author Adrian Meule, Dipl.-Psych. The difference is that they are more likely to get back on track quickly.

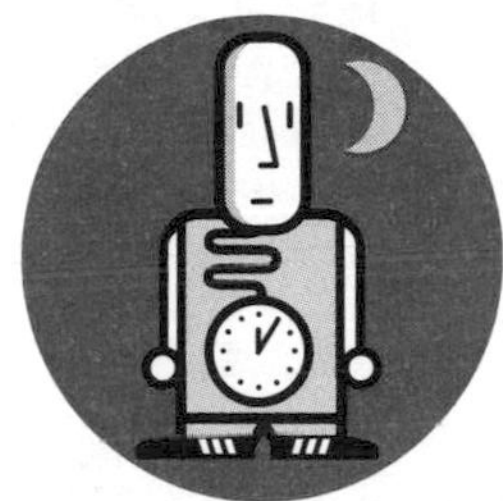

You Play *Call of Duty* until 2 A.M.

A new study in the *American Journal of Clinical Nutrition* reports that scant sleep can cause you to overeat fatty foods. When people slept only 4 hours a night for 5 days, they took in nearly 300 calories more than when they slept 9 hours a night. Too little shut-eye may increase your appetite by short-circuiting your brain's sense of reward.

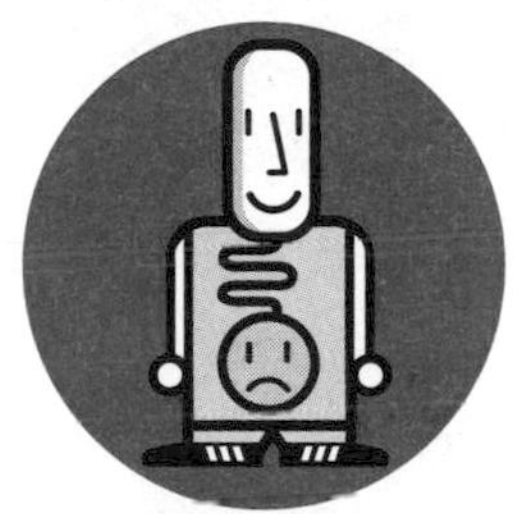

You're Too Darned Optimistic

If you're like most people, you wildly overestimate the number of calories you burn during exercise. According to a study in the *Journal of Sports Medicine and Physical Fitness*, people thought that a workout incinerated about 900 calories when it actually burned just 300.

The Slow Way to Big Biceps

Your muscles can lower more weight than they can lift. That's why eccentric (or negative) reps, which lengthen muscles, can spark new growth. Adding the dumbbell clean improves total-body power. Here's how to do it.

Select dumbbells that are 5 to 10 pounds heavier than what you'd typically use for 5 rep sets. Hold them at your sides and stand with your ankles, knees, and hips slightly bent **(A)**. "Cheat" the dumbbells to the top position with a clean: Explosively stand up straight while bending your elbows to draw the weights to your shoulders **(B)**. Take 5 seconds to lower the weights **(C)**. Do 3 sets of 5 reps, resting 90 seconds between sets.

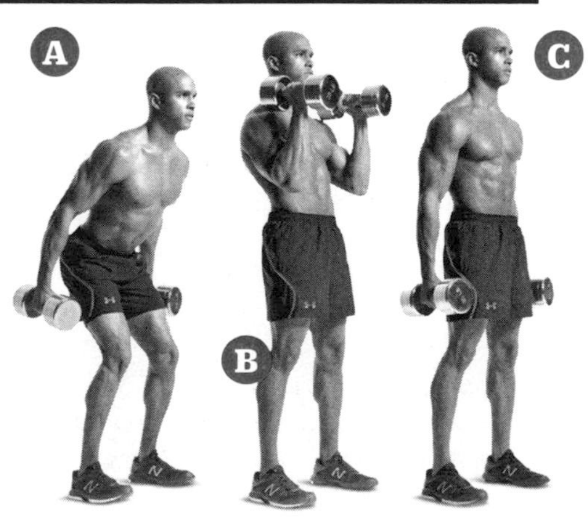

AMAZING FEAT OF FITNESS

Scale a Rope

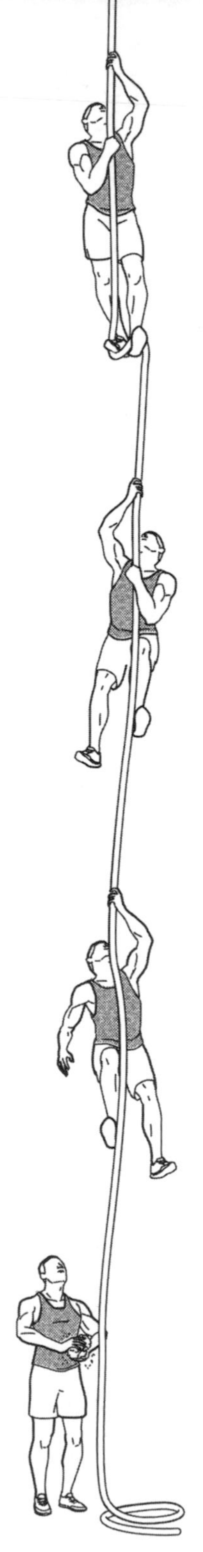

You never even got halfway up in junior high phys ed? Hold your head up. That's simply because you weren't taught properly. Here, try these tips from Marcus Bondi, Guinness World Record holder for rope climbing, and then go rescue a cute damsel.

Step 1: Prep Your Paws

Chalk up to prevent rope burn. No chalk at the gym? Buy it at a sporting goods store. If you don't like the powdery feel, use fingerless climbing gloves with split-grain leather palm reinforcement.

Step 2: Launch the Climb

Stand facing the rope with your feet shoulder width apart, knees bent. Grab it with your dominant hand as high as you can without locking your elbow. Contract your shoulders and tighten your abs for power. In one motion, pull yourself up while kicking with your opposite knee up and out. Gaze up to your next grip so you don't grab air.

Step 3: Shoot Up the Rope

Using the momentum from the first pull, grab the rope with your free hand about a foot above your original grip. Covering a shorter distance at first helps your body adjust to and move with the swaying rope. Pull yourself up again, this time kicking upward with your opposite knee for momentum. The goal is to establish a rhythm of short bursts of movement: Reach and brace, pull and kick, repeat.

Step 4: Step It Up

If you can't scale the rope with your arms only, use a foot lock to enlist your legs. Form a step with your feet by wrapping the rope under one foot and over the other. Push off this step. Once your hands regrip the rope, create another step and proceed.

Step 5: Control Your Descent

Grip and release the rope with the middle of your inner thighs for support. Your arms shouldn't extend outward from your body more than 90 degrees. Don't drop; even 3 feet of sliding can seriously burn your hands and thighs.

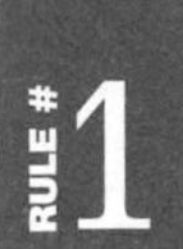

Keep your hands off the stair-climber. For every 10 pounds of weight you support on the rails of a stair-climbing machine, you burn 7 percent fewer calories.

Make Pushups Metabolic

DO PUSHUP JACKS.

From the up position, hop your legs out to the sides—like a jumping jack—as you use your arms to lower your body. Then jump your feet back to the regular position while you push up. Once those get too easy, do the same, but this time jump your arms out as well, as shown here.

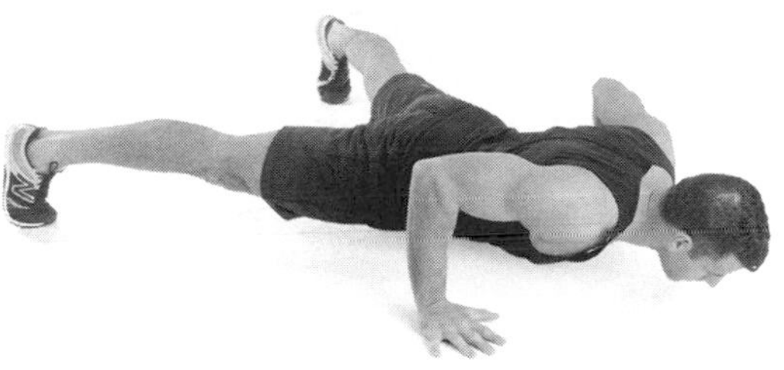

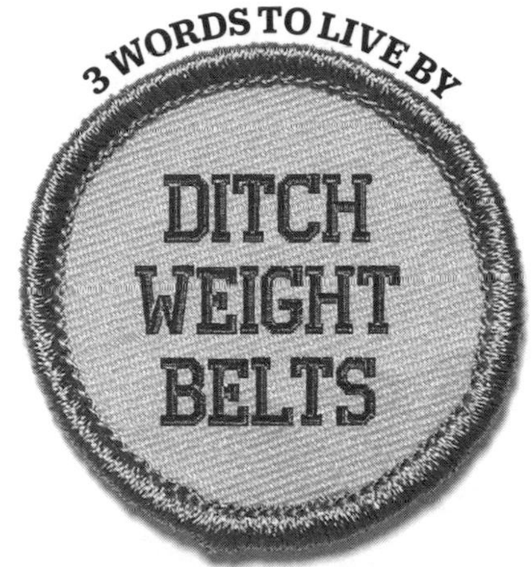
3 WORDS TO LIVE BY
DITCH WEIGHT BELTS

How to Build Hand Strength with the Sports Pages

Spread a sheet of newspaper flat on a tabletop. Place your hand in the center of the sheet and draw the paper in with your fingertips without lifting your hand from the table. Then squeeze the ball of paper tight. Two or three sheets a day is enough to build a powerful grip.

Punch a Speed Bag

Go at it like Mayweather for an intense total-body workout.

1. Put Up Your Dukes

Close your fist as if you're holding a hammer. You'll be hitting the bag with the butt end of your fists, where the hammer's handle would be sticking out. Raise your fists to ear level, knuckles pointed inward, elbows above your chest.

2. Face the Bag

Place your feet shoulder width apart and your body square to the bag, which should be at about eye level. Stand on the balls of your feet and tighten your core for stability.

3. Give It a Punch

Focus on the bag's hinge. (Looking at the bag will make you dizzy.) Strike the bag with your fist. The bag should hit the mounting platform three times—forward, back, forward—before you strike it again.

4. Find Your Rhythm

Once you're able to strike the bag effectively, close your eyes. Practice until you find the rhythm (1-2-3, 1-2-3, 1-2-3). If you listen rather than look, you're more likely to master it. Now mix things up—hit the bag twice with each hand, then three times, then once again. This will challenge your coordination and work your upper body harder.

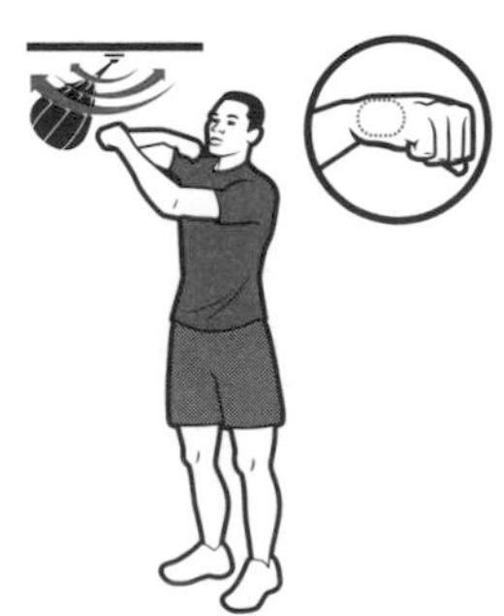

Make Your Own **MEDICINE BALL**

Turn an old basketball into an awesome piece of workout gear.

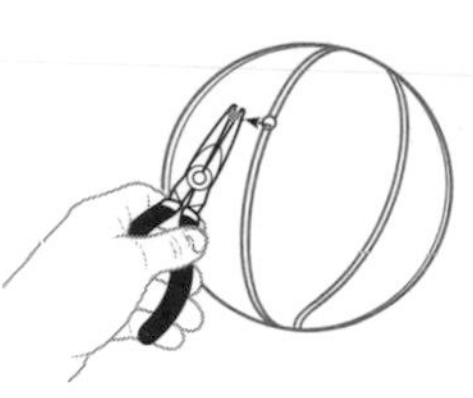

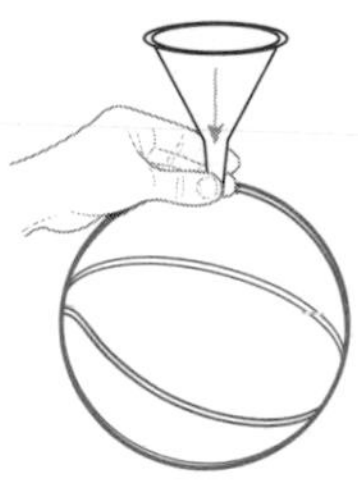

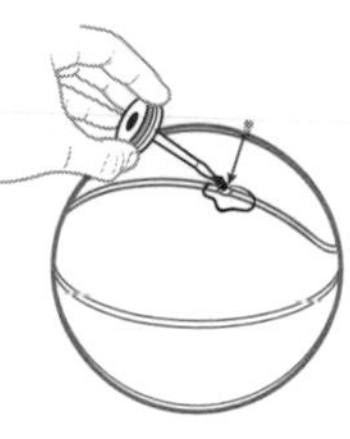

Step 1

Use a pair of needle-nose pliers to remove the rubber plug from the basketball. Set the plug aside.

Step 2

Insert a funnel with a tip small enough to fit into the air hole. Fill the ball entirely with fine-grain play sand. A 50-pound bag will make three medicine balls.

Step 3

Brush rubber cement in and around the rim of the air hole. Immediately plug the hole with the rubber stopper, using the needle-nose pliers to push in the stopper if needed.

Step 4

Brush more rubber cement over the stopper. Allow it to dry.

Barbells for Brains

Strength training for 60 minutes three times a week for 6 months can help improve short- and long-term memory performance and attention as you age, according to a Brazilian study published in *Medicine & Science in Sports & Exercise*. The need to focus on technique when doing different lifts provides a cognitive challenge you may not get while doing a repetitive exercise like running, says Gary Small, MD, director of the UCLA longevity center and coauthor of *The Alzheimer's Prevention Program*.

RULE # 2

Between sets, take 20 to 30 seconds to stretch the muscle you just worked. Boston researchers found that men who did this increased their strength by 20 percent.

Hide Valuables from *Gym Rats*

Thwart locker room thieves by making a simple safe. Find a tennis ball and use a box cutter or utility knife to cut a 2-inch slit into the ball. Squeeze the ball to open the slit and then insert any small valuables, such as a watch, a ring, or cash. Stash the ball inside your gym bag.

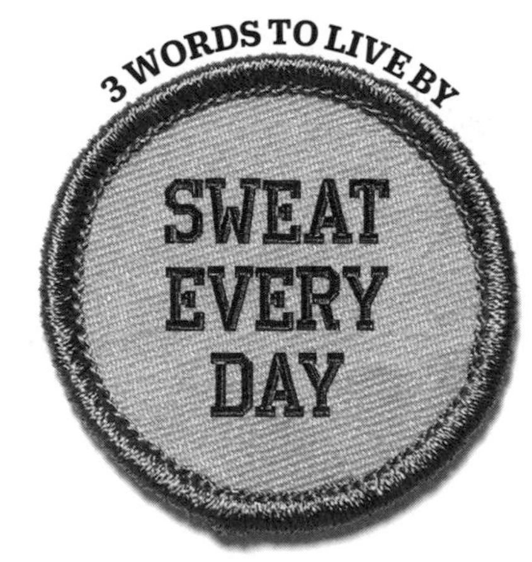
3 WORDS TO LIVE BY
SWEAT
EVERY
DAY

Escape a Botched Bench Press

You went without a spotter and you can't finish that last rep? Trainer Bill Hartman, PT, CSCS, has your exit plan.

1. If you insist on going solo at the bench, remove the collars from the bar. The risk of having to rerack the bar if the weights slip is eclipsed by the potential benefit of saving your rib cage when your muscles give out.
2. If you do find yourself failing, use your remaining strength to carefully lower the bar to your chest—but don't let it rest there, or else you may injure your ribs. Keep as much upward pressure going as you can so you aren't crushed.
3. Inch your dominant hand toward the end of the barbell so that the weight gradually slides off the opposite end.
4. As the one side of the bar dumps the weight, the unevenly weighted bar will quickly make the weights on the other side dump off as well. Keep a firm grasp on the bar so it doesn't rocket skyward.
5. Push the empty bar to the rack and breathe a sigh of relief.
6. Next time you approach the bench, ask for a spotter!

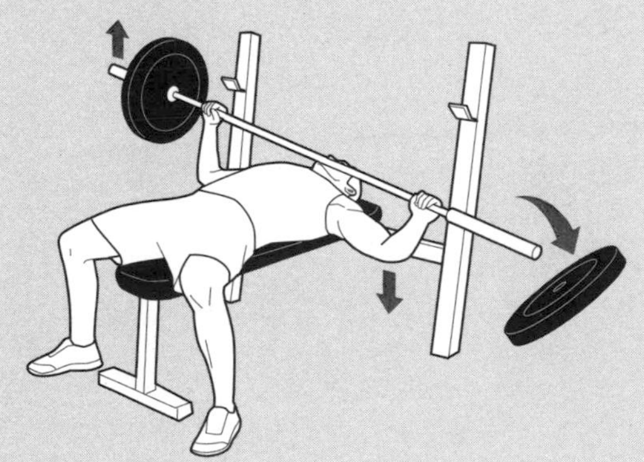

RULE #3

If you have to skip a workout, do this for 10 minutes: 30 seconds on and 30 seconds off of pushups, jumping jacks, squats, hip thrusts, and lunges. That's enough to spark some sweat and keep you honest. Skipping just one workout can raise your odds of missing another the following week by 61 percent, according to UK researchers.

AMAZING FEAT OF FITNESS

The Human Flag

Pregame: First become f . . . ing strong. This move is the ultimate test of upper-body strength, core stability, and total-body muscle control.

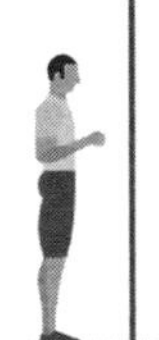
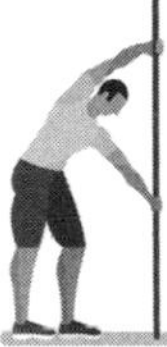
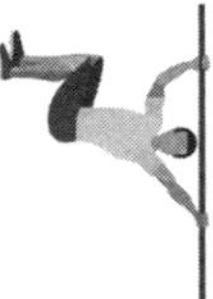
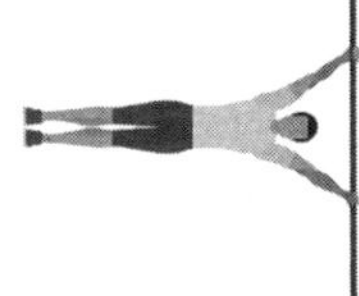

1. **Find a vertical pole.** It should be sturdy enough to hold your body weight but thin enough to grasp securely.
2. **Set your grip.** Grab it toward the bottom with your nondominant hand using an underhand grip, and higher up with your dominant hand using an overhand grip.
3. **Lock and load.** Lock your bottom elbow, leaning your body away from the pole. Press hard with your bottom arm, squeeze tightly with your top arm, and lift your legs up with your knees bent.
4. **Finish strong.** Contract your core and extend one leg at a time.

The No-Hassle, Fast-Muscle Workout

A PAIR OF DUMBBELLS AND A BENCH ARE ALL YOU NEED TO DROP UNWANTED FAT AND ADD EYE-CATCHING SIZE.

The biggest obstacle between you and the body you want might come from an unexpected source: your gym, says Craig Ballantyne, CSCS. That's because crowds can slow your workout—and your results. After all, every second you spend waiting for the chinup bar, cable station, or squat rack is less time you have for working your muscles or boosting your calorie burn.

Don't waste another minute in the gym. This fat-burning, muscle-building workout designed by Ballantyne requires only a single set of dumbbells and an adjustable bench. The order in which you perform the exercises—along with the number of reps for each—allows the same pair of dumbbells to challenge each muscle equally. The upshot: There's never been a simpler way to chisel a better body.

Directions

Perform each workout (A, B, and C) once a week, resting at least a day between sessions. Within each workout, alternate sets between exercises of the same number (1A and 1B, for example) until you complete all sets in that pairing. (In other words, follow a set of the first exercise with a set of the second exercise.) Rest 1 minute between 1A and 1B, but perform exercises 2A and 2B back-to-back, with no rest.

After you've done a set of each exercise pair, rest for 1 minute and then repeat the cycle until you've completed all the prescribed sets.

Workout A

1A: Dumbbell Chest Press

3 SETS OF 8 REPS

Lie on your back on a flat bench and hold a pair of dumbbells above your chest with your arms straight. Lower the dumbbells to the sides of your chest, pause, and then push them back up to the starting position.

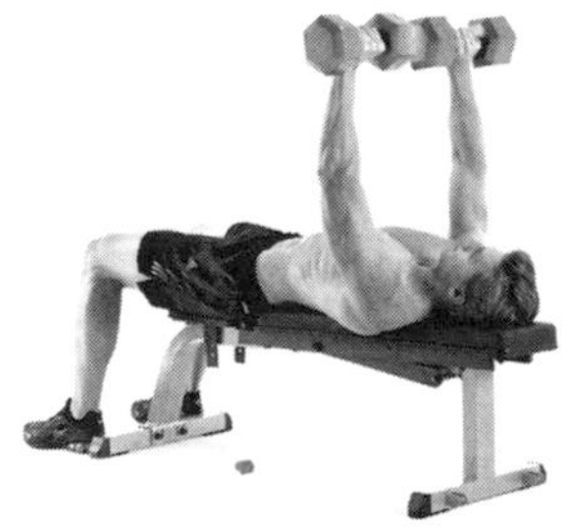

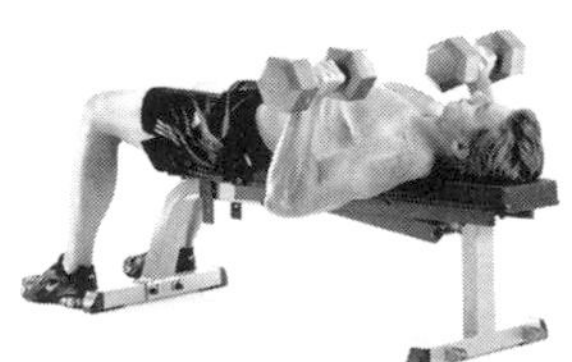

1B: Dumbbell Bent-Over Row

3 SETS OF 12 REPS

With a dumbbell in your right hand, place your left hand and left knee on a flat bench. Keep your back flat and let your right arm hang straight down, with your palm facing in. Pull your arm up to the side of your chest by bending your elbow. Pause and return to the starting position. Do 12 reps with each arm.

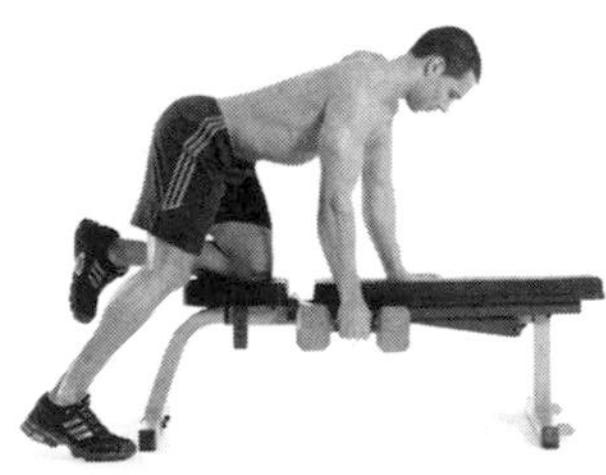

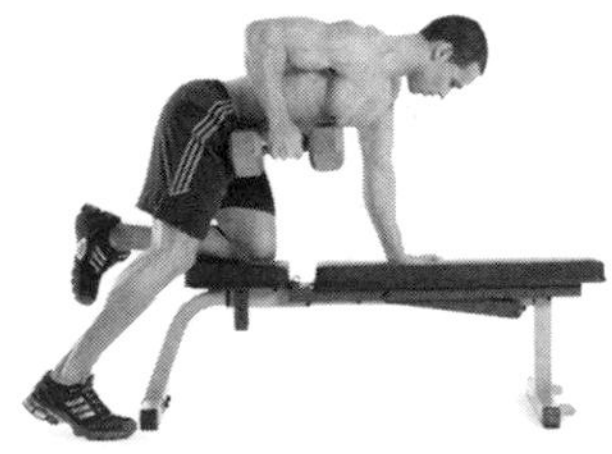

2A: Dumbbell Incline Press

2 SETS OF 5 REPS

Lie on a bench with the backrest set at a 45-degree incline. Hold a pair of dumbbells above your chest with your arms straight and your palms turned toward your feet. Lower the dumbbells to chest level and then press them above your chest, back to the starting position.

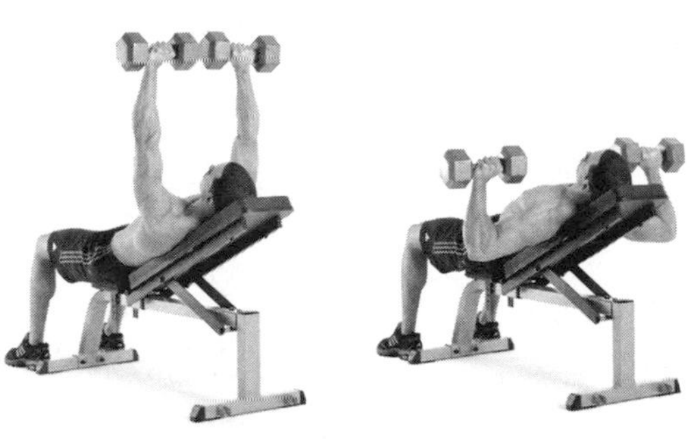

2B: Dumbbell Squat

2 SETS OF 15 REPS

Holding a pair of dumbbells at your sides, stand with your feet just beyond shoulder width apart. Push your hips back and squat as deeply as possible, keeping your lower back naturally arched. Push back up to the starting position without rounding your back. Your upper legs should be at least parallel to the floor, or even lower.

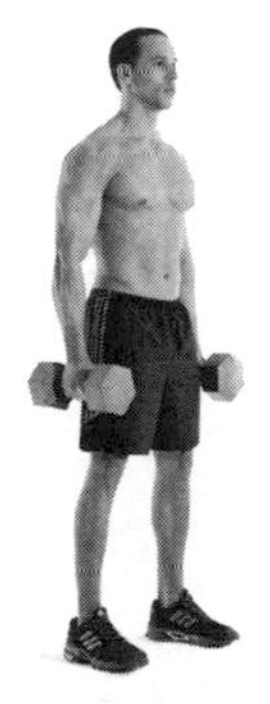

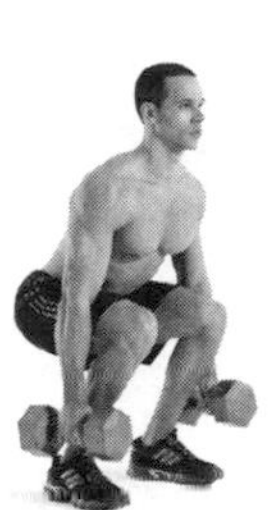

Workout B

1A: Dumbbell Split Squat

3 SETS OF 8 REPS

Hold dumbbells at your sides and stand with your right foot forward and your left foot back. Lower your body until your front knee is bent 90 degrees and your rear knee nearly touches the floor. Return to the starting position. Do 8 reps, switch legs, and repeat. That's 1 set.

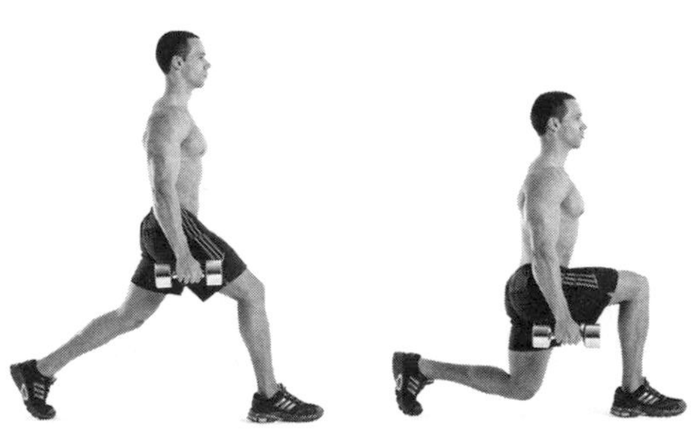

1B: Single-Arm Standing Shoulder Press

3 SETS OF 12 REPS

Stand holding a dumbbell at eye level with your arm bent, palm forward, and your other hand on your hip. Press the dumbbell straight overhead and then lower it to the starting position. Do 12 reps on one side and repeat with your other arm. That's 1 set. Lower the dumbbells to around ear level to avoid shoulder stress.

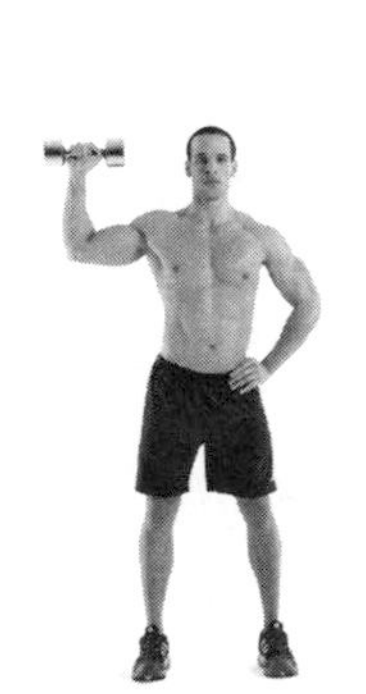

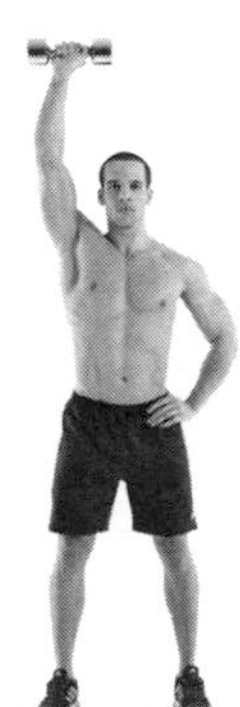

2A: Dumbbell Romanian Deadlift

2 SETS OF 10 REPS

Hold a dumbbell in each hand in front of your thighs, palms facing your body. With your knees slightly bent and feet shoulder width apart, bend at your hips and lower your torso until it's nearly parallel to the floor, without rounding your back. Pause and then rise to the starting position.

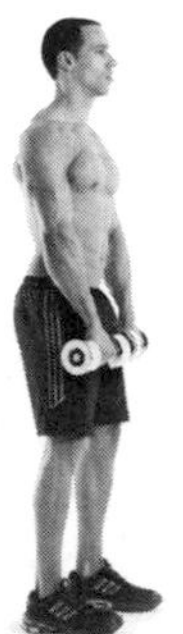
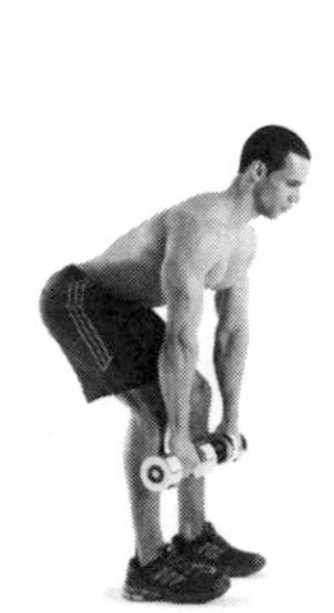

2B: Dumbbell Swing

2 SETS OF 20 REPS

With your feet shoulder width apart, hold a dumbbell's handle with both hands. Extend your arms in front of your chest. Next, slightly bend your knees and swing the dumbbell between your legs. Bring the dumbbell back up to chest level as you rise. That's 1 rep. Keeping your arms straight adds more work to your shoulders.

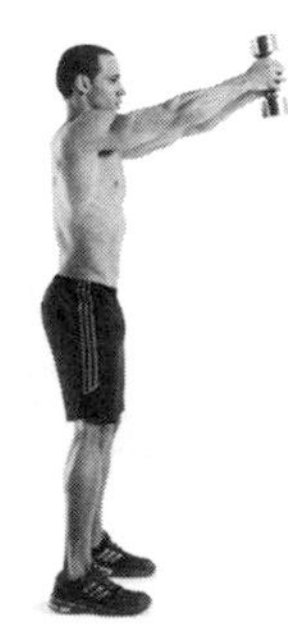
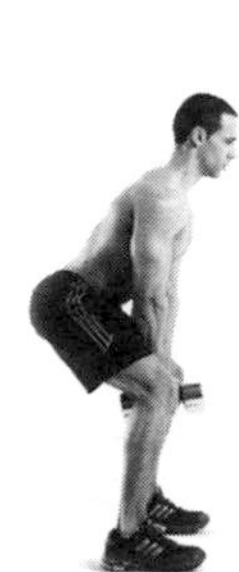

Workout C

1A: Dumbbell Step-Up

3 SETS OF 8 REPS

With a dumbbell in each hand, stand facing a bench. Place one foot on the bench and lift your body up to the standing position without letting your opposite foot touch the bench. Lower your body slowly and repeat. Complete 8 reps, switch legs, and repeat. That's 1 set. Avoid touching the bench, to keep all the tension on your working leg.

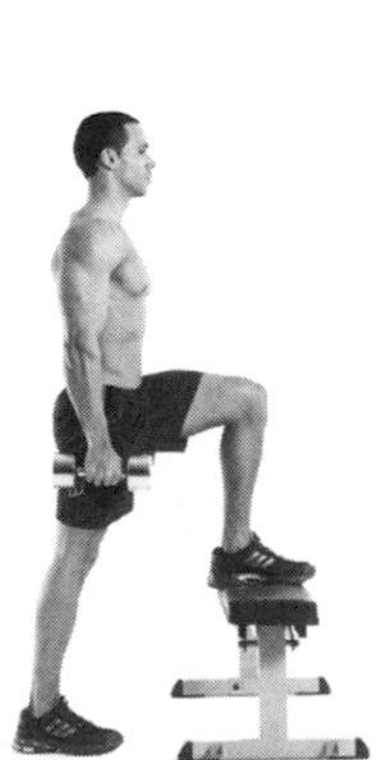
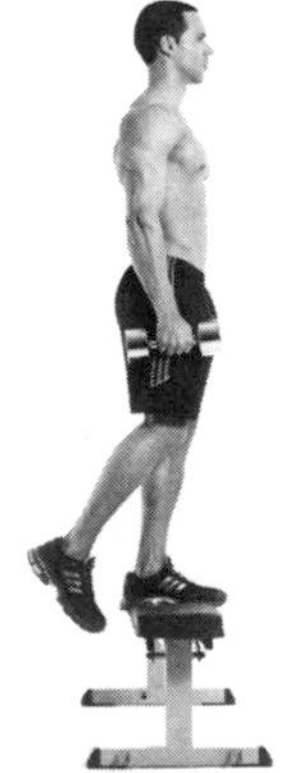

1B: Chest-Supported Incline Row

3 SETS OF 12 REPS

Grab a pair of dumbbells and lie chest down on a 45-degree incline bench. Let your arms hang straight down, palms facing each other. Row the dumbbells to the sides of your chest by bending your elbows and squeezing your shoulder blades. Pause and lower the weights.

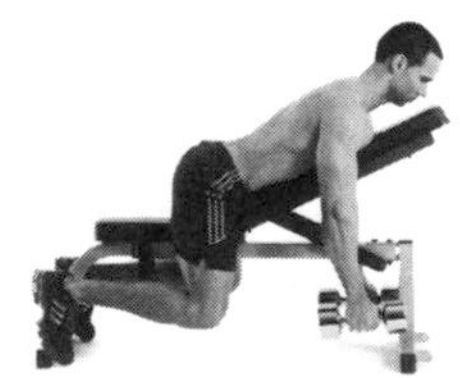
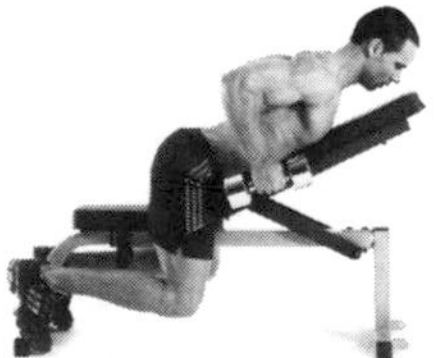

2A: Dumbbell Curl

2 SETS OF 10 REPS

Grab a pair of dumbbells with an underhand grip and hold them at arm's length next to your thighs. Curl the dumbbells toward your chest as far as you can without moving your upper arms. Pause, and slowly lower the weights to the starting position.

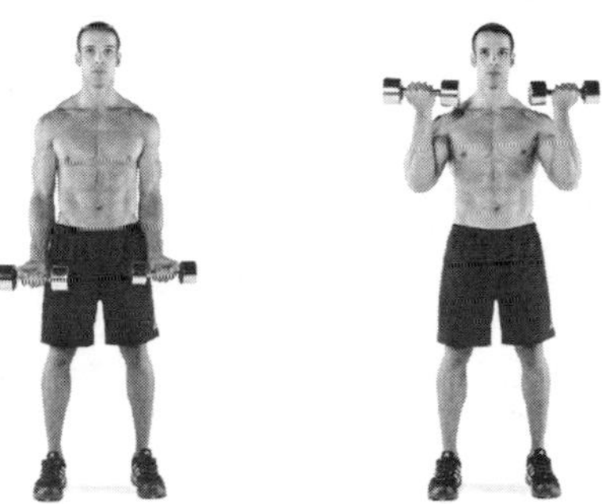

2B: Lying Dumbbell Triceps Extension

2 SETS OF 12 REPS

Lie faceup on a bench, holding a pair of dumbbells with your arms extended above your chest, palms facing each other. Without moving your upper arms, bend your elbows and move the weights toward your ears until your forearms are past parallel to the floor. Straighten your arms back to the starting position and repeat.

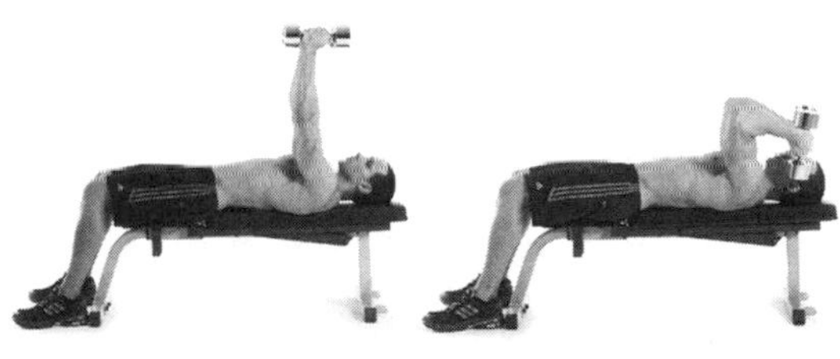

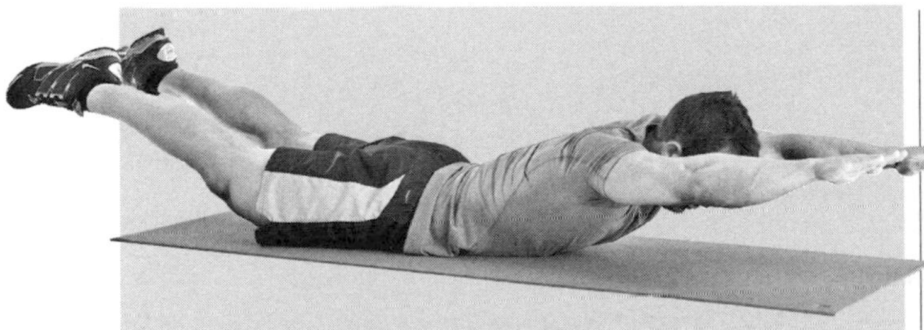

End Back Pain

For every set of abdominal exercises you do, perform a set of lower-back exercises to ensure balanced muscle and improve posture. The Superman is a great lower-back exercise you can do anywhere: Lie facedown on the floor with your arms and legs extended as if you were flying over Metropolis. Now raise your hands and legs so that only your hips remain in contact with the floor. Hold for a few seconds, lower, and repeat for 10 reps.

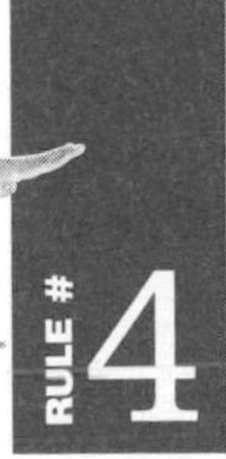

Doing 31 minutes of resistance training will keep your metabolism elevated for 38 hours, according to a University of Wisconsin at La Crosse study.

BUILD BIGGER BICEPS

- To work your biceps harder, bend your wrist backward slightly—and hold it that way—while doing dumbbell curls.
- Your arms will look bigger if you also work your triceps. Dips blast them best.

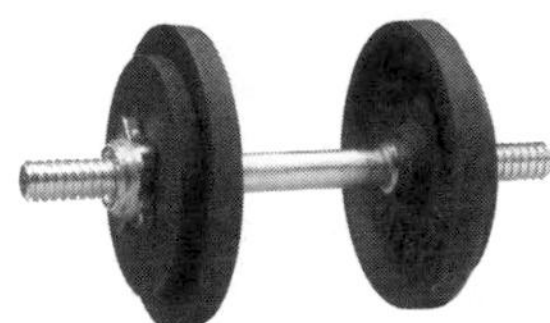

MUSCLE IN A BAG

The shifting sand inside a sandbag makes this muscle tool harder to balance and sling around. That's a good thing, because it forces your muscles to work together, triggering faster all-around growth, says Josh Henkin, CSCS, inventor of the Ultimate Sandbag Training System. You can buy a great sandbag from Henkin or make one yourself. Here's a circuit that'll kick sand in your face.

Perform the following exercises as a circuit, doing as many reps of each as you can in 30 seconds before moving on to the next one (use a 30- to 70-pound bag). Rest 30 seconds between moves. Do the circuit three times . . . if you can hack it!

1. Side Lunge and Snatch

Hold a sandbag in front of your thighs. Lunge to your left, touching the sandbag to the floor. Quickly stand up, flipping the bag onto your forearms as you press it overhead. Return to standing and then lunge to your right. Continue alternating sides. "Keep your weight over your heel," says Henkin. "That will force your hamstring and glute to activate, so you'll lift from your hips instead of your back."

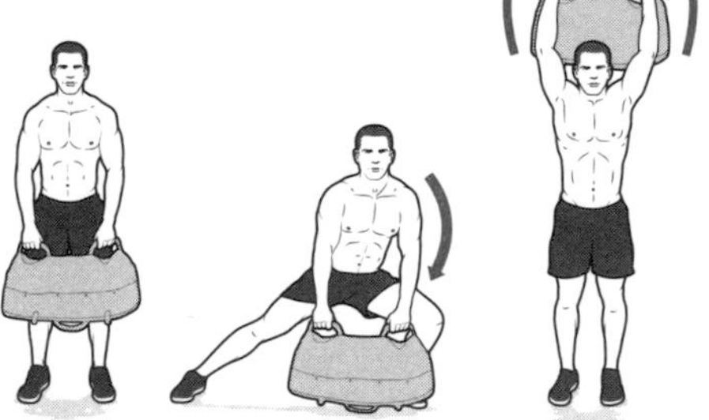

2. Pushup with Sandbag Drag

Place a sandbag on the floor and assume a pushup position so the bag is to your right. Grab the bag with your left hand and drag it underneath your chest to your left side. Do a pushup. Now drag the bag back to your right side with your right hand. Do another pushup. Continue alternating sides. "Brace your core to avoid rotating your body as you drag the bag," says Henkin.

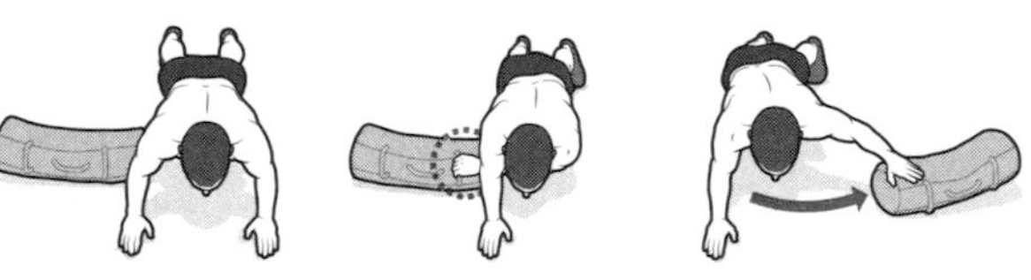

3. Rotational Reverse Lunge and Balance

Hold a sandbag in front of your thighs. Step back with your right foot and swing the bag to the outside of your left thigh. Stand up, raising your right knee as you flip the bag over your forearms to catch it at chest level. Pause and return to the starting position. Repeat, switching legs halfway through the set. "To increase difficulty, go into your next lunge without pausing," says Henkin.

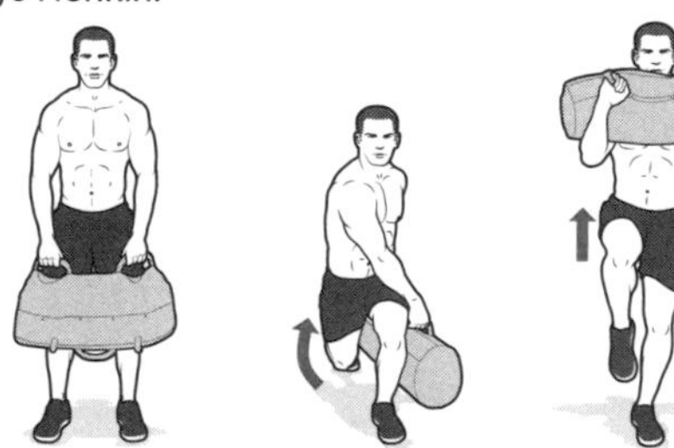

4. Single-Leg Row

Holding a sandbag at arm's length, raise your right leg behind you as you lower your torso until it's nearly parallel to the floor. Pull the bag to your chest, pause, and then slowly lower it. Switch legs after 15 seconds. "It's harder to hold on to a sandbag than a dumbbell or a barbell," says Henkin, "so you'll work the muscles in your forearms in addition to those in your back."

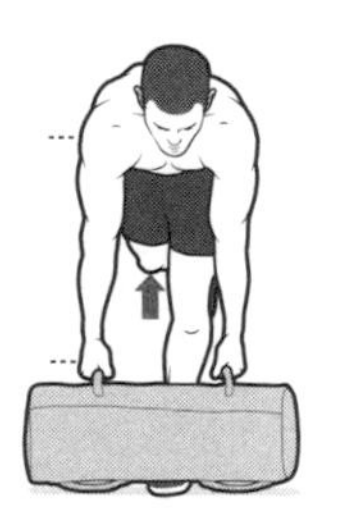

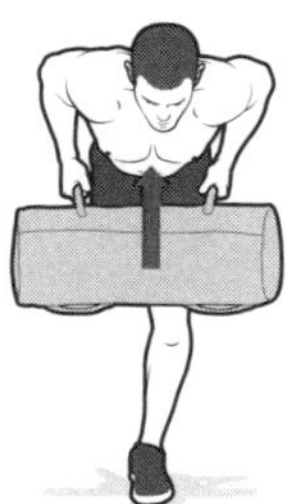

DIY Sandbag

Don't want to drop $100 or more on a commercial sandbag? Here's how to make one for $50 or less.

What You'll Need

100 pounds of play sand (available at most hardware stores)
4 large garbage bags
Duct tape
2 sturdy duffel bags (canvas or military)

Put It All Together

1. Pour 30 pounds of sand into the first garbage bag (use a bathroom scale to weigh it) and seal the top with duct tape, leaving enough room for the sand to move around.
2. Place the first garbage bag in a second one and seal them both with duct tape.
3. Place the double-bagged sand inside a duffel and zip it shut; you can duct-tape the zipper for added security.
4. Repeat the process to make a 70-pound sandbag.
5. Grab the ends of the bag to perform the exercises.

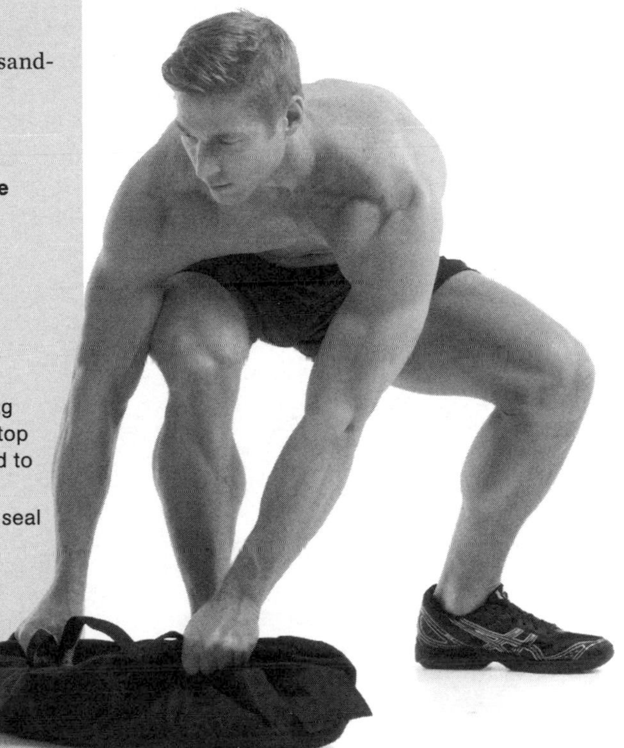

Weight Loss Made Simple

+ DO THIS:				
Go for a brisk 20-minute walk.	Stand during three 10-minute phone calls.	Play vigorously with your kids or pet for 15 minutes.	Spend 15 minutes washing dishes.	Take 10 minutes to straighten up one room.
— NOT THIS:				
Sit for your entire lunch hour.	Put your feet up on your desk.	Watch TV before dinner.	Head straight to the couch.	Go straight to bed.
= EQUALS				
49 extra calories burned.	33 extra calories burned.	82 extra calories burned.	27 extra calories burned.	21 extra calories burned.
212 TOTAL EXTRA CALORIES BURNED				
METABOLISM BOOST: ABOUT 10 PERCENT				

Turn a Towel into a Barbell

THE KEY TO A MORE RIGOROUS TOTAL-BODY CHALLENGE COULD BE FOLDED UP IN YOUR BATHROOM CLOSET, SAYS *MEN'S HEALTH* TRAINING ADVISOR BJ GADDOUR, CSCS.

1. The Move: Pushup Hold

WHAT IT TARGETS:
Chest and back
WHY IT WORKS: *It's a traditional pushup, but isolated holds make it more challenging.*

HOW TO DO IT:

1. Get down on all fours. Wrap the towel around your upper back and under your armpits, grabbing the ends. Lie on your stomach.

2. Holding the ends of the towel, assume the bottom of a pushup position. Push up against the towel as hard as you can, continuing to breathe and tensing all your muscles, for 4 seconds. Lower your body, but not all the way down to the floor, to rest briefly. Repeat the move for a total of 30 to 60 seconds without ever lowering your body completely to the floor.

MAKE IT HARDER:

Narrow your feet in the pushup position and perform the move on one leg, switching sides at the halfway mark.

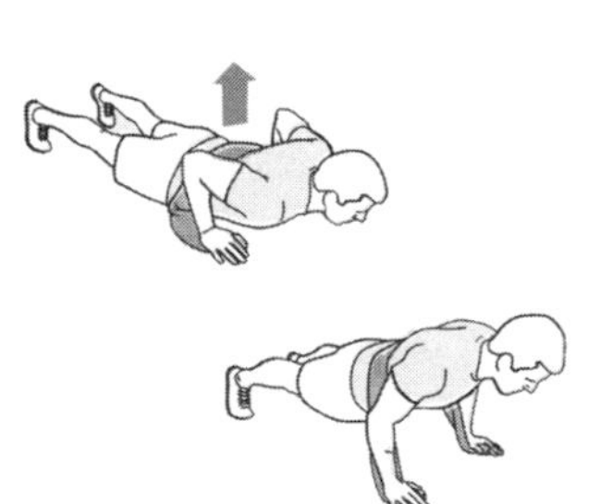

2. The Move: Seesaw Push-Pull

WHAT IT TARGETS:
Shoulders, chest, and arms
WHY IT WORKS: *Moves your arms through their full range of motion.*

HOW TO DO IT:

1. Hold the towel taut at your chest; your arms should be shoulder width apart and elbows bent 90 degrees. Keep your hips and shoulders square and your heels pressed into the floor as you tighten your abs and glutes.

2. Simultaneously push with your left arm until it's straight (like a chest press) and draw back your right arm until your right hand reaches your armpit (like a row). Pause and hold for 2 seconds. Then push with your right arm and draw back with your left. Alternate for 30 to 60 seconds total.

MAKE IT HARDER:

Sink into a deep squat; then perform the exercise. That way you're better able to engage your lower body.

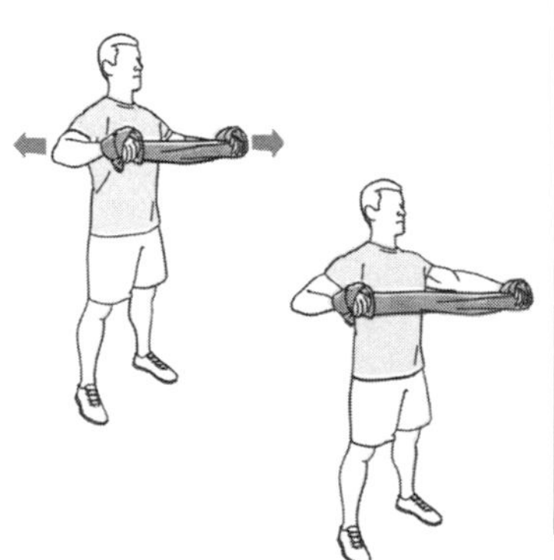

3. The Move: Split Squat and Biceps Curl

WHAT IT TARGETS:
Arms and legs
WHY IT WORKS: *Upper and lower body work together.*

HOW TO DO IT:

1. Assume a split stance, your right leg forward with your right foot on the middle of a towel. Grab the ends of the towel and pull it taut.

2. Pull up on the towel ends as you slowly lower your hips. When your back knee is a few inches from the floor, pause. Hold for 2 seconds, keeping your legs tensed and your weight on your front heel.

3. Reverse the move, now pulling on the towel as you rise. Repeat the move for 30 to 60 seconds total, switching sides at the halfway mark.

MAKE IT HARDER:

Hold your squat continuously for 30 to 60 seconds. Repeat the exercise until exhaustion.

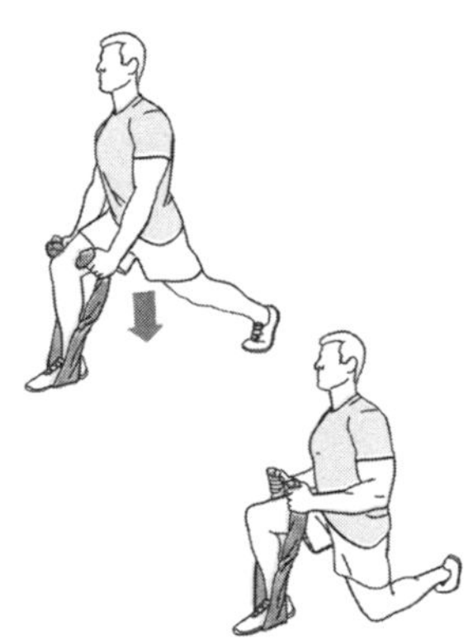

Put Your Spare Tire to Work

Zach Even-Esh, owner of Underground Strength in Edison, New Jersey, and Jason Hartman, CSCS, a strength coach with the US Army Special Forces, explain how to build your own sprinting sled.

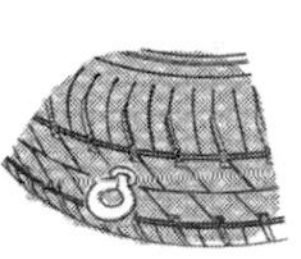

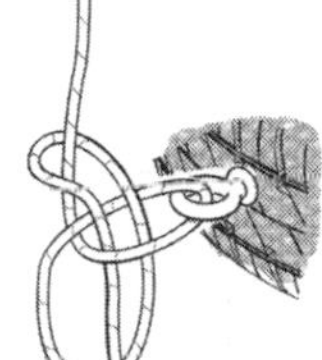

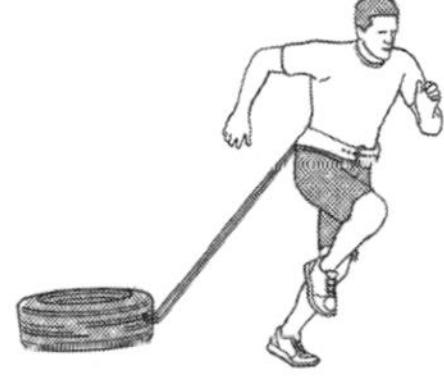

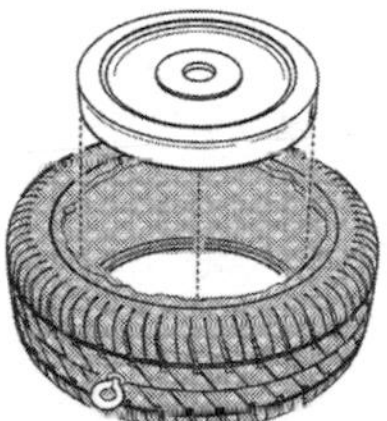

1 Find Recycled Rubber

Ask your mechanic for an old pickup-truck tire. He'll likely have tread-bare rubber he'll unload for free. Buy nylon rope (15 feet) and an eye bolt (big enough to run the rope through) with a nut and washer.

2 Make Room for Your Anchor

In the center of the tire tread, drill a hole that's slightly smaller than the bolt. Insert the eye bolt into the hole from the outside of the tire; then secure it from the tire's interior, using the washer and nut.

3 Rope Yourself into Things

Run the rope through the eye bolt's hole and tie it with a bowline. Tie another bowline (see page 41) at the rope's other end and wrap it around your waist. Position the rope tail behind you.

4 Turn Muscles into Mush

Warm up with lunges and short jogs. Then do five 30-yard, all-out sprints, resting 1 minute between each. Afterward, power walk 30 yards forward and backward five times, resting a minute after each round.

BONUS:
Make a Tire That Tires You

For a tougher tow, use a utility knife to trim an inch or two off the entire diameter of the upper sidewall to widen the opening. Then set a 45-pound weight plate inside the tire. Commence grunting.

Massage Sore Muscles

To relieve pain, don't just randomly poke and rub; grab your balls and follow along.

1. Your lower back aches from sitting.

Place a tennis ball between your right side (a few inches above your hip) and a wall. Shift your weight to your left leg and bend your right knee. Turn away from the wall so the ball rolls toward your spine. Turn back. Repeat five times. Move the ball an inch lower and repeat. Once you reach your tailbone, work your left side.

2. Your chest is tight from weight lifting.

Do this after a shower, when your muscles are loose: Place a tennis ball between a doorjamb and your chest, an inch below your collarbone. Roll the ball horizontally toward your sternum and back five times. Drop the ball an inch and repeat down to your lowest rib.

3. Running gives you foot twinges.

While seated, press a golf ball into the pad of your foot and roll it side to side 10 times. Gently roll the ball from the center of your toes to the center of your heel, then to the right and left of the center tendon; repeat five times. Turn your foot in; roll the ball from your big toe to your heel five times.

How To Start a Fire

Incinerate your nutritional indiscretions with these activities (for a half hour).

Vinyasa Yoga
135 Calories
= A baked potato
= An English muffin
= 27 Cheez-Its
= 3 Dove milk chocolate Promises

Brisk Walking
143 Calories
= 1 ounce of BBQ potato chips
= ½ cup of ice cream
= A Starbucks 16-ounce cappuccino
= A Budweiser 12-ounce bottle of beer

Shooting Hoops
184 Calories
= 3 ounces of ham
= Red Lobster Cheddar Bay biscuit
= Keebler Sandies Pecan Shortbread cookies

Downhill Skiing
245 Calories
= 10 baked onion rings
= 1 cup of chow mein noodles
= 1 fried chicken thigh
= 1 slice of yellow cake

Swimming
286 Calories
= 1 plain hot dog
= 1 McDonald's Grilled Ranch Snack Wrap
= 1 small egg bagel
= 1 small Wendy's vanilla Frosty

Cycling
327 Calories
= 1 slice of homemade pumpkin pie
= 1 cup of baked beans with beef
= 1 Pizza Hut slice from a large, hand-tossed cheese pizza

Jogging
367 Calories
= a 10.6-ounce chocolate milkshake
= 1 small Burger King fries
= 6 to 8 cheese nachos
= 1 small Quiznos Chicken Caesar salad

Circuit Weight Training
477 Calories
= 2 pancakes with butter and syrup
= 1 Jamba Juice Blackberry Bliss Power Smoothie
= 1 Ruby Tuesday Petit Sirloin

Pound the Heavy Bag

Want to punch up your training? Learn to work the bag. Here's your tutorial from Jason Strout, co-owner of Church Street Boxing Gym in New York City, where Lennox Lewis has sparred.

1. Fight in Your Weight Class

If the bag wobbles from side to side after you throw a punch, go with a heavier bag. You'll have a better workout.

2. Adjust Your Stance

Stand at arm's length from the bag with your feet shoulder width apart for balance. If you're right-handed, place your left foot slightly in front of your right so your left heel and right toe are aligned. Stay on your toes and keep your knees slightly bent—that's how you'll spring into your punches.

3. Throw a Powerful Punch

Aim for the middle of the bag; otherwise it'll spin and you'll risk hurting your wrists. When you jab, keep your shoulder, elbow, wrist, and knuckles aligned. After the punch, pull your arm back just as quickly to boost your cardio workout. Be sure to add crosses and hooks. Work in small combinations: jab-cross, jab-cross-hook, jab-hook-cross. Keep the routine basic, but focus on your form.

4. Do More with Less

Pound away for 10 minutes and you'll work up a sweat, but you'll also miss out on a more intense workout: short, quick, powerful punch combinations for 3-minute rounds. Rest 30 seconds between rounds; do five rounds total. For an added workout, jump rope between sets to keep your cardio up.

Bonus:

WRAP YOUR HANDS FOR A BOXING WORKOUT

Avoid bloody knuckles with Ringside Quick Boxing Hand Wraps ($6, ringside.com). You won't have to worry about a complicated gauze-and-tape technique. You can wear them inside boxing gloves, like the durable Title Gel Intense Bag/Sparring Gloves shown above ($100, titleboxing.com).

Install Pullup Rings

THIS SETUP HAS A UNIQUE ADVANTAGE OVER A PULLUP BAR: BECAUSE YOUR HANDS AREN'T IN A FIXED POSITION, RINGS ALLOW FOR NATURAL, PAIN-FREE MOVEMENT THROUGHOUT THE EXERCISE. PLUS, YOU CAN DO YOUR REPS IN THE GREAT OUTDOORS.

WHAT YOU'LL NEED

Two tow straps
Two full-strength carabiners
Two 4" lengths of PVC pipe (1½" diameter)
Athletic tape
Two 12" chains

Find Sturdy Support

Look around the backyard for a tree with a thick branch that can safely support your body weight. The branch doesn't have to be parallel to the ground, but it should clear the dirt by about 15 feet.

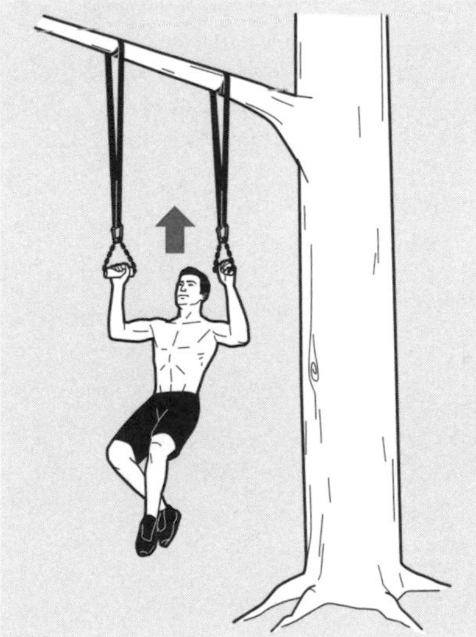

HOW TO MAKE IT

1. Fling the tow straps over the branch and then wrap them around the branch as needed so the ends of the tow straps hang evenly. They should stop about a foot higher than you can reach.
2. Hook a carabiner through the end of each tow strap.
3. Wrap the PVC pipes in athletic tape. To make each handle, thread a chain through the pipe and hook the ends of the chain onto the carabiner.
4. The handles should be as high as you can reach. If they're too high or too low, readjust the number of times you loop the tow straps around the branch.

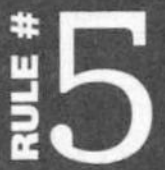

RULE # 5

Never wear a sponsored race T-shirt emblazoned with the squashed-together logos of the sponsors unless you plan to sweat in it.

Fact:

Laughing 100 times is the psychological equivalent of exercising on a rowing machine for 10 minutes.

Best Four-Legged Running Partners

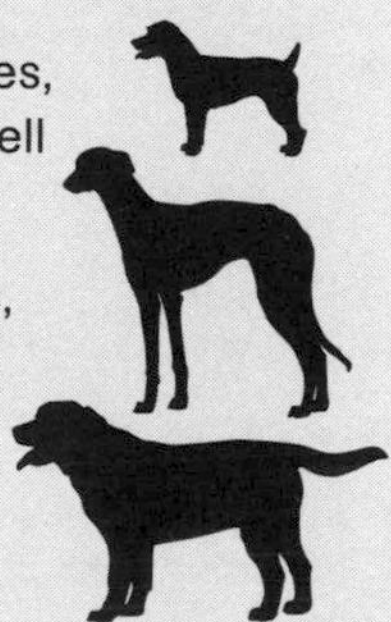

LONG RUNS: Weimaraners, Goldendoodles, German shorthaired pointers, Jack Russell terriers

SHORT FAST RUNS: Greyhounds, beagles, golden and Labrador retrievers

TRAIL RUNNING: Border collies, Belgian sheepdogs, Labrador retrievers

The Cannon Ball Workout

SCULPT A STRONGER, LEANER, MORE ATHLETIC BODY WITH THIS BALLISTIC, FAT-FRYING, OLD-SCHOOL MUSCLE TOOL—THE KETTLEBELL.

Fifteen years ago, very few people outside eastern Europe had ever heard of kettlebells. Today these weights are in almost every gym in America, and "kettlebell workouts" is the sixth most Googled exercise term on the planet. No wonder: "Kettlebells are more user-friendly than barbells or dumbbells," says kettlebell pioneer and StrongFirst.com chairman Pavel Tsatsouline.

"You don't need as many to hit every muscle, and they offer distinct advantages for boosting mobility and all-around strength." Follow these rules to get the most out of every rep.

TRAINING RULE 1:

Understand How They Work

Unlike a barbell or dumbbell, a kettlebell has a load that's offset from its handle. "That amplifies the ballistic forces in quick, dynamic movements, effectively making the kettlebell feel heavier than it actually is," Tsatsouline says. It also places greater demand on your stabilizing muscles, core, and coordination, leading to bigger (and much faster) gains.

TRAINING RULE 2:

Know When to Use Them

"Kettlebells are ideal for explosive, total-body exercises, such as swings and snatches," says Tsatsouline. They're also good for the overhead press because you get a good stretch at the bottom and a perfect lockout at the top. As for the triceps extension, biceps curl, and other moves that hit smaller muscle groups, a kettlebell also works just as well as a dumbbell does.

TRAINING RULE 3:

Focus on Your Form

A kettlebell's off-balance design makes good technique even more important. "Keep your wrists straight," Tsatsouline says. Bending your wrists raises your risk of strain and doesn't let you transfer power as effectively between your body and the bell. Also, keep your weight on your heels and your shoulders pulled down and back. "That increases your stability and allows you to generate more power," says Tsatsouline.

Anatomy of a Kettlebell

A. HANDLE: The most common spot to hold—especially for ballistic moves like swings and snatches.

B. HORNS: Hold these (the sides of the handle) for goblet squats and when the bell is upside down.

C. BASE: The heaviest part of the bell and where the mass is centered.

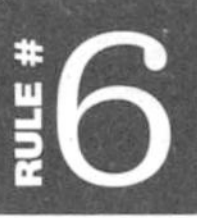

Every pound you lose feels like 5 fewer pounds to your knees.

POWER MOVES

TWO KETTLEBELL EXERCISES EVERY MAN SHOULD MASTER

1. Kettlebell Single-Arm Press

A kettlebell is best for this move because "you can start the lift lower, which is safer for your shoulders," Pavel Tsatsouline says. "At the top it pulls your arm back slightly, improving mobility."

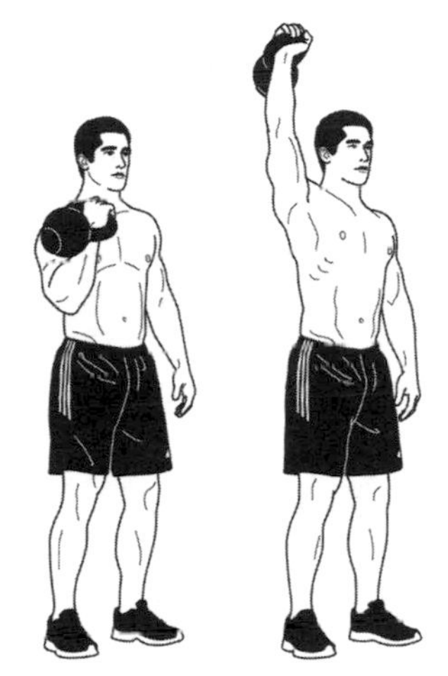

Stand with your feet shoulder width apart and hold a kettlebell in front of your shoulder with your palm in, elbow tucked, and the weight resting on the top of your forearm. Press it straight up, rotating your arm so your palm faces forward. Do equal reps on both arms.

2. Kettlebell Swing

This classic move offers serious power-building and six-pack benefits. You'll burn about 14 calories a minute (the same as running 6 miles an hour), say University of Wisconsin researchers.

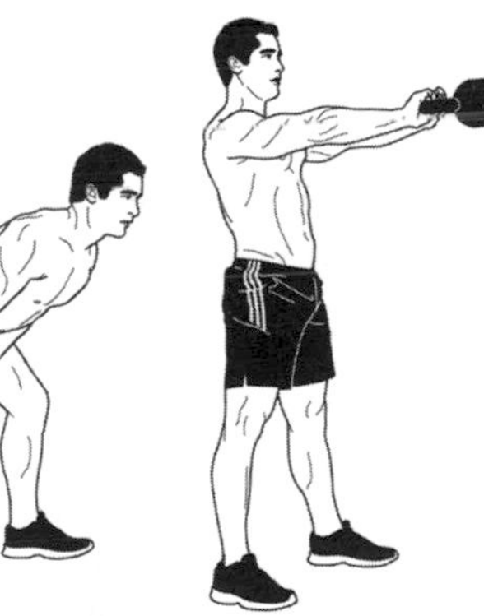

Set a kettlebell on the floor, spread your feet slightly beyond shoulder width, and grab the handle. Hike the bell between your legs and then thrust your hips forward as you swing it to chest level. Swing it back between your legs. That's 1 rep. Continue swinging without stopping.

RULE # 7 **Whenever it's practical, walk. For every hour of brisk walking, you add an hour to your life.**

Improve Your Running Form

Lean Forward

Good running form is a slight forward tilt—about three degrees, not too far forward, not too far back. Allow your eyes to guide you to the properly tilted and aligned neck and torso. Let your gaze settle on the horizon. Keep your chin tucked instead of letting it jut out.

Be on the Ball

Landing on your heels means you're overstriding. Harvard researchers found that forefoot strikers have fewer injuries than heel strikers. Flick back your heel quickly after contact; visualize pawing the ground with the balls of your feet.

Relax Your Arms

Runners often hold tension in their arms and hands, which sends it into their shoulders. To avoid this, run with your thumb and first two fingers touching lightly as if holding delicate potato chips that you don't want to break.

Swing Right

When running, your arms should swing back and forward, not across the midline of your body. If they do, you'll rock from side to side. If you feel tension in your neck and shoulders, drop your arms straight and shake them out to relax your muscles.

Make a Muscle Cramp Vanish

STOP YOUR WINCING WITH THIS SIMPLE TRICK FROM TOP PHYSICAL THERAPIST BILL HARTMAN, CSCS, PT.

Don't Stretch

Cramps are caused by your muscles contracting uncontrollably, and your natural reaction when a cramp sets in is to try to stretch your way out of it. Resist the urge to elongate the muscle. Stretching only puts your muscle through more strain, which could lead to more pain.

Flex Instead

Leverage the intelligent approach: reciprocal inhibition (RI). This is a nervous-system phenomenon that you can activate yourself. When you contract the muscle on one side of a joint hard enough, the opposing muscle—the one cramping, in this case—will stop firing, easing the cramp. The following cramps are the most common. The next time one strikes, put RI into action with these moves.

CRAMP	YOUR MOVE
Bottom of your foot	Lift your toes toward your shin.
Calf	Bend your ankle, bringing your foot toward your shin.
Hamstring	Sitting or standing, fully extend your lower leg.

Finish Your First Marathon in an Upright Position

- ***Pick a flat course.*** The best marathons for first-timers are flat and scenic. Do your homework at www.runnersworld.com
- ***Get sticky.*** Slather Vaseline or sports lubricant anywhere you might chafe; underarms, nipples, and inner thighs are our favorites.
- ***Climb over the wall.*** Mile 20 is where most runners "hit the wall" and feel complete physical and mental exhaustion, says Budd Coates, a four-time qualifier for the Olympic Marathon Trials. Put your family there so you'll get a mental boost.
- ***Stay loose.*** When you run a long race, you can inadvertently build tension in your shoulders, arms, and fists, which saps energy. To keep your fists relaxed, pretend you're holding a potato chip between your thumb and index finger. And don't break it.
- ***Wear disposable clothing.*** It's often chilly in the early morning wait before the start of the race. To stay warm, cut the toes off a pair of long tube socks and pull them over your arms. A plastic garbage bag with head and arm holes cut out is a great wind and rain breaker to wear while waiting for the gun. Both are cheap, so you won't feel guilty about chucking them during the race.
- ***Stop side stitches.*** If you feel stabbing pain in your side while running, tighten your abdomen, say our friends at *Runner's World*. You can also rub out the pain with your two middle fingers or exhale forcefully when the foot on the opposite side of the stitch hits the ground.

Make the Perfect Preworkout Protein Shake

Your muscles need a precise balance of nutrients to make the most of a workout, says Alan Aragon, MS, a nutritionist in Thousand Oaks, California, and a *Men's Health* advisor.

Build Your Base

You want enough quality protein to maximize muscle protein synthesis and minimize muscle breakdown during a workout. You also need carbs for energy and a little fat to help you absorb nutrients. Start with $1\frac{1}{2}$ scoops of protein powder (about 30 grams) and 12 ounces of fat-free milk instead of water. This yields roughly 240 calories, 40 grams of protein, 16 grams of carbs, and 3 grams of fat. Toss in some fruit for flavor, or a tablespoon of peanut butter or almond butter for a creamier shake. These will boost calories, carbs, and fat, but they're good for your overall diet.

Keep It Smooth

Buzz the concoction in a blender. Add ice if you like your shakes thicker. If you're using a shaker bottle, prevent clumping by pouring about a cup of the milk into the bottle before adding the powder. Shake it up until the powder is well incorporated, add the rest of the milk, and shake again until smooth.

Time It Right

Drink your shake within the hour prior to your workout. This is the best time to fuel your muscles for high-intensity training. (To cool off after a workout, try the delicious Muscle Power Shake recipe above.)

Muscle Power Shake

Down this protein- and carbohydrate-rich recovery shake after a tough workout. It tastes like a Creamsicle, but without the added sugar.

BLEND THIS:

1 scoop vanilla protein powder
1 orange
¼ orange peel
1 tablespoon walnuts
2 tablespoons flaxseed meal
1 cup water
½ cup orange juice
3 ice cubes

Per serving: 399 calories, 32 g protein, 14 g fat, 39 g carbs

The Grapefruit Diet

In a study in the *Journal of Nutrition and Metabolism,* people who drank about $\frac{1}{2}$ cup of unsweetened white grapefruit juice before every meal for 12 weeks lost 13 pounds and 2 inches off their waists; they also consumed up to 30 percent fewer calories a day.

Fact:

Arnold Schwarzenegger sported a 57-inch chest during his 1970s bodybuilding heyday.

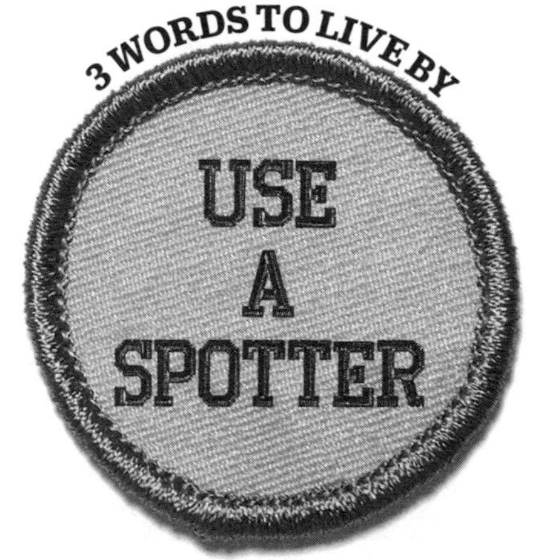
3 WORDS TO LIVE BY
USE
A
SPOTTER

Push Yourself to New Heights

The next time you do an overhead press, don't just stand there—give yourself a push. The push press can help you build serious lower-body power, according to a study by British researchers. When participants performed the move, which adds a partial squat to the overhead press, they exerted the same amount of force into the ground as they did during a barbell jump squat. The takeaway: By swapping your regular shoulder exercise for the push press, you receive the benefits of two moves for the price of one. Just 3 to 5 sets of 3 to 5 reps once a week will do the trick.

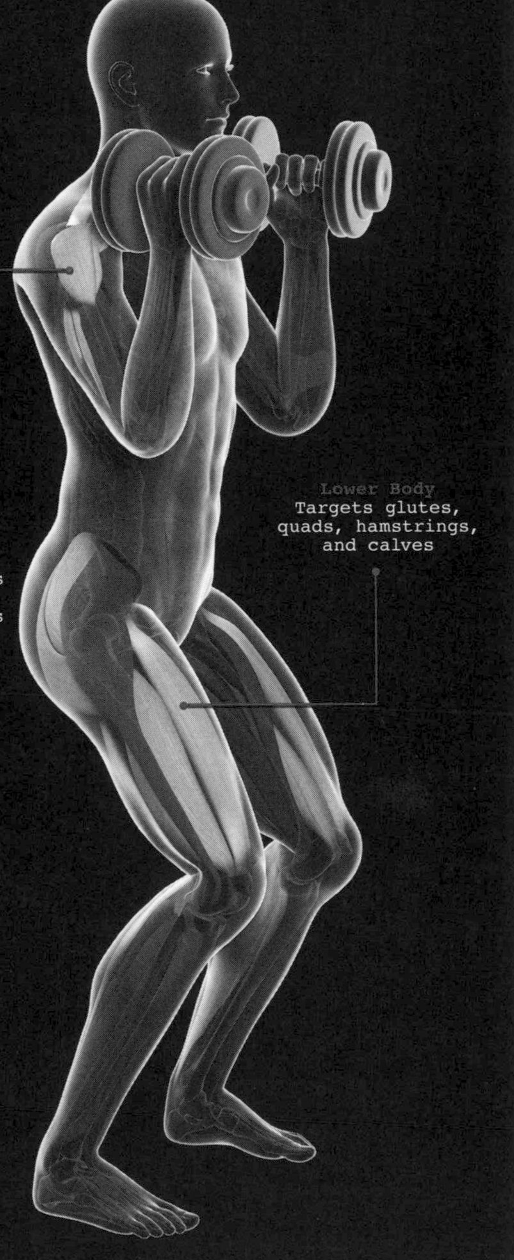
Upper Body
Targets triceps and front and middle deltoids
Lower Body
Targets glutes, quads, hamstrings, and calves

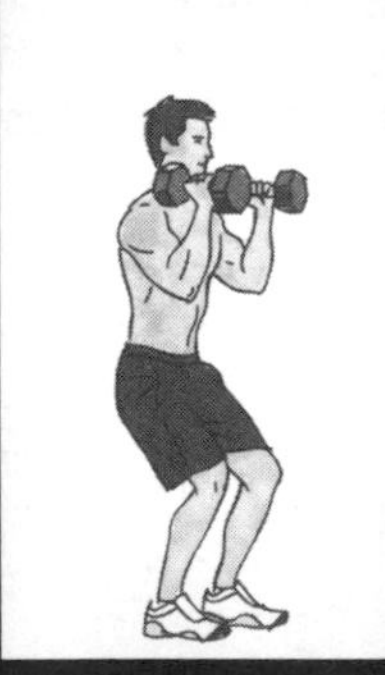

Step 1

Hold dumbbells in front of your shoulders; dip your knees.

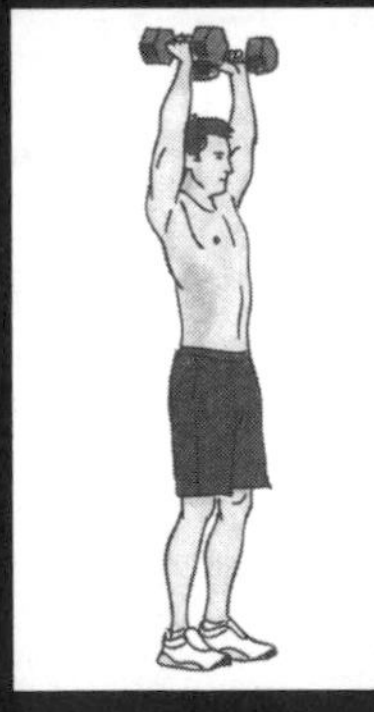

Step 2

Push explosively with your legs and press the weights up.

Seven Stupid-Simple Ways to EAT LESS

1 GRIN YOURSELF THIN

To maintain a healthy weight, do something to make yourself smile. Scientists in Brazil say serotonin, the "happy hormone," reduces appetite, and raised levels of it make you more likely to burn fat.

2 CRACK SOME NUTS

In an Eastern Illinois University study, people who were given shelled (that is, naked) pistachios ate 211 calories' worth while those who had the in-shell variety (you crack 'em open) consumed only 125 calories in the same sitting.

3 PUT A FORK IN IT

Your nondominant hand, that is. You'll be more mindful of what you're eating and end up consuming less. (Using chopsticks works, too, especially if you're not a pro.) Have plenty of napkins on hand.

4 USE A CHEAT PLATE

With the Portion Plate ($12, theportionplate.com) you see partitions for meat (a quarter of the plate), whole grains (another quarter), and fruits and vegetables (half the plate), along with pictures of foods in the proper serving sizes to guide you. You'll also feel younger.

5 ADD BISON TO YOUR PROTEIN HERD

Grill up a 3-ounce buffalo steak every now and then. It has only 148 calories and 4 grams of fat. Plus, the 26 grams of lean protein in that bison steak can keep you satisfied enough to decline dessert.

6 BE AN EARLY BIRD

Late risers not only eat more calories (almost 200 more at dinner and another 375 after 8 p.m.) but also eat more unhealthily than those who wake up around 8 a.m., according to a Northwestern University study.

7 EAT WITH A WOMAN

Men consume 37 percent less when they eat with a wife or girlfriend than when they dine out with their buddies, according to researchers at the State University of New York at Buffalo.

RULE #8

Work opposing muscle groups—your biceps and triceps, for instance—back-to-back for a faster workout. While one muscle is working, the other is resting.

Best Move for a V-Shaped Torso

The standing bent-over row activates more muscle across both your upper and lower back, say Canadian scientists. But you have to do it right or risk a herniated disk. Never round your spine; instead, keep the natural arch in your back when you bend over. Hold dumbells with a neutral grip at arms length. Raise the dumbbells to the sides of your chest, pulling your shoulder blades down and together as you perform the move.

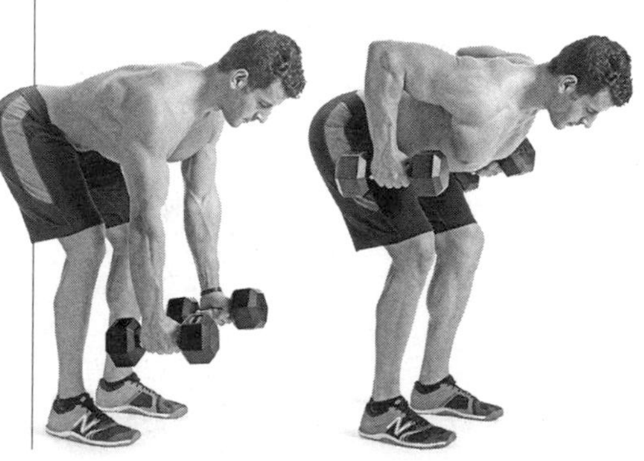

Slim in Seconds

1 Sit or stand as tall as you can.

2 Keep your head up and your chest high.

3 Retract your shoulder blades as if you're holding a pencil between them.

4 Contract your abs and obliques as if they're creating a corset around your midsection.

Don't Crunch to Lose Weight

Why? The exercise is inefficient as a fat-burner. It takes 250,000 crunches—that's 100 a day for 7 years—to burn 1 pound of fat.

RULE # 9

Barefoot running on soft beach sand strengthens your calves, arches, and Achilles tendons and restores proper mechanics to flat-footed runners.

Pull Off the Perfect Swimmer's Flip Turn

Conserve energy and improve your freestyle lap times.

A. Start your flip just at the end of the lane marker, 3 to 4 feet from the wall, for a smooth transition.

B. Take one last stroke, suck in a big breath, and tuck your head and your arms into your gut. Your butt will come out of the water slightly.

C. Bend your knees, bring them over your butt, and make contact with the wall with the balls of your feet.

D. Explode off the wall, arms extended toward the other end of the pool. Use a corkscrew motion to power yourself out of the turn.

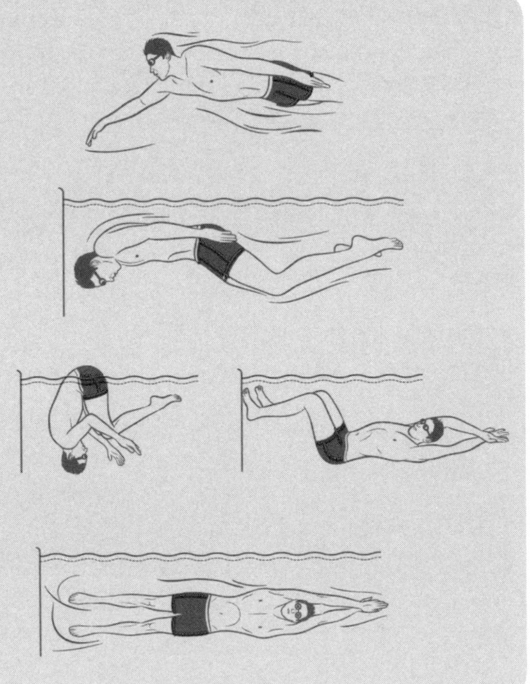

31 Days to a Flat Gut

1 WEEKEND	2 MONDAY	3 TUESDAY	4 WEDNESDAY	5 THURSDAY	6 FRIDAY
Eat eggs for breakfast. A study in *Nutrition Research* found that people who egg it up consume fewer total calories the rest of the day.	Stand up whenever you read or take a phone call at work. (You can also use a stand-up desk.) Standing burns 1½ times more calories than sitting does.	Grab a pen. People who kept a food log for at least 3 weeks lost 3½ pounds more than those who didn't, a University of Arkansas study found.	Chew food slowly and completely: You'll take in nearly 12 percent fewer calories than if you scarf it.	Don't eat meals in front of the TV. In a University of Massachusetts study, people who did that took in nearly 300 more calories a day.	Weigh yourself each week. Three out of four successful dieters do this, the *American College of Sports Medicine Health & Fitness Journal* reports.
7/8 WEEKEND	**9 MONDAY**	**10 TUESDAY**	**11 WEDNESDAY**	**12 THURSDAY**	**13 FRIDAY**
Dog-sit for a neighbor. But don't just sit—take Brutus for a walk. You'll burn 61 calories in 15 minutes. (Better yet, make it an hour.)	Want to blow off today's workout? Bad idea. Miss one now and you're 61 percent more likely to skip one next week, says a study in *Health Psychology.*	At lunch, have an apple instead of apple juice. Chewing triggers satiety, so you'll likely consume nearly 15 percent fewer calories, notes the journal *Appetite.*	Added sugars lead to added lard, so cut them out. This week, drop the sweetest offenders—soda, baked goods, cereals, candy, fruit drinks, and ice cream.	Mix a shake: Consuming 55 grams of whey protein a day for 23 weeks can leave you 4 pounds lighter than if you'd eaten those calories in carbs, USDA scientists say.	Open the fridge and put produce at eye level. You're 2.7 times more likely to eat healthy food if it's in your line of sight, say scientists at Cornell University.
14/15 WEEKEND	**16 MONDAY**	**17 TUESDAY**	**18 WEDNESDAY**	**19 THURSDAY**	**20 FRIDAY**
Reward yourself with a great Saturday night dinner, but don't make it an all-weekend feed, or you may binge later, University of Texas researchers warn.	Clean the house. People with the most spic-and-span abodes have the highest levels of physical activity, research from Indiana University reveals.	If you think you're too busy to work out, think again: An 11-minute workout can help you burn more fat all day, a Southern Illinois University study found.	Make pushups work harder for you. Do an iso-explosive pushup: Hold your body in the down position for 3 seconds and then push up explosively.	Don't let the bread basket hit the table. An Eastern Illinois University study found people ate 85 percent more bread when they were offered seconds.	Have some minty gum before your workout. The peppermint scent boosts sprinting speed and gym strength, says the *Journal of Sport & Exercise Psychology.*
21/22 WEEKEND	**23 MONDAY**	**24 TUESDAY**	**25 WEDNESDAY**	**26 THURSDAY**	**27 FRIDAY**
Eat beta-glucan for breakfast. This oat fiber can help regulate appetite for up to 4 hours, according to a study in the *Journal of Nutrition Research.*	Pee often. A study in the journal *Obesity* found that people who drank two 8.5-ounce glasses of water before each meal lost an extra 4.5 pounds in 12 weeks.	During your workout, rest for no more than 60 seconds between exercises to keep your metabolism-boosting hormones high for the duration.	Fill your plate from the stovetop. You'll likely eat up to 35 percent less than if you shovel it from a serving dish on the table, say Cornell University researchers.	Keep your treadmill set to a minimum incline of 2 percent to painlessly boost workout intensity. Increase the incline further to burn even more calories.	Toss a half cup of chickpeas into your next pot of winter soup. You'll tack 6 more grams of flab-fighting fiber onto your bottom line.
28/29 WEEKEND	**30 MONDAY**	**31 TUESDAY**			
Walk to talk. Turn up your cell phone ringer and leave the phone in a far-off corner of the house to force yourself to stand up and go to it when it rings.	Drinking 2½ cups of fat-free milk in the a.m. instead of the calorie equivalent in juice can lower calorie consumption by 8.5 percent, says an Australian study.	Cheers! Drink a 12-ounce Guinness Draught instead of a Bud to save about 20 calories and gain the same antioxidants found in wine.			

RULE # 10

Work out in the morning if you can. A British study found that people who exercised at 6:45 a.m. pushed themselves longer than people who worked out at 6:45 p.m.

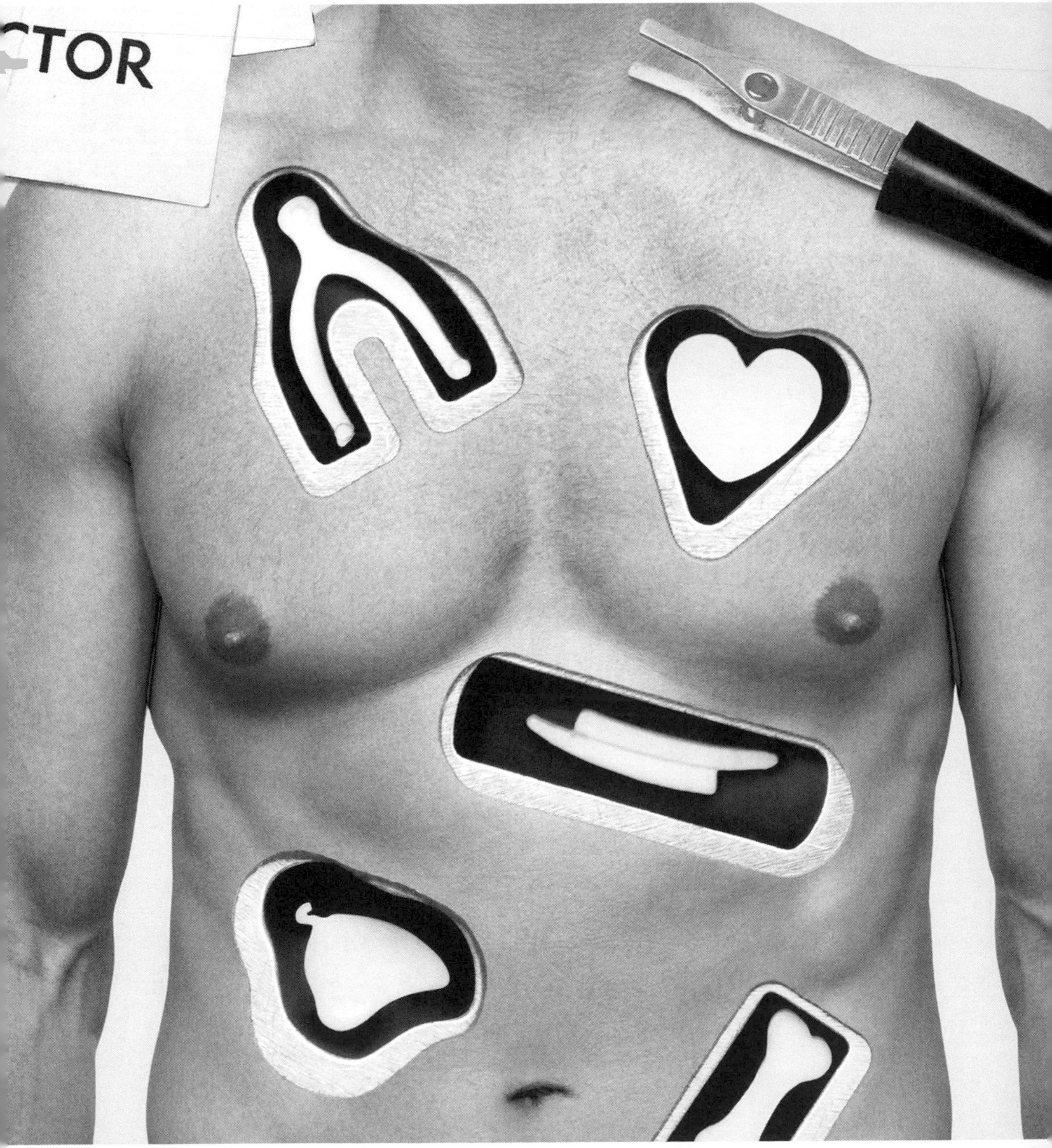

CTOR

Stealth Health

Beat Back Pain, Fight Brain Drain, Save Yourself from Choking, and Dozens of Other Tips and Life-Extending Tricks

It's no great secret that women are a lot better than men when it comes to seeking health care. Unless he has a piece of rebar sticking out of his abdomen or a really bad rash in a really unfortunate place, a man is unlikely to rush off to see a GP and would rather DIY for first-aid. According to stats from the Centers for Disease Control and Prevention, men are 80 percent less likely than women to go for regular doctor visits. Gentlemen, we can do better, and it wouldn't take much. If only docs would invest in examination gowns that covered your ass, you'd be much more inclined to visit them. Until then, we've pulled all the crucial medical information you need to stay relatively healthy in one handy chapter. Our lawyers require us to tell you that this advice should not replace proper medical care, but seeing as you're unlikely to visit your doctor anytime soon, we figure this stuff might actually cover your ass a bit better than that gown.

13 SIMPLE HOME HEALTH REMEDIES

DON'T WASTE TIME RUNNING TO THE DRUGSTORE WHEN YOU HAVE THESE HANDY FAST FIXES.

Athlete's Foot

Sprinkle baking soda on your feet and between your toes, or apply a paste made with 1 tablespoon of baking soda and lukewarm water. Wait 15 minutes, then rinse and dry your feet thoroughly.

Burns on the Roof of Your Mouth

If hot pizza scorched the roof of your mouth, use an over-the-counter cough lozenge with benzocaine to cut the pain. If you don't have any, try using sugar.

Canker Sores

Hold a wet tea bag on these sores; the tannin from the tea acts as an astringent.

Charley Horse

Arch your toes back toward your body while gently rubbing your calf. Start behind the knee and slide your hand down the muscle to the heel, then repeat. Rub along the length of the muscle, not across it.

Heartburn

Chew a stick of sugarless gum. The increased saliva will help your stomach acid flow, and it will also coat and protect the esophagus.

Hoarseness

Your vocal cords need rest, so don't speak. To get rid of the frog in your throat take a 5-minute hot shower, drink warm herbal tea with a slice of lemon, and avoid caffeine, smoke, alcohol, and large, fatty meals.

Indigestion

Mix one of the following items in a glass of water for an emergency antacid: 1 teaspoon of apple cider vinegar (to increase stomach acidity) or ½ teaspoon of baking soda (to ease bloating). Then take a walk. A postmeal stroll can help you digest your food up to 50 percent faster.

Ingrown Toenail

Soak your foot in warm water to soften the nail. Then roll a small piece of cotton to the thickness of a candle wick, soak it with iodine, and place it between the skin and the tip of your nail. Wrap the toe with gauze, tape it, and change the dressing daily until the nail grows out.

Itchy Eyes

Probably due to allergies. A cold washcloth held over closed eyes will shrink blood vessels and reduce redness.

4 SIMPLE STEPS TO WEIGHT CONTROL

- Always be aware of your weight.
- Never skip meals.
- Never let yourself become ravenously hungry.
- Indulge (sensibly) in what you like.

RULE # 1

Avoid kidney stones if you never want to experience pain on par with childbirth.

How? Drink at least eight glasses of water a day, limit your salt consumption, and drink plenty of fat-free milk for the calcium that binds with the stone-causing minerals and ushers them out of the body.

Nosebleed

Sit up so that gravity will lower the vein pressure inside your nose. Tilt your head forward slightly to keep blood from running down your throat.

Rashes

Rub a paste of crushed vitamin C tablets and water on your skin.

Sore Feet

Pour a handful of uncooked beans into your slippers and walk around for a few minutes. The rolling beans create an instant massage. Then hold your feet under the bathtub faucet; run the water on hot 1 minute, cold the next. Alternate for 10 minutes, ending in a cold rinse. To prevent future pain, spread marbles on the floor and pick them up with your toes.

Sunburn

Take an oatmeal bath. Wrap a cup of oats in cheesecloth and hang it from your faucet so that the bathwater runs directly over it as the tub is filling. No one knows exactly how the oatmeal works to soothe the pain, but you will feel better.

60

Percentage your sperm count may increase if you replace two servings of processed red meat each week with fish. Seafood's high omega-3 content and absence of growth hormones may help your sperm thrive.

Source: Journal of Nutrition

4 Health Mistakes You Make Daily

You Brush after Breakfast. Acidic foods like fruit and juice can weaken enamel. Brushing after eating these foods may lead to discoloration, cracks, and chips. Instead, swish with water and wait 40 minutes for the calcium in your saliva to demineralize weakened areas of your teeth. Then brush.

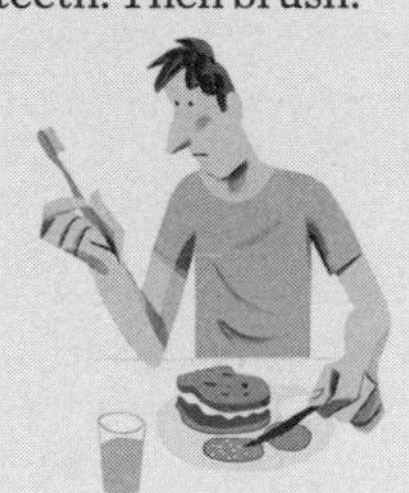

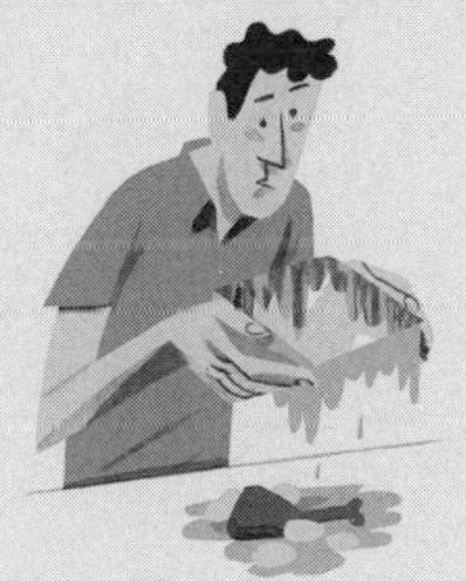

You Microwave Your Lunch in Plastic. Even if the plastic is BPA-free, phthalates can leach into your food, potentially altering hormones. Instead, transfer food to glass before nuking it.

You Drive Home after Happy Hour. People with a blood alcohol concentration of .01 percent—well below the .08 legal limit—are 46 percent more likely to cause a crash than drivers who are totally sober, according to a UC San Diego study. Cut your BAC by 30 percent by eating before drinking.

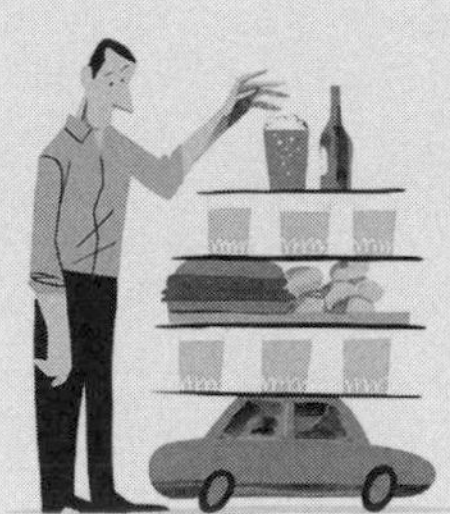

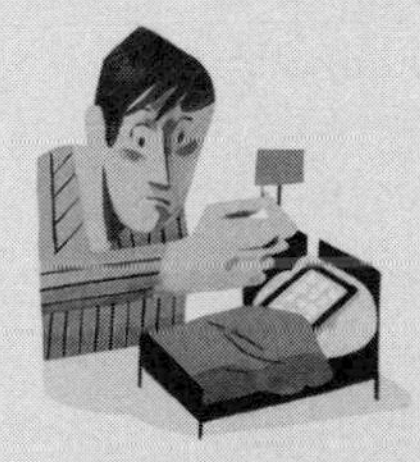

You Check Your Work E-Mail before Bed. Managers who use their smartphone for work after 9 p.m. wake up groggy, a University of Florida Study found. Other studies suggest too little sleep can raise your odds of dying of stroke. Power down by 9 p.m. and turn off e-mail notifications.

The Worst Things You Can Put in Your Mouth

Chewing tobacco. Natch.

Pens and pencils. Chewing on them causes tiny stress fractures in teeth.

A Red Savina habanero chile pepper. It's the world's hottest pepper, rated at 500,000 units on the Scoville heat scale. Jalapeños by comparison top out at only 5,000.

Ice. Ice is crystal; so is tooth enamel. Chew ice and the ice usually wins.

A frozen margarita. Take two kinds of alcohol, add a lot of sugar and salt, and freeze the mixture, and you have a tasty drink that's bad for your liver, heart, arteries, blood sugar, blood pressure, energy level, and digestion. Bottoms up!

Nails. You're on a roof replacing some shingles and you casually put two nails in your mouth . . . and then you slip. ER docs we know say they've seen punctured tongues, cheeks, even lungs.

Cooked food from street vendors. Significant undercooking and cooling of hamburgers, chicken dishes, and beef kabobs raises the risk of food poisoning.

Toothpicks. Rooting around your mouth with a toothpick can sever or loosen the ligaments that attach teeth to bone.

The No-Blow Way to Clear a Stuffy Nose

Blowing your nose hard seems like the manly thing to do, but it's stupid, because it can force mucus and germs deeper into your sinuses. Do this instead:

- **Apply wasabi.** Add anything spicy to your food to blast open nasal passages.
- **Steam clean.** Take a long, hot shower or apply a warm washcloth to your forehead, nose, and cheeks.
- **Lube up.** Spritz some saline spray up your nose to keep mucous membranes moist.
- **Just breathe.** Don't blow; exhale gently through your nose into a tissue.

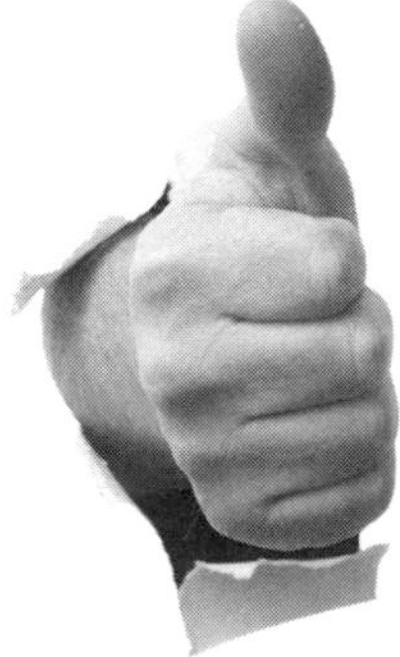

Soothe a Smashed Thumb

Next time you mistake your thumb for a three-penny nail, squeeze it. Lift the appendage above the level of your heart and squeeze the tip for up to 5 minutes to reduce swelling, bruising, bleeding, and pain. Ice it afterward.

Fact:

The average guy takes only 6 seconds to wash his hands, which is 14 seconds short of what the CDC recommends.

HOW TO OBLITERATE A *Bad Mood*

Force a smile when you're stressed. Even fake smiles reduce stress, a University of Kansas study found.

Take a stroll when you're bummed out. A study in the journal *Environmental Science and Technology* reports that you can improve your mood with just 5 minutes of exercise outdoors in nature.

Crank up Mozart when you're pissed off. Scientists in Germany found that people who listened to classical music before experiencing conflict showed less aggression and reported lower levels of residual anger. People who listened to aggressive tunes, say, Mastodon's "The Motherlode," felt like punching someone out.

Check Your Pillow

A good pillow supports your head and neck as you move during the night. Fold your pillow in half; if it doesn't return to its original shape when you release it, go shopping.

Have a Cold One

A hot shower may feel good, but a cold one revs up your body. German researchers found that cold baths increased disease-fighting white blood cells, improved circulation, and boosted testosterone for the Spartans who took them regularly.

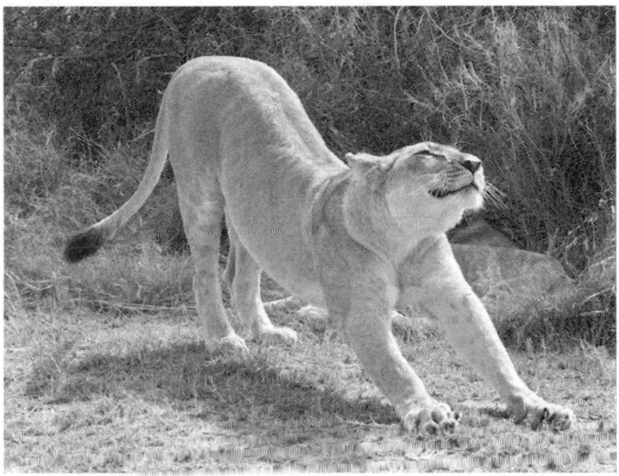

Purr-Fect Your Posture

Stretch like a cat for 30 to 60 seconds when you roll out of bed each morning. It's like hitting a reset button on your body. Get on all fours on the floor and curl your back toward the ceiling like a frightened cat. Hold for 10 seconds, then bend in the opposite direction, lowering your belly button toward the floor. Catlike stretching first thing in the morning improves posture, promotes blood flow, and relieves body tension, according to the Mayo Clinic. And better posture is an instant age eraser.

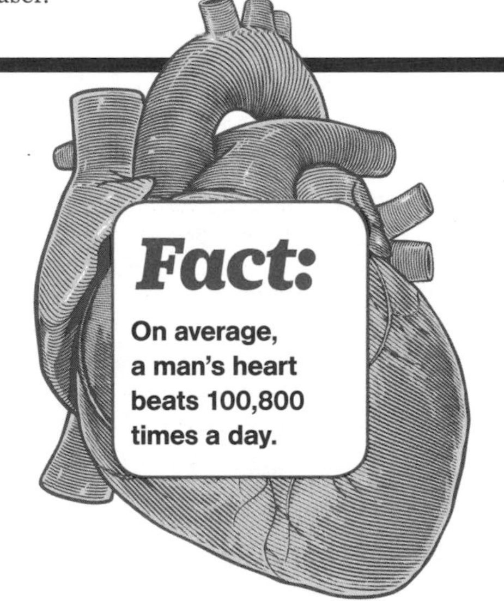

Fact:

On average, a man's heart beats 100,800 times a day.

10 Ways to Grow Gray Matter

Brain researchers name their top exercises for intelligence:

1. Taking dance classes
2. Doing yoga/meditating
3. Learning a musical instrument
4. Reading
5. Studying a foreign language
6. Playing chess
7. Juggling
8. Taking advanced courses
9. Learning complex skills
10. Cognitive training games

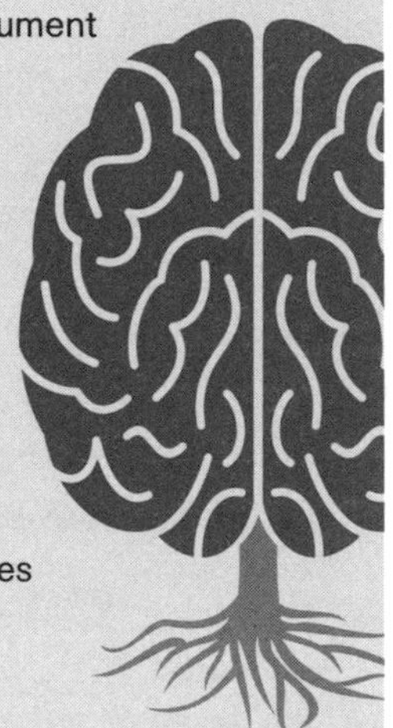

Go Mole Hunting

The more moles you have, the higher your melanoma risk. Are you getting yearly skin screenings with a dermatologist? Didn't think so. Well, book it, Dano. And in between screenings, snap photos of your moles and log them in an app, like UMSkinCheck, that sorts them from head to toe. "A new mole that keeps growing and comes to look different from the rest should be shown to a doctor," says Julia A. Newton-Bishop, MD, a professor of dermatology at the Leeds Institute of Cancer and Pathology in the UK.

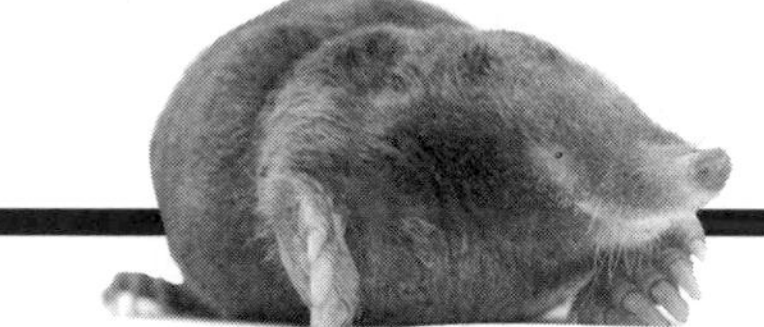

What Does a D.O. Do?

Same thing as an MD, mostly. Doctors of osteopathic medicine have the same education and are licensed in all states. Many DO's may still have more holistic treatment philosophies than old-school doctors, and some may be better versed in preventive medicine.

Relieve a Blow to the Groin

On *Jackass* it was considered funny. In real life, however, a bash to the balls can be more than wind-sucking painful; it can lead to the loss of a testicle. Knocked in the nuts? Do this:

1. Put your jewels on ice to reduce swelling and pain.
2. Make a testicle cradle. Take a rolled up T-shirt and put it underneath the testicles with one end of the roll resting on each thigh to support the scrotum.
3. Take Tylenol for pain relief. Avoid aspirin, which promotes bleeding.
4. If you are swollen and black and blue, go to an ER and ask for the urologist on call.

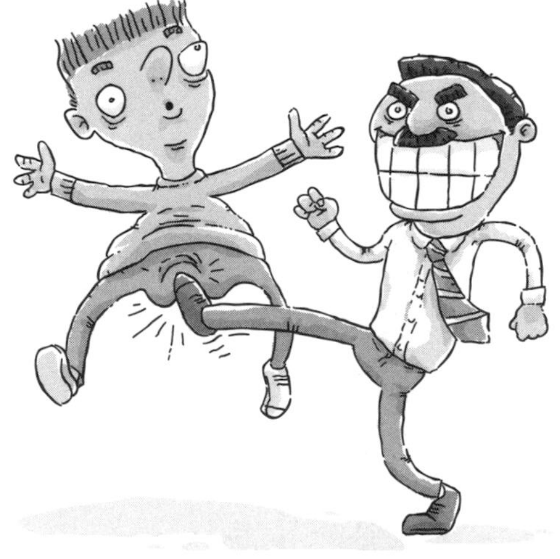

How Beer Makes You Fat

1. You take a swig.
2. Within seconds, the beverage passes through your esophagus and into your stomach.
3. Twenty percent of the alcohol is absorbed from your stomach into your bloodstream; the rest is absorbed from your intestines.
4. The alcohol travels through your blood to your liver, where it's broken down. During this process, waste products called acetate and acetaldehyde are created.
5. Acetate and acetaldehyde signal your body to stop burning fat. At the same time, your body starts making fat from another waste product of alcohol, acetyl CoA.
6. Your body can effectively process only 0.5 to 1 ounce of alcohol per hour. So the more you drink, the longer your body is inhibited from burning fat. And the more fat builds up from the excess acetyl CoA. (A 12-ounce beer contains about 0.6 ounce of alcohol.)
7. Sorry to bum you out.

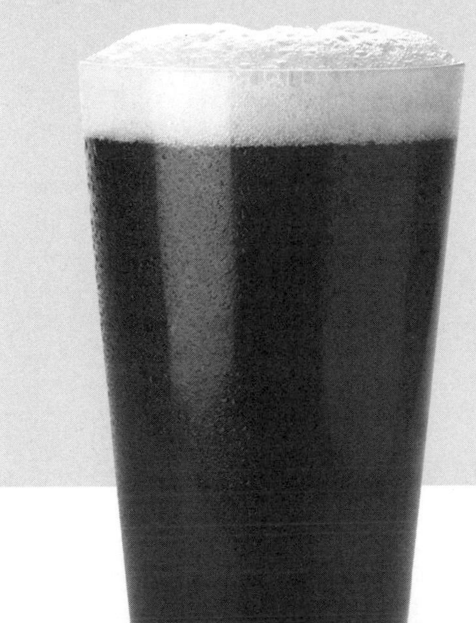

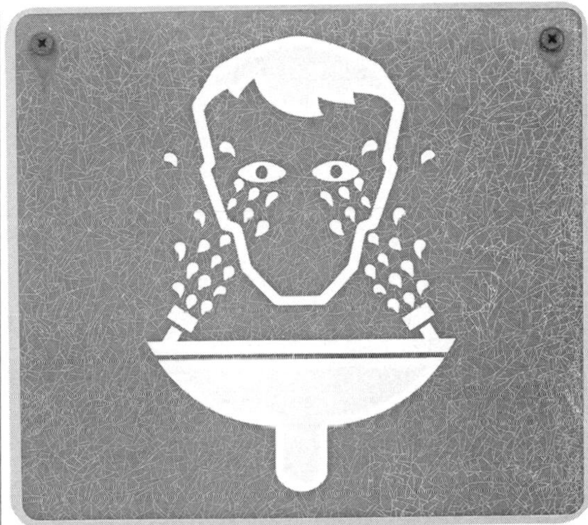

Clear Grit from Your Eye

If your tears won't flush the speck from your eye, sweep out the grime with your eyelid. Pull your top lid down over the lower one; the lower lashes will act as a broom, sweeping the speck out from under the upper eyelid. A gentle stream of water from a water bottle may work, too.

Take a Knee

Studies show that people who attend church regularly live 3 years longer on average than heathens do.

Fact:

Particles expelled during a sneeze can travel up to 103.6 miles per hour.

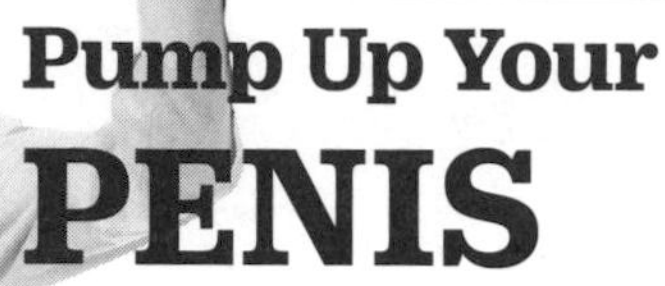

Pump Up Your PENIS

Move your hips around as if you were using a Hula-Hoop. Seriously. Do this for a few minutes each day and you'll increase flexibility in your pelvis and improve circulation in the whole region, which is key to firm erections. Ukelele and grass skirt optional.

Fact:

Doctors can now grow skin for burn victims using the foreskins of circumcised infants. One foreskin can produce 23,000 square meters, which would be enough to tarp every Major League infield with human flesh.

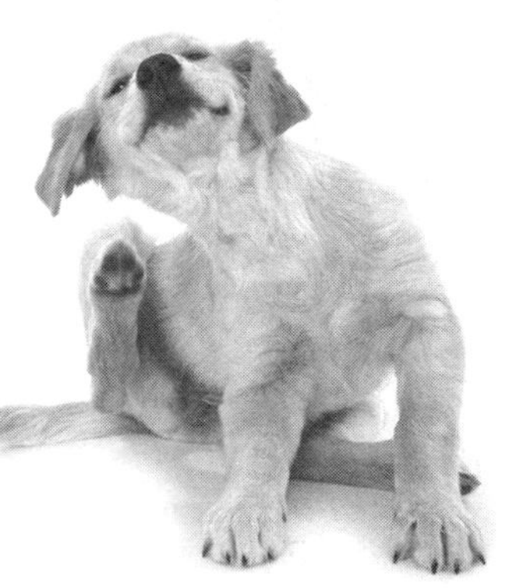

Why Scratching Feels So Good

Uncommon Knowledge: There is actually a Center for the Study of Itch at Washington University in St. Louis. The director of the center, Zhou-Feng Chen, PhD, tells us scratching hurts so good because "it may activate your reward system." Pain may also play a role: If scratching hurts your skin, the pain can help quell the itch because the two sensations are competing. The downside: Too much clawing can cause injury. If that's you, firmly rub the area with a chilled cotton T-shirt instead.

RULE # 2

The best way to prevent back pain is to strengthen your core. Seventy-five percent of all lower-back problems can be prevented by building your abdominal muscles.

The Earlobe Heart Test

Studies have shown that deep vertical creases running down the middle of the earlobe indicate a tendency toward heart disease.

10 BEST FOODS FOR YOUR HEART

1. Nuts
2. Fish
3. Oats
4. Avocados
5. Black beans
6. Flaxseed
7. Green tea
8. Watermelon
9. Spinach
10. Red wine

The Wheel of Misery

Hurtin' buckaroo? Before you start whining, check out this ouch ranking from Paul Christo, MD, a pain medicine specialist at Johns Hopkins:

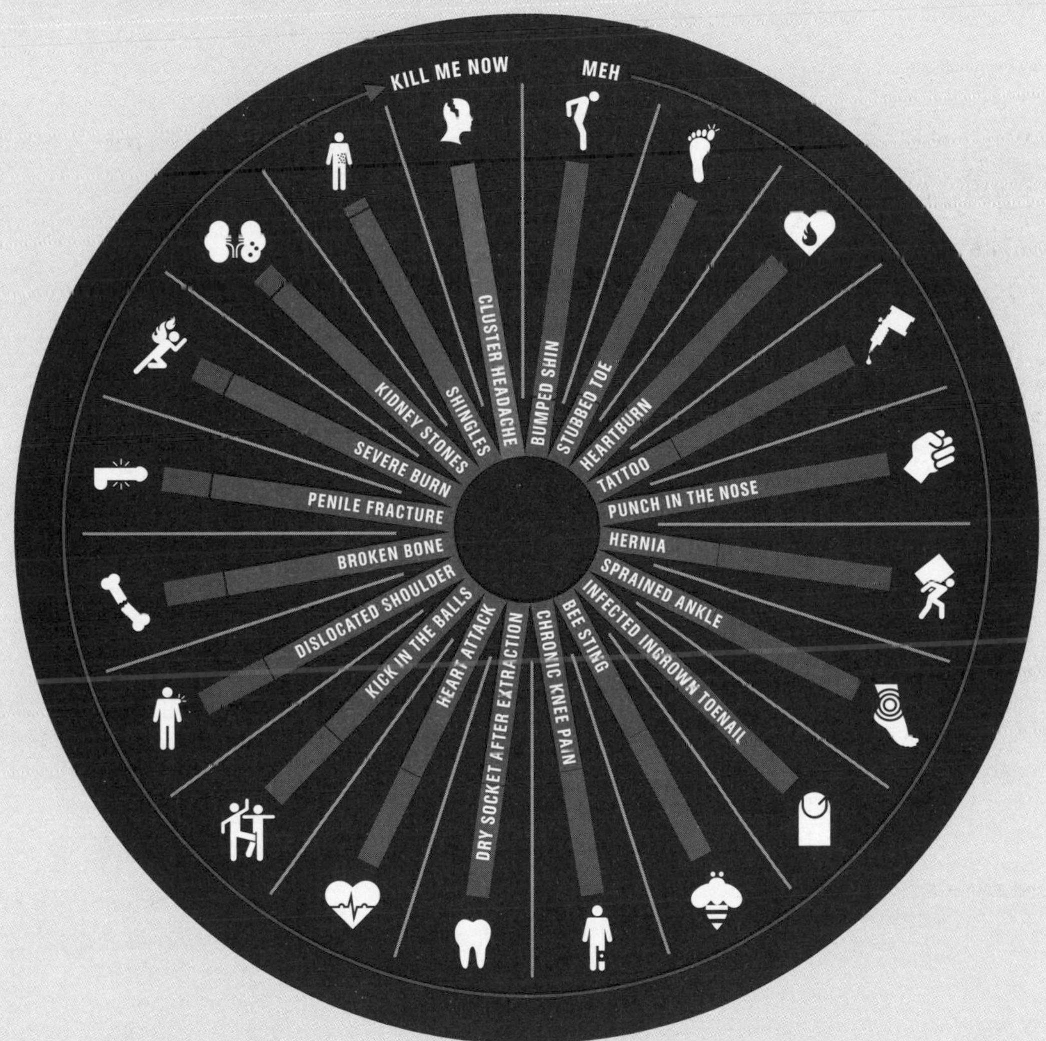

Fact: **Sudden, sharp pain in the balls could be testicular torsion, where the testicle twists and cuts off blood supply. If not treated quickly, it could result in the loss of a testicle.**

Train Your Brain

From the following letter sequences see how many words of three or more letters you can form in 3 minutes. Your goal is 18 for A and 20 for B, says Gary Small, MD. The benefit: You're training your brain to sift quickly through information.

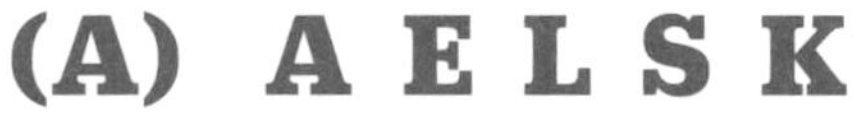

(B) T R E I O A

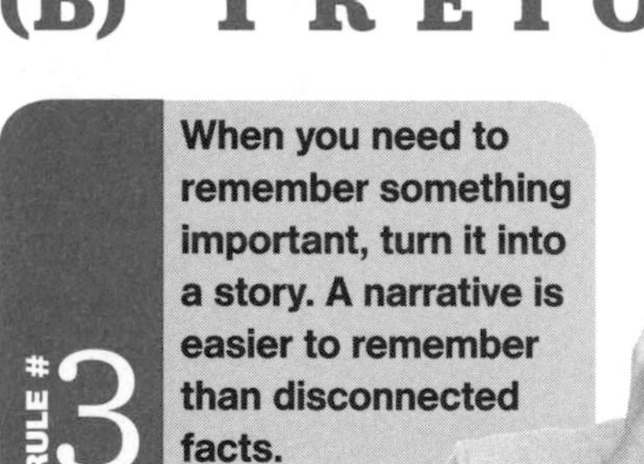

RULE #3
When you need to remember something important, turn it into a story. A narrative is easier to remember than disconnected facts.

Hiccup Tricks

Hiccups are spasms of the diaphragm, the muscle separating the chest and the abdominal cavities. As far as science can tell, they are perfectly useless, but most of us began to hiccup in the womb and continue to do so, usually at inopportune times, throughout life. Next time you're afflicted with hiccups just as you're called on to summarize your corporation's 5-year plan, try some of these cures offered by the *Journal of Clinical Gastroenterology.*

- Yank forcefully on the tongue.
- Lift the uvula (the little boxing bag at the back of your mouth) with a spoon.
- Tickle the roof of your mouth with a cotton swab back at the point where the hard and soft palates meet.
- Chew and swallow dry bread.
- Gargle with water.
- Hold your breath.
- Compress the chest by pulling the knees up or leaning forward.
- Bend over and drink water upside down.

STEAK STUCK?

Give Yourself the Heimlich

Choking on a piece of porterhouse is a cruel way for a man to die, especially if he's a vegetarian. But it's the sort of thing that happens 2,000 times a year in the US. If something becomes lodged in your windpipe, don't wait around for a waiter to notice you're turning blue. Give yourself the Heimlich maneuver. Clench a fist and place the thumb side against your upper abdomen, just below your rib cage. Grasp the fist with your other hand and thrust inward and upward a few times. If that doesn't work, lean forward over the back of a chair or side of a table, pressing it into your upper abdomen. Push yourself quickly downward, forcing air out of your lungs. Repeat until you're shooting steak bullets across the table.

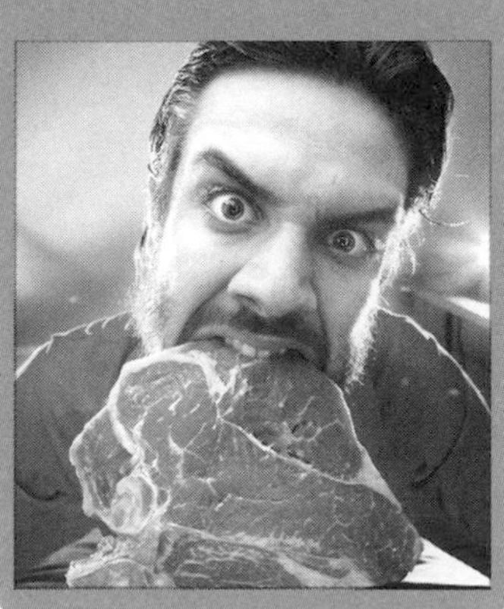

The Rest of Us Are Conducting Penicillin Research

Only 50 percent of Americans clean out their refrigerators once a month, and 70 percent keep home refrigerator temperatures at the recommended 40°F or lower, according to a USDA survey.

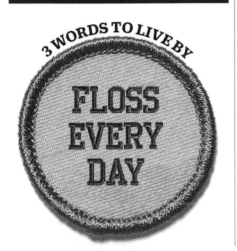

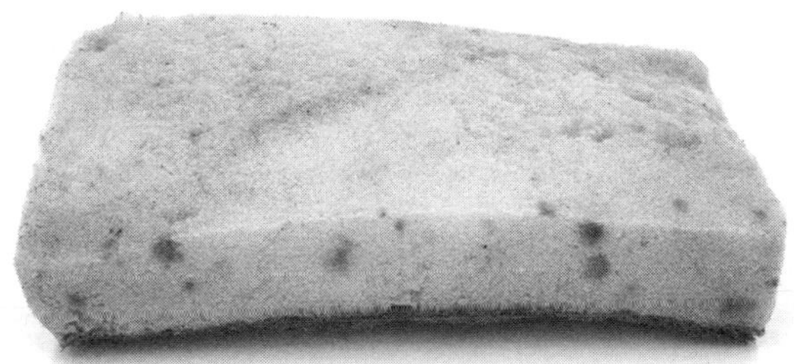

3 WORDS TO LIVE BY
FLOSS
EVERY
DAY

Beat Bad Sponge Bugs

Sponges are home to millions of bacteria; cleaning your kitchen with them often does more harm than good. Keep a stack of clean rags or towels on hand for cooking and cleanup. Once a week, soak sponges overnight in a cup of water mixed with a few spoonfuls of bleach.

Power Up with Nuts

Superpowers: Boost testosterone, build muscle, burn fat

Secret weapons: Protein, monounsaturated fat, vitamin E, niacin, magnesium

Battle: Obesity, muscle loss, wrinkles, cardiovascular disease

Sidekicks: Cashew and almond butters

Fact:

Smoking can shorten your penis by up to a centimeter. Lighting up calcifies blood vessels, stifling erectile circulation.

When to Toss It

Vitamins—3 years. If there's no expiration date. Over time, active ingredients lose their potency.

Contact lens case—3 months. To reduce risk of eye infections from parasites and fungi that can live there.

Pillow—1 year. Dead mites and their shit can make up 10 percent of a 2-year-old pillow's weight.

Toothbrush—3 months. Old, frayed bristles do an inferior job and harbor bacteria, increasing risk of gingivitis.

Bed sheets—1 to 2 weeks (wash). Germs from your mouth and skin can multiply and can cause gastro and respiratory infections.

Smoke alarm—5 to 10 years. Technology is always improving, so your alarm shouldn't be outdated. (And remember to test it monthly.)

Mattress—9 to 10 years. That's about the time the coils flatten out. Lumps and lack of support can stress your back.

Erase a Black Eye

Control swelling, promote healing, and appear like less of an animal with this plan from Gary Dorshimer, MD. As head team physician for the Philadelphia Flyers, this doc has treated his share of shiners.

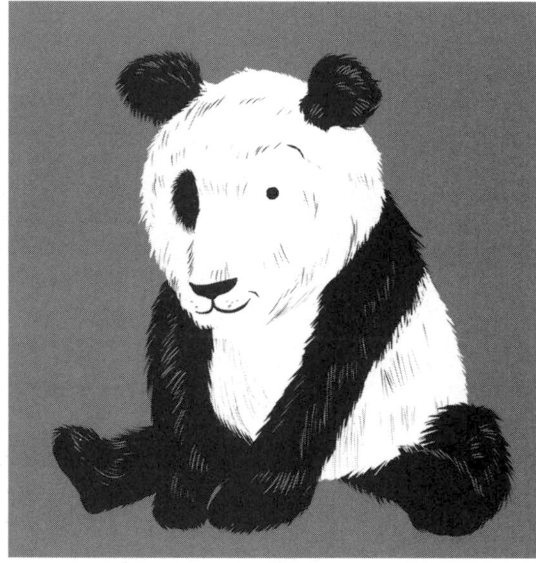

A. Cool It!

Apply a cold compress to your eye to slow blood flow and curb swelling. Grab a bag of cold (not frozen) peas or a cold, damp washcloth. Hold the compress to your eye for 5 minutes, break for 20 minutes, and repeat until the swelling stops. Use the compress for a 5-minute session three or four times a day.

B. Pop the Cap

For pain relief in pill form, stick to acetaminophen (Tylenol). Avoid anti-inflammatories, such as aspirin or ibuprofen, for the first 24 hours. They could thin your blood, resulting in more swelling.

C. Put Gravity to Work

The black and blue happens because fluid doesn't drain properly. Put an extra pillow under your head at night. The elevation eases swelling and prevents blood from pooling around your eye socket.

D. Turn Up the Heat

After 48 hours of cold compresses, switch to a warm, moist compress. Heat increases circulation, drawing white blood cells to the site of the bruise to help repair tissue. Apply the compress, 10 minutes at a time, as often as you want. It'll feel great too.

E. Put Your Finger on It

Massage around the bruise—very gently—with your fingertips. This can reduce swelling by draining fluid and increasing circulation.

Don't Be a Party Pooper

You're more likely to be sickened by salsa than by any other dips. Researchers testing different types of dips that had been contaminated by double-dippers found that salsa had seven times more microbes than the others. Turns out the runny consistency of the tomato-based snack can carry germs from a half-eaten chip into the bowl.

How to Avoid Ingrown Toenails

Never cut your toenails in a rounded shape so that the sides curl down into the skin. Leave the outside edges of the nail parallel with the skin.

Q. How do you find the healthiest dark chocolate?

A. Check the wrapper for the percentage of cacao, an indicator of the amount of antioxidant flavonols. As little as a third of an ounce a day of 70 percent cacao chocolate can improve heart health, studies show. Look at the ingredients list: Avoid dark chocolate that specifies "alkalinization" or "Dutch processing," which strips out flavonols. What you want to see is sugar and vanilla to balance out the bitterness of the cacao, and cocoa butter to hit the sweet spot of creaminess.

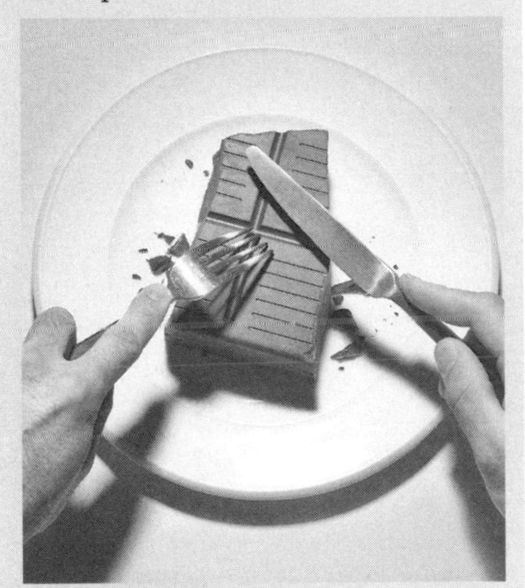

MED SCHOOL VOCABULARY TEST

sar·co·pe·ni·a

Pronounced *sahr kuh pee nee uh*, it's the loss of muscle tissue that accompanies aging and regularly lifting nothing heavier than a fork. From the Greek, it means, literally, "lack of flesh." The average guy starts to lose 1 percent of his muscle mass per year after age 30 unless he does something about it. Skeletal muscle is a major user of calories, so as you lose muscle, you tend to replace it with fat. To prevent sarcopenia, get off your ass and turn to Chapter 3 for some weight-lifting workouts and eat more protein, the building block of new muscle.

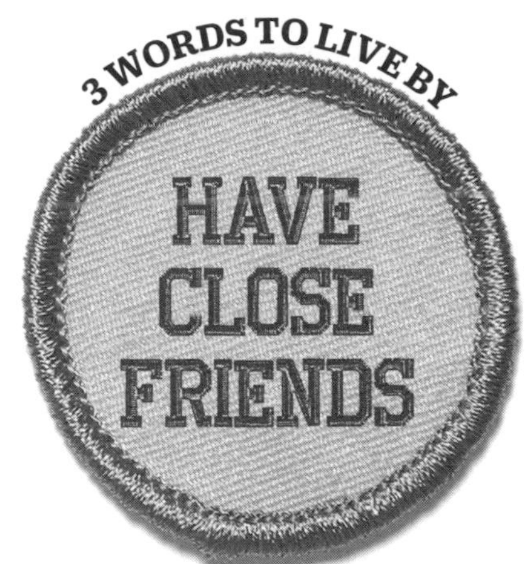
3 WORDS TO LIVE BY
HAVE CLOSE FRIENDS

The Gait Way to Living Longer

Walking can cut your risk of dying of brain cancer by about 40 percent, according to research from the Lawrence Berkeley National Laboratory. The magic minimum needed to earn the benefits, scientists say, is 12 miles a week.

Fend Off Frosty Fingers

When your hands feel like they're going numb in freezing weather, swing your arms in a circle. This will bring blood rushing to your hands and warm them up fast.

Run for *Your Back*

Running can help prevent lower-back pain, so hit the road. In fact, jogging strengthens your back-stabilizing muscles more effectively than back extensions do, says a Canadian study. "As you push with each leg during a run, the other side of your pelvis wants to drop," says study author David Behm, PhD. "Your trunk muscles contract to keep your pelvis in line." And unlike back extensions, running mimics everyday movements. To work your core more, run on an unstable surface, like sand or turf, Dr. Behm says.

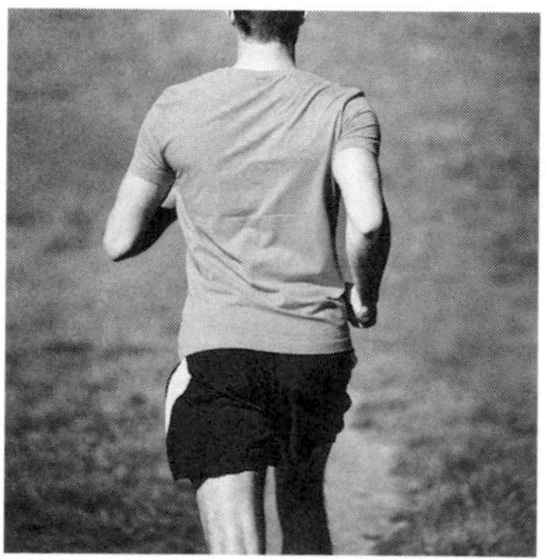

Sugarcoat a Toasted Tongue

Burned your tongue with hot food? Sprinkling some sugar on it may ease the pain.

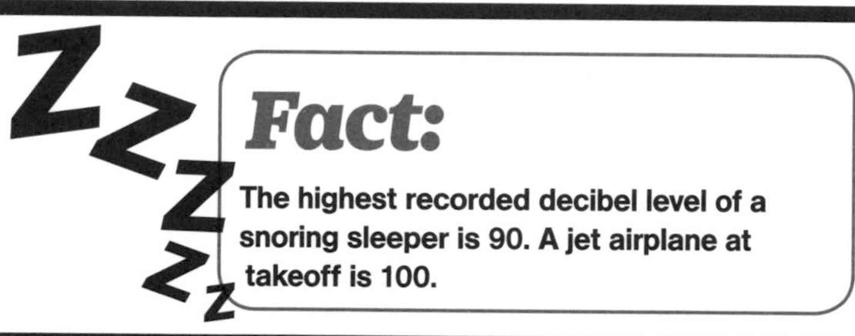

Fact:
The highest recorded decibel level of a snoring sleeper is 90. A jet airplane at takeoff is 100.

Double Up for Health

Food scientists say these culinary alliances are healthier when eaten together.

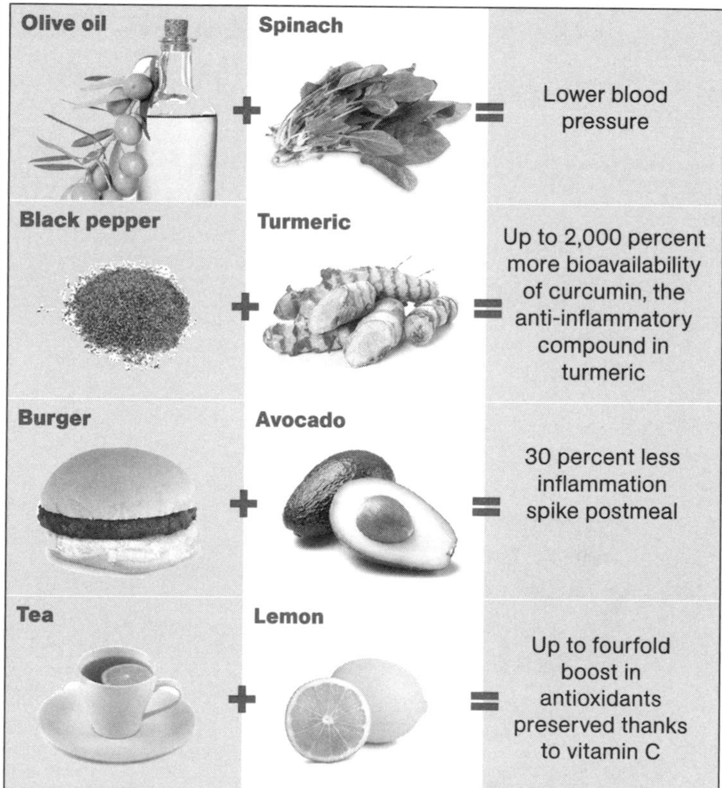

Olive oil
Spinach
Lower blood pressure
Black pepper
Turmeric
Up to 2,000 percent more bioavailability of curcumin, the anti-inflammatory compound in turmeric
Burger
Avocado
30 percent less inflammation spike postmeal
Tea
Lemon
Up to fourfold boost in antioxidants preserved thanks to vitamin C

Fast Fixes for Life's Sudden Mishaps

Curse

Swearing, or doing anything that triggers your fight-or-flight response, may provide short-term pain relief, UK researchers found. Another odd option: Punch yourself in a different body part (not too hard!), says study author Richard Stephens, PhD.

Spray

Bad bump? Baseball athletic trainers swear by Gebauer's Instant Ice spray for players hit by pitches. It numbs the skin and helps the poor guy forget the pain and return to action, says Jon Michelini, MS, ATC, head baseball athletic trainer at the University of Florida. Gebauer's Instant Ice is a nonprescription, nonflammable topical skin refrigerant. Use like ice for muscle spasm (stream spray only); minor pain and swelling from sprains, strains, bruising, and contusions; and minor sports injuries.

Smear

Mentholated lip balm can soothe minor cuts. The menthol binds to opiate receptors, triggers other receptors that make the skin feel cool, and opens blood vessels, says Paul J. Christo, MD, who teaches anesthesiology at Johns Hopkins.

Pour

When you burn yourself slightly, just run cool water over it, says William T. Zempsky, MD, a pain expert at Connecticut Children's Medical Center. Or hold a cool, moist cloth over the burn for a few minutes.

Chill

If taking aspirin upsets your stomach, try dissolving the tablets in a glass of milk. That'll prevent the tablet from lodging against the lining of your stomach and causing irritation.

The Easiest Way to Lose Weight

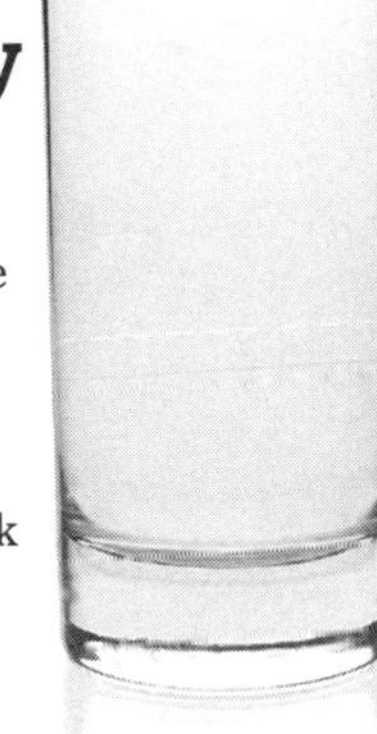

Drink two glasses of water before every meal. You'll stay hydrated, and filling your belly will cause you to eat less. Second easiest way to lose weight: Hold your fork in your nondominant hand; you'll eat less.

Go to Sleep *FASTER*

Sleep is critical to looking younger and being healthier. Instead of counting sheep to fall asleep, just wear wooly, warm socks. Swiss researchers found that people fell asleep quickest when their hands and feet were warmest. This happens because warm feet and hands cause blood vessels to enlarge, allowing more heat to escape your body, which in turn lowers your core temperature, inducing sleep. Try this, too: Drink a small glass of tart cherry juice just before going to bed. The carbs may elevate your brain's production of serotonin, a neurochemical that can help you nod off quicker, and cherry juice contains natural melatonin, the hormone that regulates sleep.

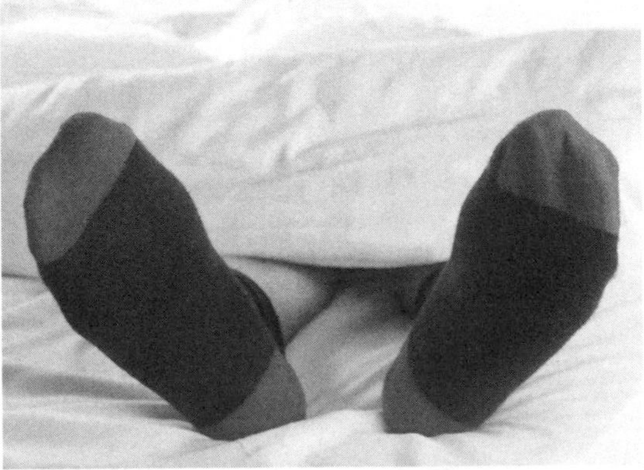

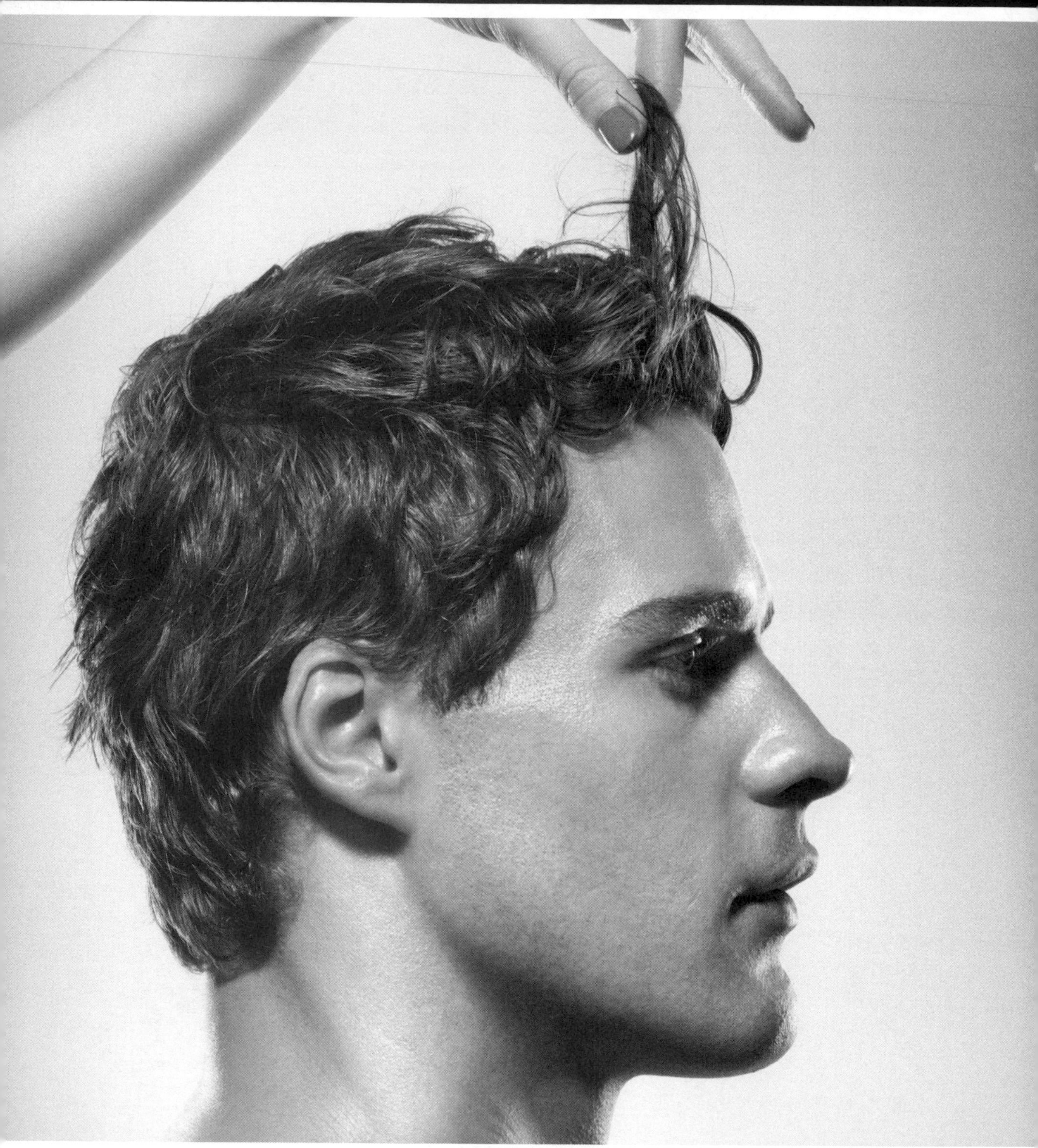

Style and Grooming

Advice and Simple Rules to Take the Guesswork out of Getting Dressed

How to look your best qualifies as Uncommon Knowledge because most men feel a bit intimidated when it comes to clothing. Few of us are born with an innate sense of style. You might be able to match the hatch with the perfect dry fly, but can't for the life of you pick a new tie to go with a suit. A sense of style, like a double-haul cast in fly fishing, is developed.

Unless your father was particularly well dressed and took you shopping with him often, you probably don't feel all that comfortable in a menswear store. But if you want to look really good, there's no getting around it: You must learn how to shop for clothes and pay attention to details.

Great style consists almost entirely of details. And that goes for manscaping, too. Skill is acquired through trial and error and attention to detail. Fortunately *Men's Health* has been helping men dress for all occasions (and keep their nails and eyebrows neatly trimmed) for decades.

Consider the following pages a handbook for upgrading your personal style so you'll look great anywhere. Turn the page for the blueprints.

The 16 Pieces of Clothing
EVERY MAN SHOULD OWN

All you need to look well dressed for any occasion in your life.

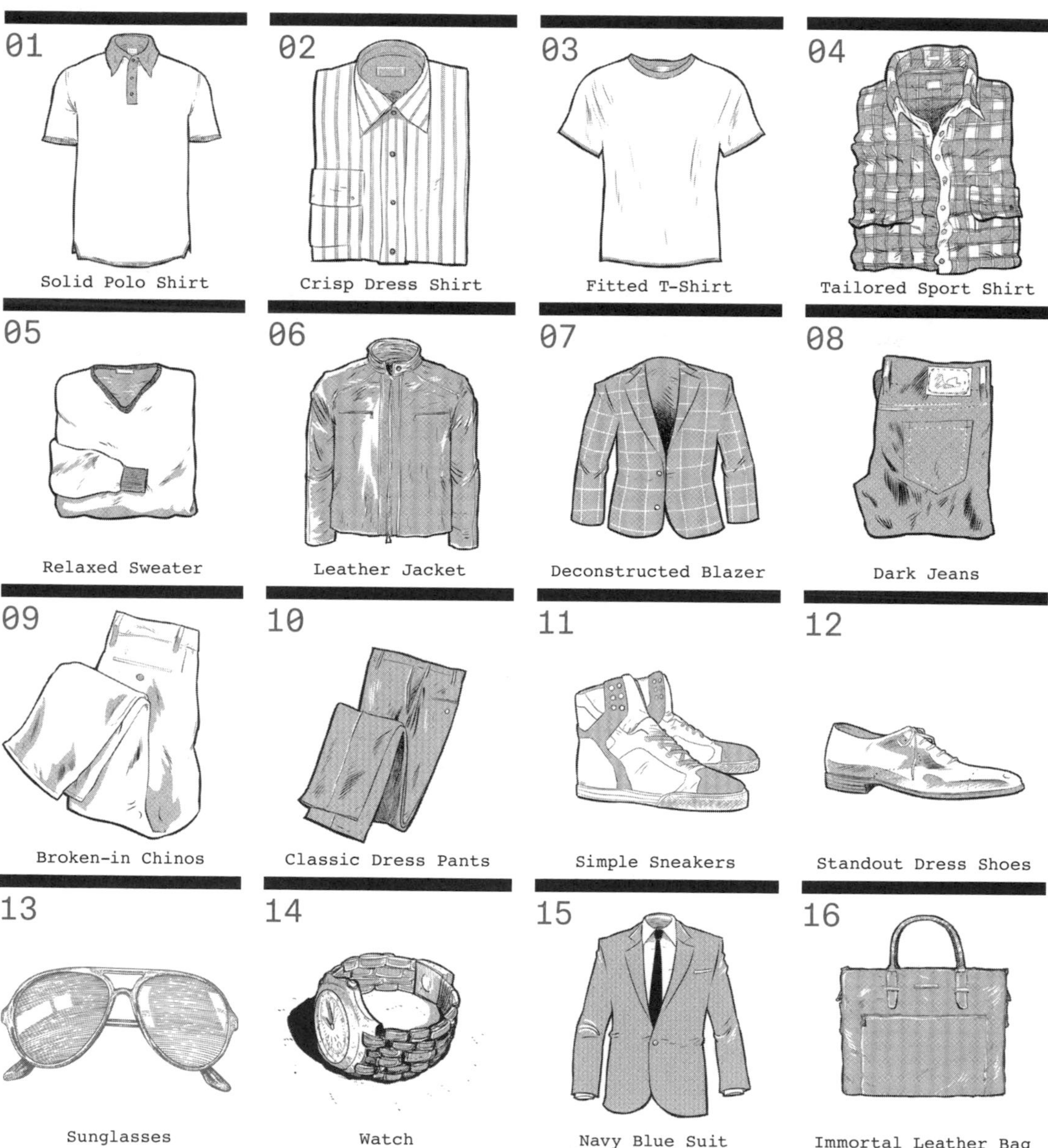

01. Plain Polos

A well-styled polo keeps your style sophisticated without the drudgery of wearing sleeves. Flex your right to bare arms: The sleeve should end about halfway down your biceps. Pair it with a sweater or tailored jacket. Let it stand alone on sunny days.

02. Crisp Dress Shirts

A white dress shirt is the building block of every man's wardrobe. It never goes out of style and works in situations from business casual to black tie. But you'll also want several crisp dress shirts in various colors (not just boring blue) and striped patterns. To stand apart from the other guys in the office, style it right:

- Fabric says something about you: Oxford cloth is democratic and preppy, while poplin is more refined and easier to dress up, yet casual enough for denim.
- Match your collar style to your face. Round or wide mugs look best with a narrow collar, while a spread collar balances a narrow face. Most of us fall somewhere in the middle—so a modified-spread collar is an ideal pick and always means business.
- With a white shirt under a charcoal suit, you can let your tie sing.

03. Fitted T-Shirts

Leave the loose fit to the free tees you earn running 5-Ks. Shoot for 100 percent cotton and a hint of stretch (for a better fit). Add a few details—like stripes—and you'll never go back to a generic three-pack. Wear under a blazer or sweater. Never tuck it in.

How to Fold a Dress Shirt

Developing a bit of skill in sartorial origami can help you stay sharp and fresh and not wrinkled, as if you just wrestled an alligator in your shirt.

1. **Lay Out the Shirt.** Fasten all the buttons, even on sleeves. Lay the shirt facedown on a wide table. (Not a bed; too soft to smooth out fabric.)
2. **Section Off the Fabric.** Pinch the fabric at the top of the shirt halfway between the collar and shoulder. Then find the same spot near the bottom and pinch the fabric. Pull taut. The resulting line is your fold point.
3. **Fold In the Sleeves.** Release the fabric at the top of the shirt and grasp the shoulder. Fold the entire section over so it rests beneath the collar. Now fold the sleeve back on itself so it lies straight down in line with the folded portion. Repeat on the other side.
4. **Flip Up the Bottom.** Grab the two corners of the bottom of the shirt and fold them up to the middle. Next, move your hands to the new bottom edges and fold those up again until the fabric is lying just under the collar.
5. **Put It Away.** To make sure the collars don't become too flat, place one shirt in the suitcase with the collar facing up. Then lay the next one facedown with the collar at the opposite end.

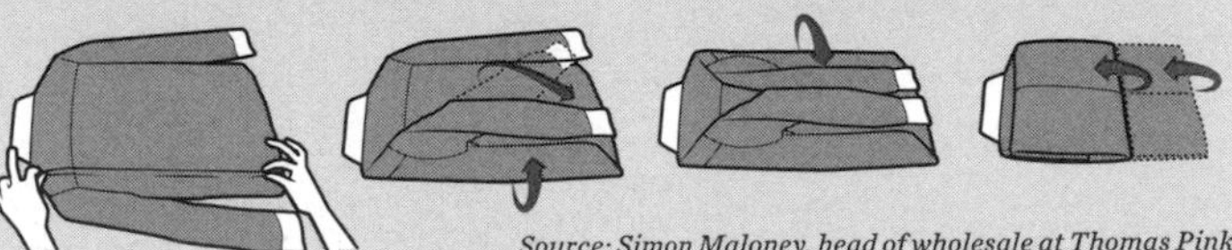

Source: Simon Maloney, head of wholesale at Thomas Pink

04. Tailored Sport Shirt

Aim for versatility: It should be short enough to leave untucked when a casual mood strikes. Let it wrinkle a bit and keep the top button undone, even if you're wearing a tie.

RULE #1

When shopping for clothes, try everything on, except for underwear. Even in Target. Make that especially in Target.

05. Sweaters

Layer for warmth in winter or chill out with a cotton-linen blend that's breathable enough for summer evenings. Just be sure to avoid the bulk:

- The thinner the knit, the closer it should fit your frame. Heavy sweaters should be loose but not boxy.
- Try a jacket. Sweater jackets, like a relaxed peacoat style, are a great alternative to a coat. Since you'll wear layers underneath, keep the fit roomy.
- Crew neck solids are a foundation piece—great with anything. Nonbanded bottoms are more forgiving on heavier midsections.
- A cardigan is the ultimate multipurpose knit. Dress it up with a shirt and tie for work, or go casual with a T-shirt and jeans.
- Stick to natural fibers. They are the most comfortable, and they let your body breathe no matter what the temperature.
- V-neck sweaters: If you own only one, make it fine gauge and solid, in either merino wool or cashmere. When you wear it with a collared shirt, keep the collar tucked in.

RULE #2

Crisp dress shirts should be ironed and tucked in—always. You should have only 1 to 2 inches of slack when you pinch it at the waist.

06. The Leather Jacket

Make sure the fit is snug and stay away from excessively shiny buttons and zippers. Soft, buttery leather trumps rigid and heavy. Test the boundaries. You could live in this thing. It works great over a T-shirt and jeans, even better over a shirt and tie.

Unstick Your Zipper

Apply a drop of liquid soap to a cotton swab and dab the zipper. Lightly tug the zipper back and forth to distribute the soap. Eventually the teeth should come unstuck.

Source: Darlene DeAndrade, expert tailor

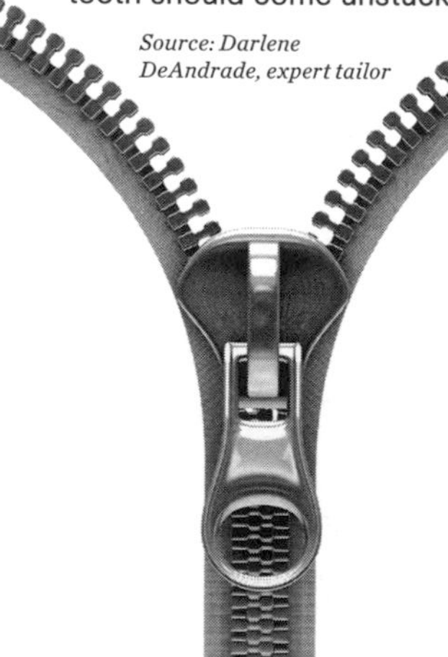

07. Deconstructed Blazer

Rethink the classic staple. Because it lacks the lining and padding of a traditional sport coat, this jacket will feel light on your shoulders. Wear anywhere you'd don a normal blazer. This is your go-to when it's hot; the lightweight fabric keeps you from drowning in sweat.

Tie On Texture

Unexpected tie fabrics, such as thick wool or chunky tweed, set you apart. Aim for a 2- to 3-inch width—about the size of your lapel. Bold colors like red go best with more subdued grays and whites. The suit or the tie, not both, should draw the eye.

RULE # 3 **Edit your closet every season. It's a toolbox, not a junk drawer.**

09. Chinos

Not every occasion is denim-friendly. Chinos combine comfortable cotton twill with the fit of your favorite jeans. They should fit like tailored pants—or even better, jeans. And pass on any chinos with pleats. Try a pair in gray or slate blue, colors that stand out but still go with everything.

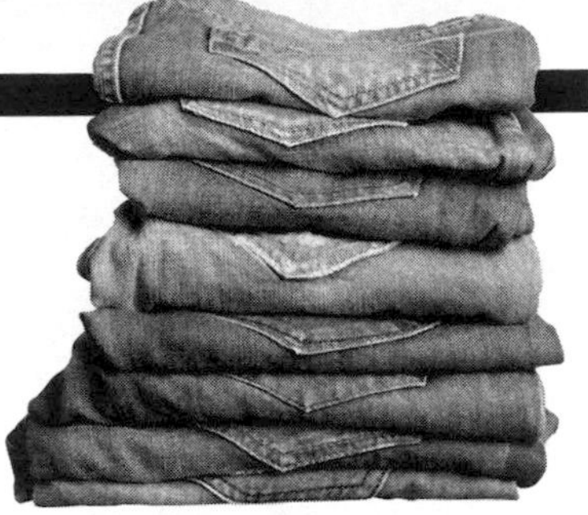

08. Jeans

Denim is the cornerstone of a man's wardrobe. Once you find the perfect fit, buy three pairs. You'll be set for years—especially dark denim. Even though jeans now arrive in a paralyzing array of washes, cuts, and styles, style experts back the straight leg as the only enduring style.

- If you're slim, going baggy won't fool anyone. Instead, accentuate your frame by going with a streamlined, straight fit that's narrow through the leg and skims your waist. Keep the jeans fitted in the seat; that way you create the illusion of bigger glutes. Pocket flaps add heft, but avoid accents like pocket stitching and flashy hardware. Lighter rinses and distressing only draw attention to your legs, making you look skinnier, so add a little depth with a dark rinse.
- If you're athletic, opt for traditional straight-cut jeans that are fitted through the waist, seat, and thighs. They'll provide ample room for well-developed quads while skimming your frame just enough to highlight your physique. Look for jeans with 2 or 3 percent Lycra so they'll stretch, but no more, or they might cling. Just steer clear of anything overly slim.
- If you're a bigger build, aim to strike a balance with a relaxed straight fit. You'll want a slightly extended rise, which means the jeans sit at, not below, the waist. That'll offer a few extra inches in the thighs and seat; and since the legs are cut straight down, your ankles won't be swimming in denim. If you can grab more than a handful of fabric at your quads, find a fit that's a little slimmer or have a tailor tighten up the pants. And choose darker colors—they do a better job of hiding extra pounds.

RULE # 4 **Match the neck of your T-shirt to the neck of your sweater. Wear V-neck T-shirts and sweaters together; the T-shirt can have a higher neck. A cardigan works with any style. But a crew-neck T-shirt with a V-neck sweater is okay only if Captain Kirk is your style icon.**

10. Classic Dress Pants

Don't go heavy; lightweight wool will hug your frame better and keep you cool in stuffy office spaces. Hike that waist up to just below your navel. These aren't your weekend jeans.

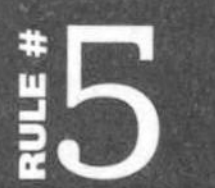

RULE #5

The length of your shirt matters—too short and it looks like a crop top; too long and nobody notices how great your pants fit. The proper shirt should fall around the top or middle of your back pocket, says Durand Guion, VP and men's fashion director at Macy's.

11. Simple Sneakers

Your running shoes are only for running. And keep your neon mesh gym shoes in your locker. Look for classic designs and neutral colors to sport outside the locker room. Keep them clean and you can pair them with dark jeans, bright chinos, or even a suit.

Q. Should I wash new clothes before I wear them?

A. You won't die if you don't, but your skin might suffer: "The dyes, resins, and finishes added to clothing can cause skin problems," says Mark Denis P. Davis, MD, a dermatologist at the Mayo Clinic. For example, synthetic fabrics are often colored with disperse dyes, which may trigger allergic reactions. Natural fabrics, such as cotton, aren't necessarily safer—they often contain irritating formaldehyde resins added by manufacturers to make the fabric resist wrinkling.

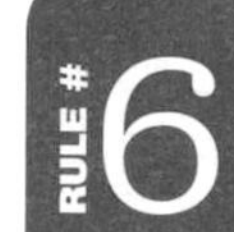

RULE #6

Match shoes and belt in color and finish. Shiny shoes = shiny belt. Suede/buck shoes = matte finish belt.

12. Standout Dress Shoes

Leather or suede. They're the uppers worth investing in. Break out from wearing dress shoes only with trousers. Your wingtips and brogues want to date around—and they'll look great with distressed denim or chinos.

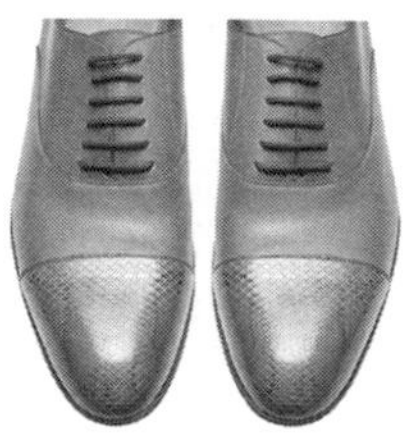

Buy Shoes That Really Fit

TIME YOUR VISIT Try on shoes in the afternoon. Your feet swell slightly during the day because walking increases blood flow down there, and you need to be sure your shoes fit your expanded feet. If you must shop in the morning, don't buy shoes that are snug.

CHECK THE FEEL Look for three key indicators of a good fit. First, your toes should lie flat in the shoe. Second, the ball of your foot—where your toes meet your foot—should sit comfortably at the shoe's widest point. Finally, your heels should slip slightly as you walk. (Too tight and you'll blister.) If you're clenching your toes to keep the shoe on, it doesn't fit.

TAKE A REAL WALK Persuade the salesperson to let you take a 2- to 3-minute stroll on a surface other than the plush carpeting of the store. Creasing along the ball of the foot is normal. Creasing along the toes means your foot is too far forward and you need more length.

Source: Kevin Vollrath, master fitter and regional sales manager for Allen Edmonds

13. Sunglasses

A perfect-fit pair will frame your face without deflating your wallet. The classic staple of sunny days? Aviators. It's hard to look bad—and easy to look badass—in them, but since styles vary, give the details close inspection and choose a set that works best for you.

- The shape of the frames should contrast with the shape of your face. See "Frame Your Face" to the right to help you pick the perfect style.
- As a rule, clean metal styles work for wider faces. Sizing tip: If you can see the temples flaring outward, the frames are too narrow for you.
- A retro style like Ray Bans are wider at the bottom, and help balance a narrow chin.
- Make it pop: Colored and mirrored lenses show you have bold confidence in your spec style.

14. A Watch

A quality time piece keeps you on time and never goes out of style, but time is money—and watches are expensive. Ask these five questions before investing:

- *What kind of movement is used?* A top-notch watch runs on mechanical movement, not quartz.
- *Is there anything special about the bezel?* The ring around the dial can be a strictly decorative front, but functional ones can move counterclockwise to measure elapsed time.
- *What is the crystal made of?* Sapphire is used in finer timepieces because it's scratch resistant. Avoid mineral crystal, which is easily scuffed, if you're buying high-end.
- *Is this a screw-down crown?* Screw-down crowns provide water resistance, which is great for when you forget to take it off in the shower—or get pushed into the pool.
- *Which metal is it made from?* The big three are steel, gold, and titanium. Titanium is lightweight and durable and lends itself to sporty timepieces. Steel is sturdy and the most versatile, so it's used across the board. Gold is mostly used in finer, pricier watches.

Frame Your Face

The trick to finding flattering sunglasses is to remember that opposites attract.

Oval: Almost any style works. Make sure your eyes are centered in the frames.

Round: Contrast curves with angular frames. Avoid anything too square.

Square: Round or minimal frames work with a prominent jawline and forehead.

Heart: Your wide forehead and narrow chin are helped by round frames.

A Tie for Every Occasion

POWER TIES (silk, wool, cashmere)

The Basic Pinstripe: Red, blue, and gold mean business.

The Solid: It's a go-to solution for that tough-to-match patterned shirt.

The Discreet Polka Dot: Key word: discreet. Avoid contrasting colors.

The Black Silk: A good, safe option for a wedding or funeral.

CASUAL TIES (silk, cotton, linen)

The Skinny: Stick with solid colors or bold stripes for this 3-inch-wide (or skinnier) noodle.

The Seer-Sucker: Wear it with a linen sport coat for a cool, casual look

The Wool Blend: It's more laid-back than 100 percent wool. Wear with a corduroy blazer.

15. Navy Blue Suit

Navy is serious and sharp, and a two-button suit is always appropriate, as long as you keep the top button secured to slim your profile. Wear a vest with the full suit or simply with dress pants or jeans for even more versatility.

Dress for Your Height

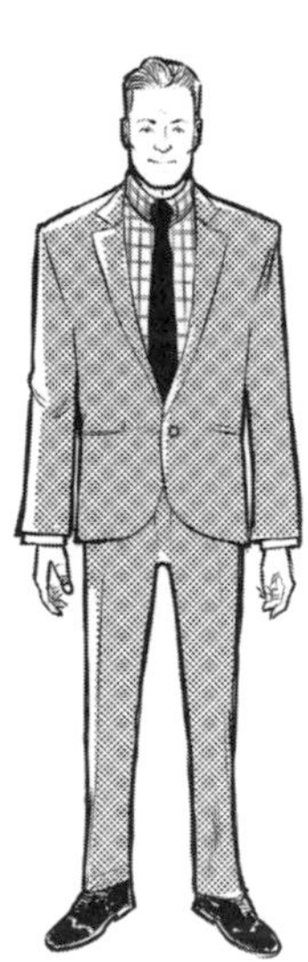

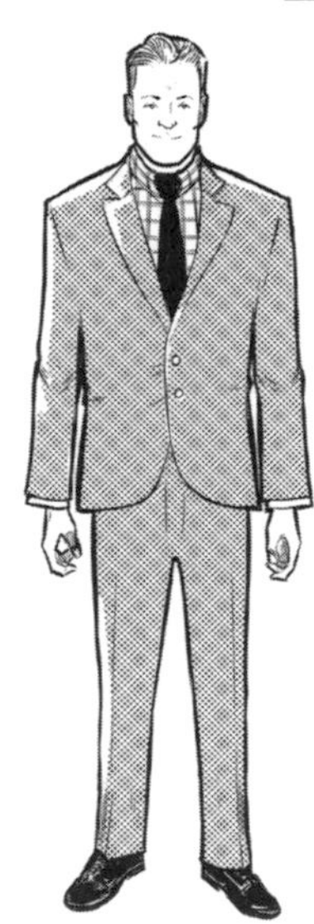

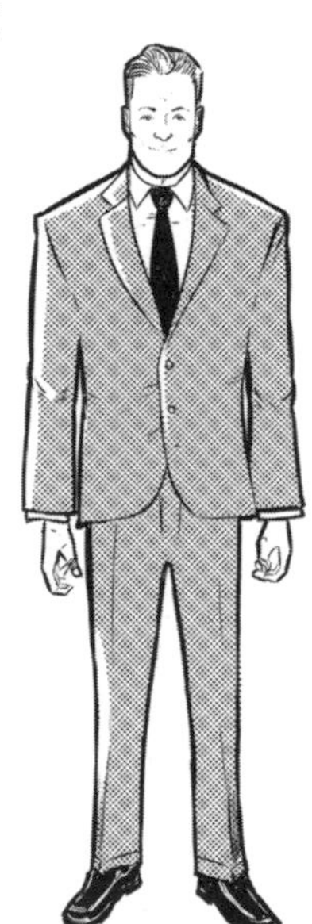

Short/One Button
A single-button suit leaves more of your shirt exposed, so you look taller.

Average/Two-Button
Truth is, nobody looks bad in a two-button suit. If you're medium height—or just content to look short or tall—make this your default.

Tall/Three-Button
Big man in a small world? This is your cut. The longer front panel leaves a shorter vertical line coming from your collar so you appear like less of a giant.

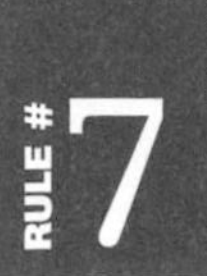

The stronger the pattern in your suit, sports jacket, or dress shirt, the weaker the pattern in your tie. And vice versa.

Get the Suit to Fit Right

1. **Strengthen the silhouette.** Have the shoulder seams set directly atop your shoulders, says Matt Harpalani of Imparali Custom Tailors in New York City.
2. **Show some hand.** The sleeves should end at the crook of your wrist. You want them short enough to leave a quarter inch of your shirt cuffs exposed.
3. **Cut it short.** Ask your tailor to take up the bottom of your jacket so it covers most of your butt.

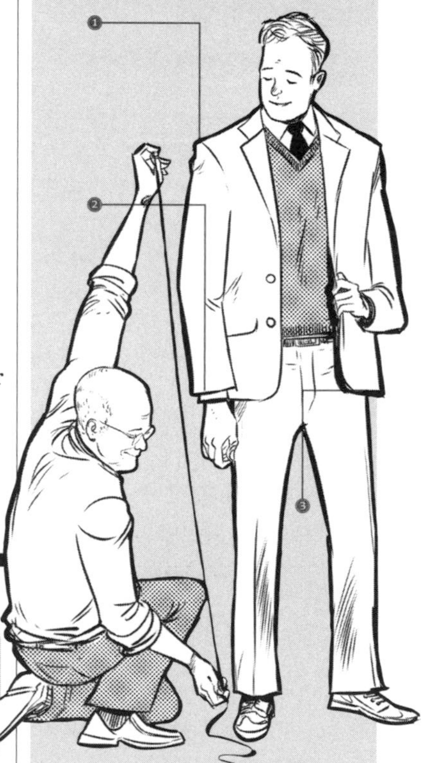

16. The Immortal Leather Bag

There's no need to schlep the kind of rock-hard briefcase your father dragged to his office. Today's cases are softer and sleeker. Look for zippers and buckles that feel sturdy. This is an investment; spend the cash now for a bag that will last the rest of your life. Canvas will cheapen the look. Smooth or pebbled leather has the opposite effect.

Q I got a tie bar. Will it work with my skinny ties?

A. The rules are simple: Your tie bar shouldn't stick out beyond the edge of the tie, says Brian Boyé, executive fashion director at *Men's Health*. You want it visible in the opening of your buttoned suit jacket, so place it between the second and third buttons of your shirt. As for tie width, remember: At its widest point, your tie should be about the same as your lapel, which is 2 ½ inches or so for the average suit.

RULE # 8

Your jacket should be neither too loose nor too tight. Your fist should fit between the top button and your body, but you can go as snug as two fingers for a modern fit.

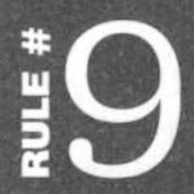

RULE # 9

Match the metal of your belt buckle to your cuff links.

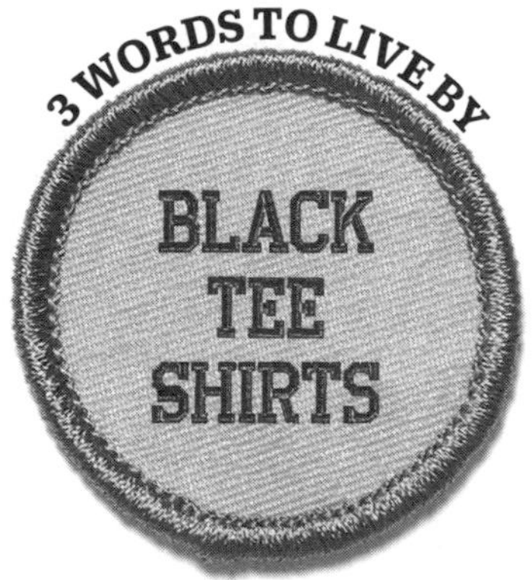
3 WORDS TO LIVE BY
BLACK TEE SHIRTS

Match a Collar to *Your Face*

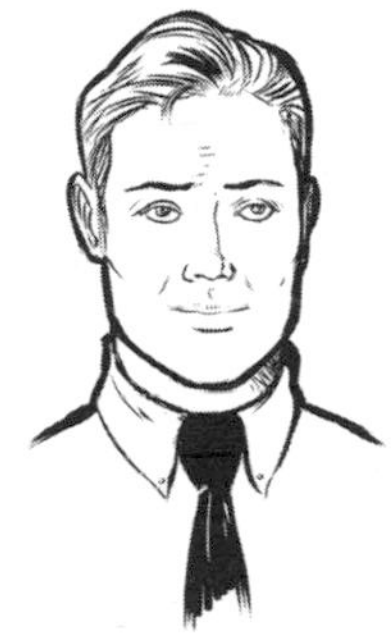

Wide Face: Narrow collars lengthen your face.

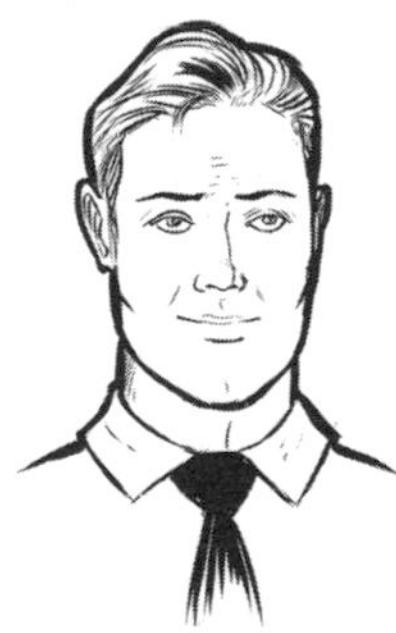

Medium Face: Go with a semi-spread collar. It's classic, and it will create the perfect cradle for a tie knot.

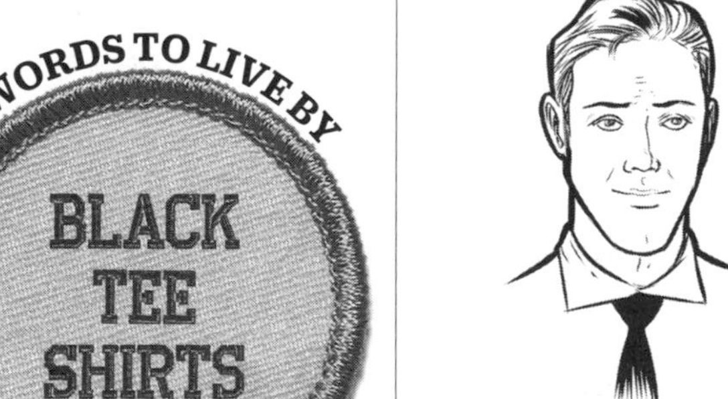

Thin Face: Have a mug like Ethan Hawke's? A spread collar can strengthen your jawline.

How to Break In a BASEBALL HAT

Transform a new cap into a well-worn lid, courtesy of Major League Baseball pitcher Paul Maholm.

Soften the brim. Most guys cup the brim with both hands and try to fold it, which results in a silly-looking pointed brim that doesn't hold. Instead, use both hands to roll the entire hat lengthwise into a burrito-like tube. After you roll it in one direction, unroll it and repeat in the other direction so that both sides of the brim receive equal treatment. Repeat two or three times until the brim becomes more flexible.

Sweat it out. Wear your hat during a workout or on a hot summer day. Baseball caps are made from cotton, so once a sweaty hat dries, it will mold to your head, creating a custom fit. Dirt scuffs and grass stains are optional.

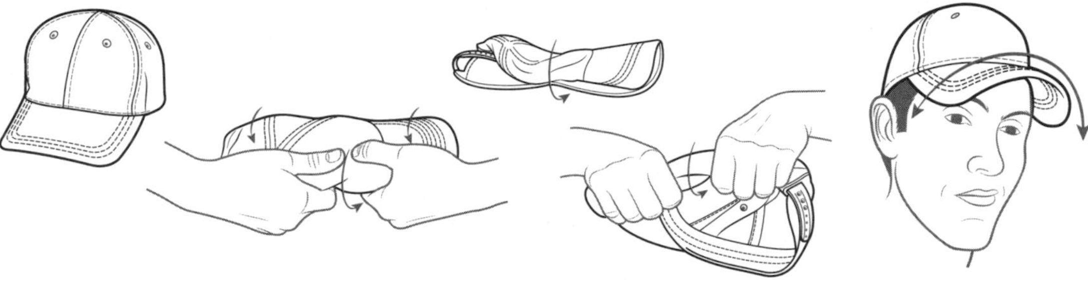

RULE # 10 **If you have on a solid suit, make sure your tie or shirt has some pattern. Wearing three solids will make you look like an undertaker or Donald Trump.**

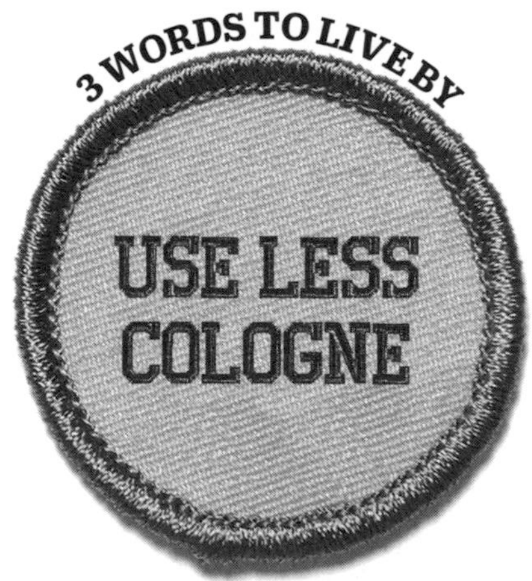
3 WORDS TO LIVE BY
USE LESS COLOGNE

Q I've seen guys look really good in a pink shirt. How can I pull that off?

A. What you're really asking is "How can I avoid hearing a coworker say, 'Check it out! Evan's wearing a pink shirt!'" Right? Start by steering clear of raspberry or bubble gum pink, says *Men's Health* fashion director Sandra Nygaard. These bright hues can make you stand out too much, and they're difficult to coordinate with other clothes. Instead, stick with the no-fail classic—a slightly muted hue, similar to a pastel, says Nygaard. If the color reminds you of a strawberry milkshake, you're on the right track. "It's subtle and goes well with all skin tones," she says. But buying the right shirt leaves you only half dressed. Give some thought to a pair of complementary pants. For a simple summer look try white, medium-wash, or light jeans. Add a chocolate-brown belt and a gold watch (or any watch with a brown or chocolate band). Then add a pair of boat shoes. Avoid loose-fitting khakis, unless you're aiming to look like a Boca Raton retiree.

RULE # 11

The tip of your tie should hit the top of your trousers. Go a little shorter for a retro look, but never go longer. EVER.

Dress like Royalty

Rich colors rule. Sapphires, emeralds, and amethysts have always been associated with royalty, from the kings of England to the shahs of Iran. But you don't need to spend a fortune to channel that power. Wearing these colors—whether in ruby cuff links or bold blue pants—says you're confident and cultured.

Your royal palette: BURGUNDY, PURPLE, GREEN, BLUE

Accessories for *A-Holes*

Accessories for men are simple. They don't scream for attention. A subtle white handkerchief in a suit pocket works well. These below, on the other hand, broadcast, "Hey, I'm an asshole."

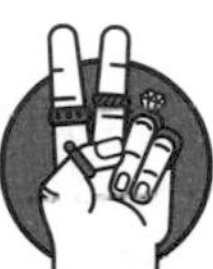

One ring is fine. But unless your name is Ozzy, keep it that way—not fussy, and never around the thumb.

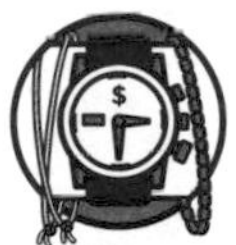

You want your watch to be the main attraction. Stick to a single bracelet, worn on the same wrist that the watch adorns—and no more.

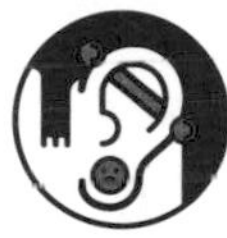

How about you stick with none? Earrings on a man are distracting, and the line between cool and corny is so fine that it's not worth the risk.

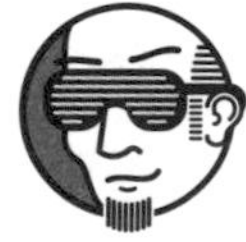

The trend toward cheap "statement" glasses works only if you're Kanye West. Resist; go with a more understated pair.

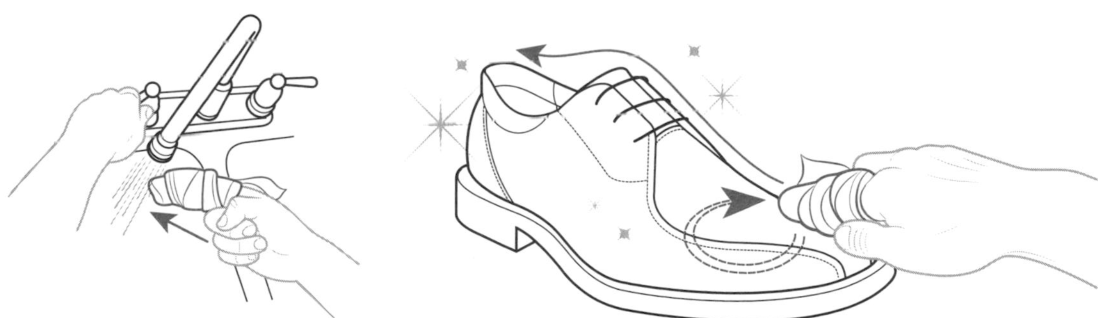

Shine Your Shoes like a Soldier

Wrap a piece of old T-shirt around your index finger and get it wet with water, which will help spread the wax. Swipe it across some polish and then rub in a circular motion, moving from toe to heel. If the polish is too thick, add more water.

Repeat the process at least twice. The first layer will look shiny, but not perfect, with some dimpling or lines on the surface. The second coat should buff these imperfections. Use less polish with each layer, continuing until the shoe shines.

Source: Jim King, national executive director of AMVETS (American Veterans)

Trim Gnarly Nose Hairs

Robert del Junco, MD, director of the St. Joseph Hospital Nasal and Sinus Center in Orange, California, helps you make the cut.

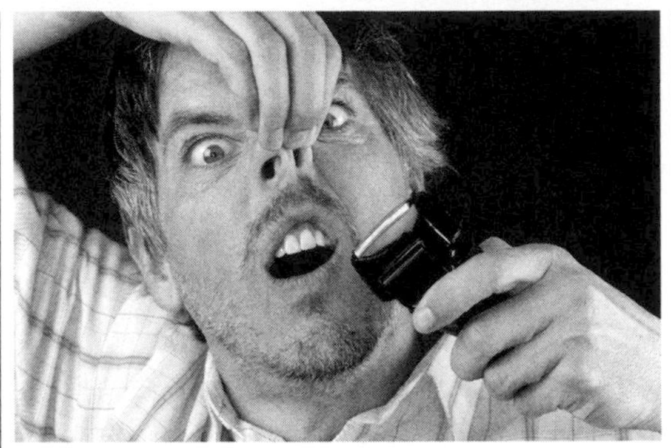

1. **Toss the Tweezers:** Don't pluck nose hairs! They block infection-causing dust and bacteria from entering your airway. That's also why you shouldn't trim them too short. Plus, a nick from scissors or a trimmer can invite microbes.
2. **Clean Your Tool:** If you're using scissors, disinfect them with alcohol, lest you transport bacteria into your nostrils. If you're using a trimmer (circular and oscillating types work well), follow the owner's manual to clean it.
3. **Don't Go Crazy:** Clip the hair no shorter than the rim of your nostril, being extra careful not to nip the inside of your nose. You'll lower your risk of a cut if you angle the trimming tool downward.

Skin Care Product: *Use Just Enough of the Stuff*

Too much is a waste of money and may do more harm than good. The coin's size indicates how much you need.

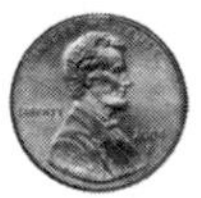

Gel: Excess hair gel can aggravate your skin, leaving you prone to acne around your hairline.

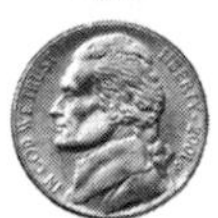

Shampoo: Too much strips your hair of natural oils. The result: flaking and itchiness.

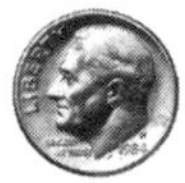

Conditioner: More than this amount plugs hair follicles, creating buildup and a flat mane.

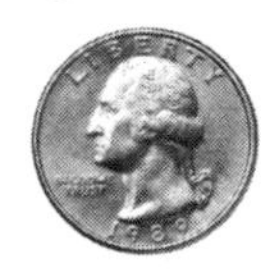

Shaving cream: Laying it on thick requires multiple razor passes, which irritates skin.

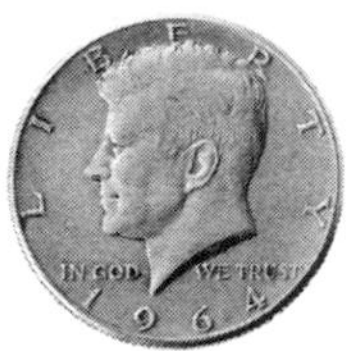

Body wash: Any more on a washcloth and you risk drying out your skin, leaving it itchy.

How to Frustrate Moths

When storing your wool sweaters for summer, have them cleaned before putting them away. And add fresh cedar blocks to your drawers, wardrobe, and even plastic storage bins to protect knitwear from moths.

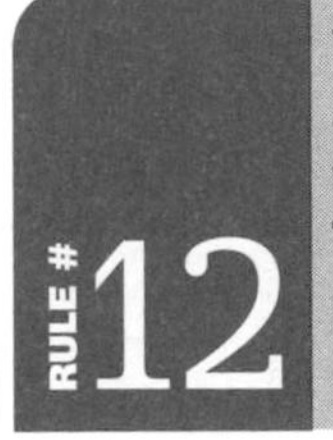

Your sweater should hug your chest. Think jacket, not bulky blanket.

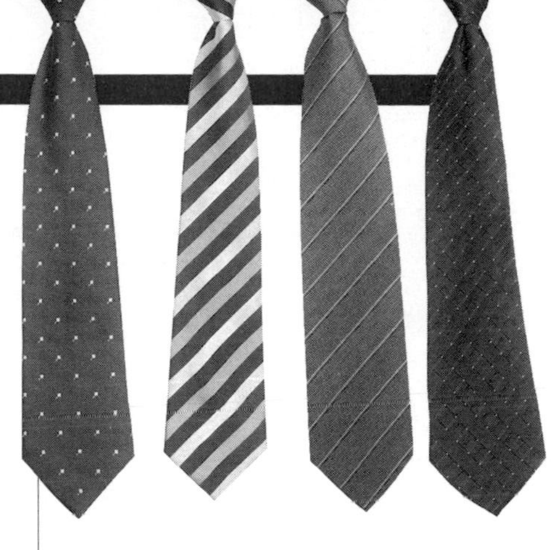

Ties, Loosen Up

As ties change, so too do the rules for matching them with shirts. Feeling confident? Then it's time you learned how to make the formal look casual.

Combine Color

In pairing colors, you can match or you can complement. If you hew to the classic, make sure your tie picks up on a dominant color from your shirt; a predominantly green shirt needs a tie that contains a similar shade. If you're a more adventurous type, seek out complementary colors. For example: Yellow works well with blue, olive looks nice on red, and charcoal adds a natural shade of contrast to tan.

The Subtle: Raw silk tweed ties make dress shirts appear less formal.

The Bold: The tie doesn't need to match the shirt, but it should complement it.

Think Texture

Tie fabrics such as nubby silk, linen, wool, and cashmere are gaining popularity and make it easy to add tactile contrast to your style. Experimenting with neckwear conveys a message to coworkers that you're creative and open to new ideas. You wouldn't break these out at a black-tie event, but they're entirely appropriate at cocktail hour or in an informal work setting.

The Subtle: Go with a tie that picks up on the dominant color in your shirt.

The Bold: Tone down a blazer with a chambray shirt and casual tie. Pair a cotton knit with a four-in-hand knot.

Own the Look

There's a right way and a wrong way to wear a tie, and the difference is in the details. Employ these three style upgrades to go from sloppy to sharply dressed.

1. Your tie should match the size of your jacket lapel in this respect. If the lapel is narrow, your tie should be narrow too. Similarly, if your lapel is wide, grab a tie with girth.
2. Feel around your neck. Your tie shouldn't be poking out from the bottom of your collar. Before you fold the collar, make sure the tie lies flat and that the top aligns with the crease.
3. If you're wearing a tie bar, place it between the second and third buttons of your shirt. It should be no longer than three-quarters of the width of the tie.

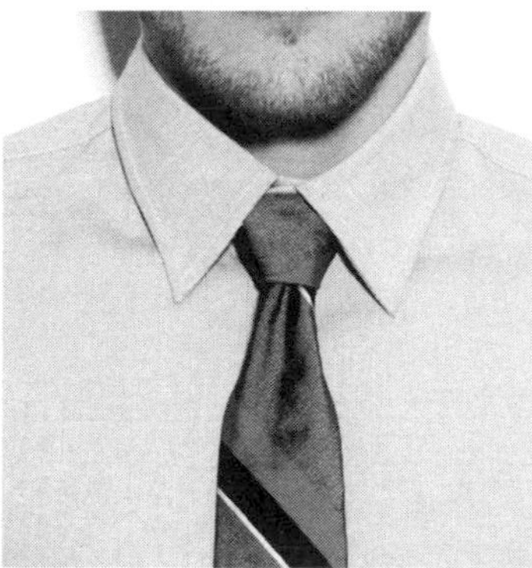

Dimple Your Tie

This one simple style move will make you a classier man, instantly.

Lay the tie flat on a table and fold it in half vertically at the point where you envision the knot and dimple. Hold the fold for about a minute until a slight crease appears. This crease will eventually help hold the dimple in place. Now tie the tie, and using your thumb, middle finger, and index finger, pinch a W right below the knot, on the fold line. Then, holding the W, tighten the tie around your neck to secure the dimple. Check yourself in a mirror. Now knock 'em dead.

Source: Simon Crompton, author and style expert (www.permanentstyle.co.uk)

Master the Half Windsor

Knotting a lightweight cotton, knit, or linen tie can be tricky. Add some heft with a half Windsor knot, suggests designer David Hart.

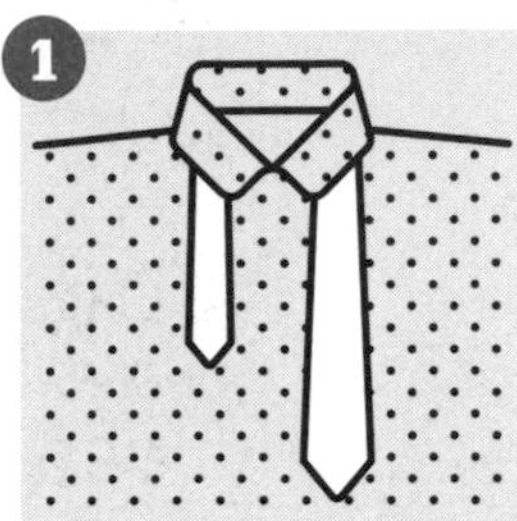

DRAPE the tie around your neck, making sure the wider end falls about 12 inches below the narrow end.

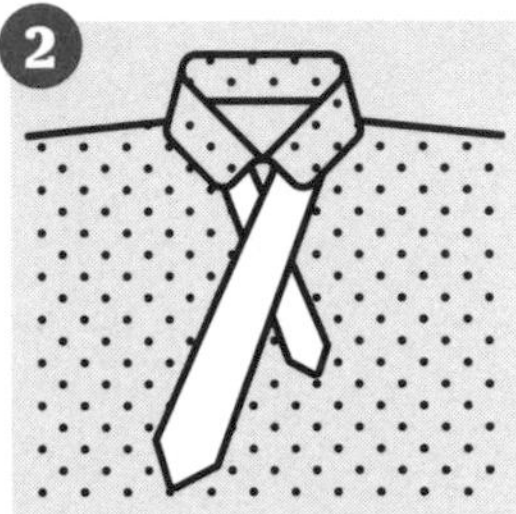

CROSS the wider end over the narrow end.

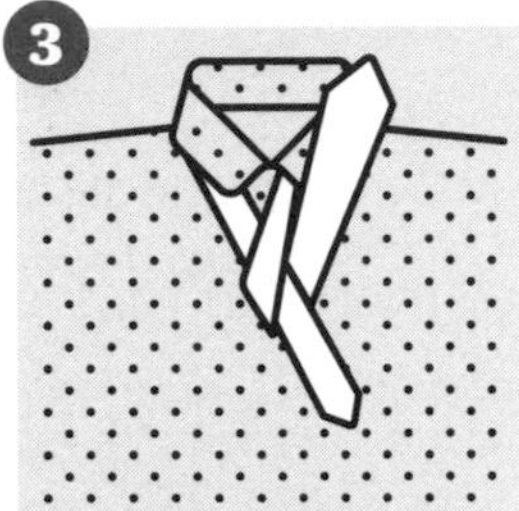

LOOP the wide end around the narrow end and lift it up.

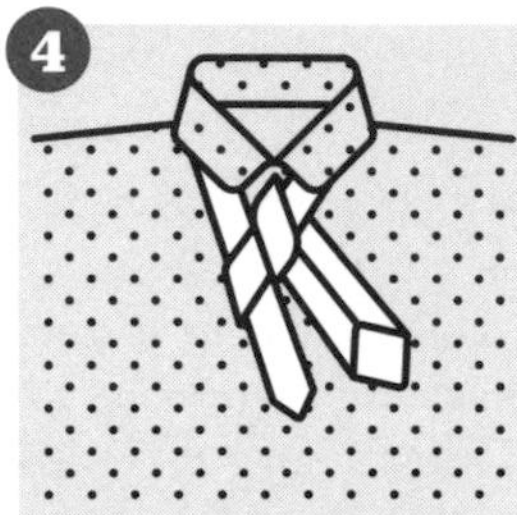

PULL the wide end through the gap between the collar and tie; move it off to the left.

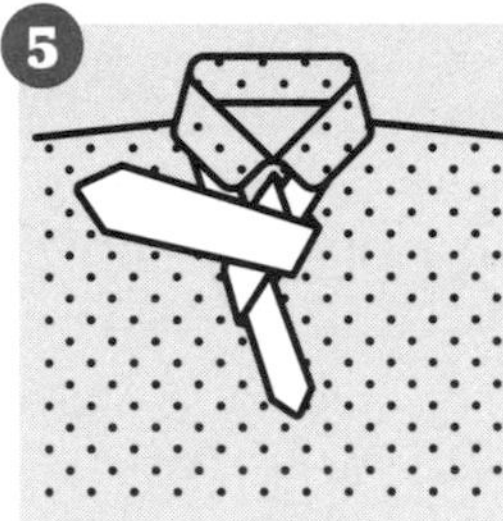

PLACE the wide end across the narrow end from left to right.

BRING it up through the gap and down through the knot in front.

WITH BOTH HANDS, tighten and adjust the knot.

Make a Statement with Eyeglasses

Eyeglasses are a huge part of your personality and style, so frame your face right. Look for glasses that match your skin tone and flatter the shape of your face. If you have light hair and a square face, blond, slightly rounded tortoiseshell frames will work well. Don't be afraid to be bold. Glasses chosen wisely will add a bit of edge to your appearance, making your look smarter, fresher, and more modern.

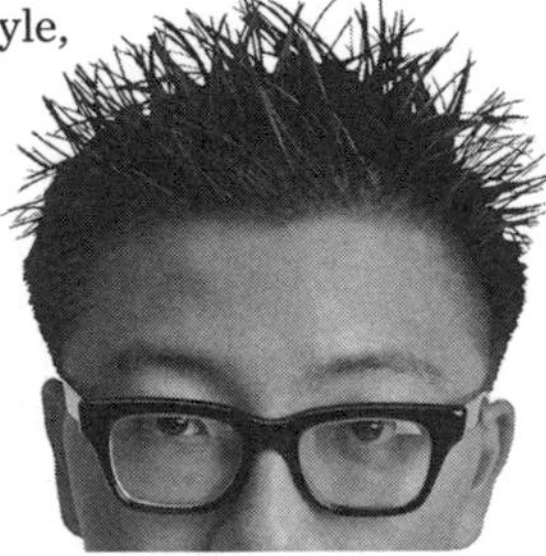

RULE # 13

Avoid nose fatigue. When applying fragrance, spritz your favorite scent on your pulse points (like your wrists and the base of your neck) and wait 10 to 12 hours before reapplying. Accidental overdose? Use a wet wipe (or a cotton ball dipped in alcohol) on the spot to lift off some of the scent. That should take the strength of the fragrance down a notch or two.

LOOK OFFICE SHARP

Today's office allows for personality and inspiration. Use these suggestions to build a wardrobe that can go anywhere—and take you places.

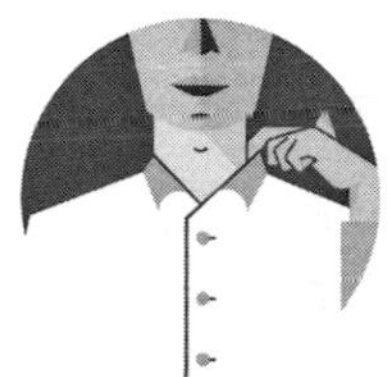

THE SHIRT

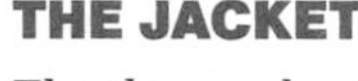

Buttoned up? One finger should fit between your neck and the shirt.

THE JACKET

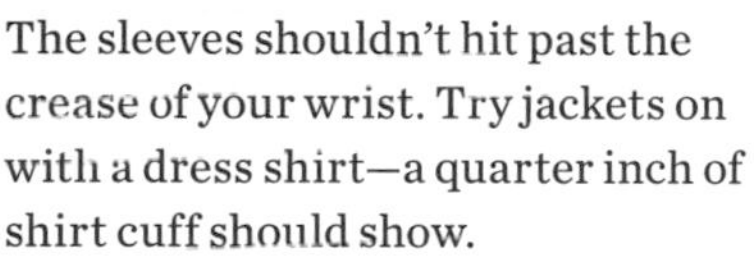

The sleeves shouldn't hit past the crease of your wrist. Try jackets on with a dress shirt—a quarter inch of shirt cuff should show.

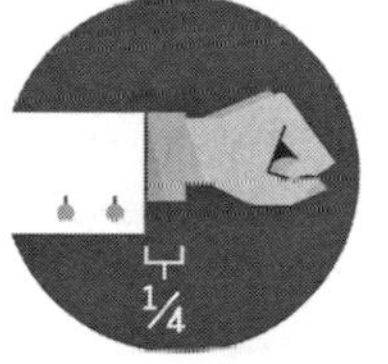

THE PANTS

Ask your tailor for half a break at the shoe. That'll keep the fit slim and straight, which makes your legs look longer.

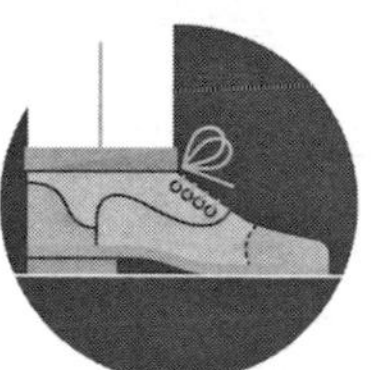

THE TIE

As a rule of thumb, our experts recommend a width of 2 to 3 inches, but this rule isn't universal. Size your ties to be proportionate to lapels.

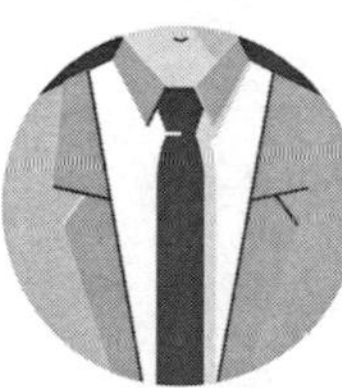

THE SHOES

No squares, and nothing too round—overstated trends will come and go. Invest in a pair with a slim toe. The skinnier the suit, the slimmer your shoe's point.

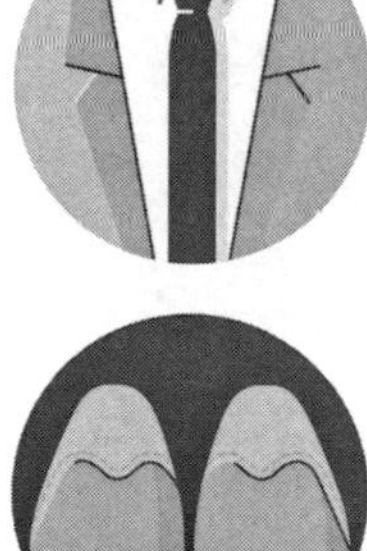

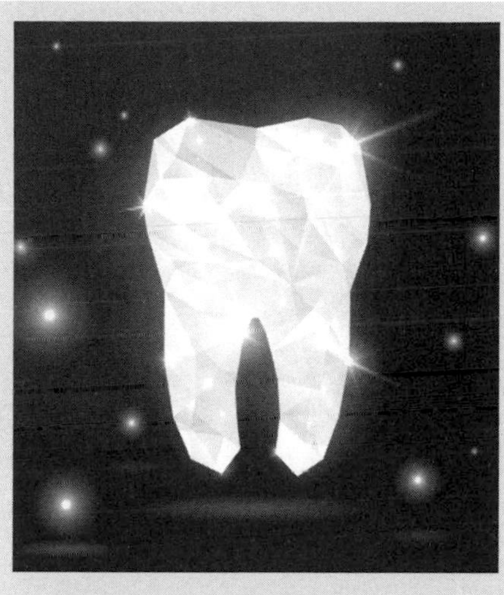

Whiten Up

Having a whiter smile is engaging and inviting. But popcorn kernels and spinach stuck up in even the whitest of grills won't melt her heart. Brush and floss and make sure your toothbrush is fresh. After the bristles are worn down, it doesn't clean teeth properly. To whiten teeth, choose gel trays instead of strips because strips don't distribute the whitening paste evenly. Teeth are usually darkest near the gumline, where strips can't reach. In a pinch, rinse with apple cider vinegar. Swishing around two parts water to one part apple cider vinegar is a natural and organic way to maintain a healthy smile.

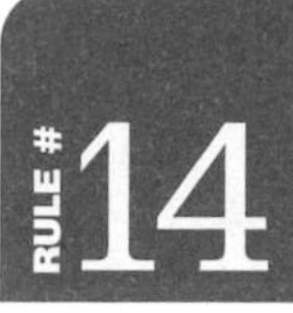

RULE # 14

Shirt and tie patterns should differ in scale. A shirt with large checks looks best with a tie that has either smaller checks or thin stripes. The reason? Patterns of similar size will compete with each other. Giving each one its own platform tells people you're different . . . but that you still know how to dress.

Fold the Perfect Pocket Square

There are dozens of ways to fold a pocket square, and most of them are, well, square. Don't bother trying to master them all. These three techniques are the only ones you need to know.

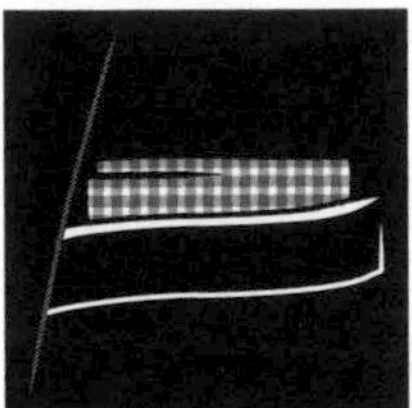

The Straight Fold

Lay the pocket square flat. Bring the left side to the right side. Fold the bottom toward the top, but stop short of lining the ends up flush. Fold the fabric in thirds horizontally so it fits your suit pocket.

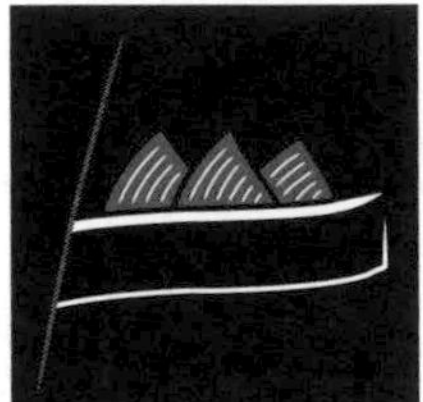

The Three Point

Fold a silk square as if you're making a triangle, but don't fold it exactly in half. Instead make two side-by-side peaks. Now bring the left side of the folded edge up and to the right of the peak, to make a third peak. Then bring the right side of the folded edge across to the left.

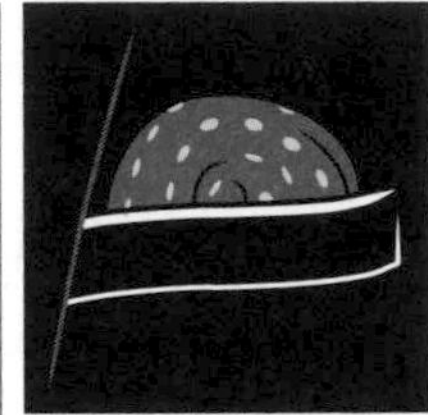

The Puff

Lay the pocket square flat. With one hand, pinch the square's center; pick it up. With your other hand, fold the fabric in half, bringing the hem to the center. Place it in your pocket with the fold exposed. Adjust it to desired puffiness.

How to Break In a Pair of Jeans

You can achieve that well-worn comfort that normally takes months to achieve in just a day.

Start Here:

Avoid loose-fitting denim. Tight jeans will break in faster because of the constant friction with your skin when you move. In fact, the more frequently you wear them, the better.

Do This Next:

Fill a couple of nylon stockings with 10 ounces each of fresh coffee grounds, and then set them aside in a 5-gallon pail until later, when you change out of those jeans.

Finish It Off:

Pour hot water over the stockings until the pail is about ¾ full. Add your jeans; let them brew for 15 to 20 minutes. Rinse in lukewarm water.

Source: Eric Schmidt, director of operations, Denim Therapy

Look Younger Instantly

Mess up your hair.

Rub a dab of styling cream between your hands and apply it from the crown out for a youthful, unstudied vibe. Thinning hair? Try clipping it close or shaving it all off—that'll keep people guessing your DOB.

How to Look Good in a Suit

An ill-fitting suit can make you look like the uncle who's been wearing the same one to family funerals since 1986. Nail these six style points and you'll look tailor-made.

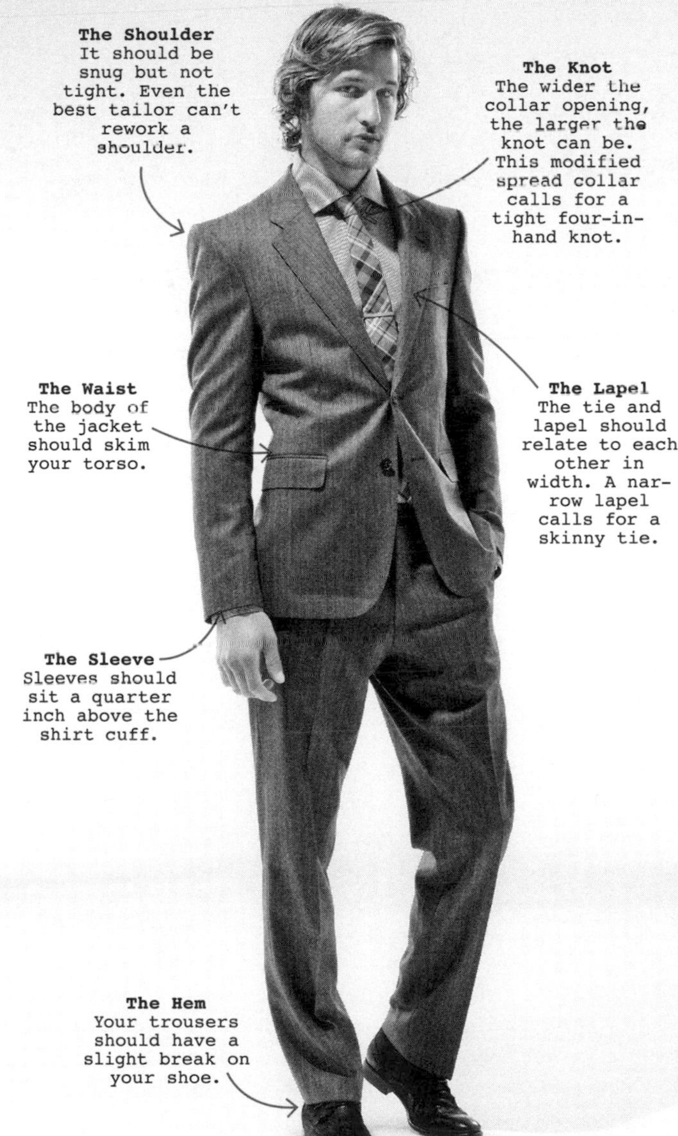
The Shoulder
It should be snug but not tight. Even the best tailor can't rework a shoulder.
The Knot
The wider the collar opening, the larger the knot can be. This modified spread collar calls for a tight four-in-hand knot.
The Waist
The body of the jacket should skim your torso.
The Lapel
The tie and lapel should relate to each other in width. A narrow lapel calls for a skinny tie.
The Sleeve
Sleeves should sit a quarter inch above the shirt cuff.
The Hem
Your trousers should have a slight break on your shoe.

RULE # 15

The bottom button of your suit jacket or sport coat always stays undone. PERIOD.

Q How can I get rid of the dark circles under my eyes?

A. Keep your paws off your peepers. Every time you rub the skin under your eyes, you open up little packets of soft pigment that are deposited into your skin to give it a darker appearance, says Bruce Robinson, MD, professor of dermatology at Mt. Sinai Medical Center. Here's what to do to look bright-eyed:

In the morning: A facial moisturizer with sunscreen can protect the delicate skin under your eyes.

In the evening: Lay off the tequila shots. Excess alcohol and salt can make your cells retain extra water, leading to the a.m. puffiness that makes dark circles look even more pronounced.

At bedtime: Use a cream with vitamin C or caffeine.

A Man's Guide *to Footwear*

A good pair of shoes is an investment you'll own for years. And these days almost every style is available at multiple price points. Stock your closet with these styles and no matter what you can afford, you'll walk away in shoes that fit your fashion sense and financial comfort zone.

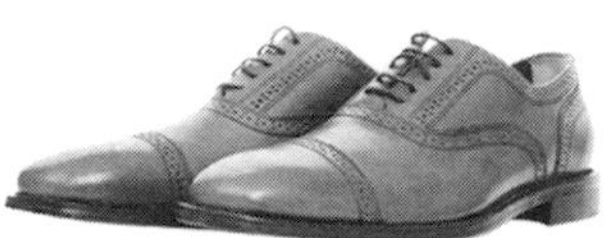

1 The Dark Brown Oxford

Nothing ruins a look like a pair of clunky, square-toed shoes. They look dated even if you just bought them, and your whole outfit falls flat. The fix? A pair of dark brown leather oxfords with a round toe. They're modern and sophisticated, and go with nearly everything.

Works best with: Business or casual dress. Think navy, gray, and charcoal suits; tweed jackets; work-appropriate jeans; corduroys; khakis; and gray flannel.

Keep them new: Have shoes resoled when your heel is wearing thin—and don't let it wear down to the leather, because you'll end up paying more.

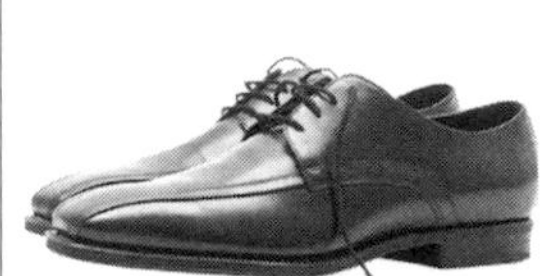

2 The Slim Black Oxford

Don't bother with black patent leather shoes you'll only wear a few times in your life, unless you're a red carpet regular or constantly getting married. Instead, opt for a pair of narrow black leather shoes—they're just as polished and elegant but also look good with your work clothes. Two birds, one shoe.

Works best with: Tuxedos, dark jeans, and navy, gray, and black suits.

Keep them new: Use cedar shoe trees (when you're not wearing them, silly). And remember: No one has ever regretted having leather shoes polished.

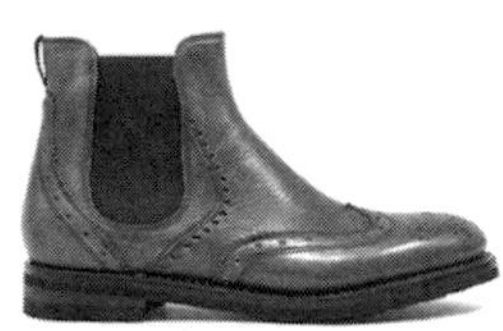

3 The Chelsea Boot

When it's so cold you can feel the wind through your laces, it's time to switch to Chelsea boots. Since they're laceless, they keep your feet and ankles warm, but unlike most boots, they're dressed up enough for the office.

Works best with: Jeans and cords. Or dress them up with dark jeans, a button-down or sweater, and a tweed jacket.

Keep them new: If there's snow on the ground, there's probably salt too, which ruins leather. Remove stains with a 50/50 mixture of white distilled vinegar and water, and wipe dry. Use a water and stain protective spray.

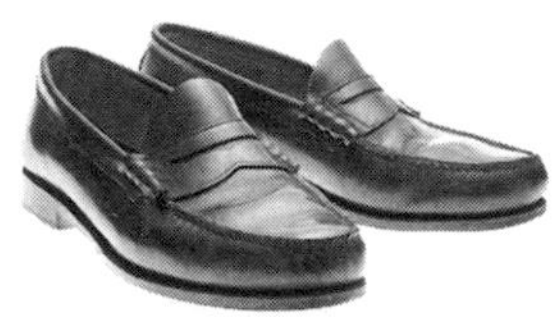

4 The Loafer

The two biggest complaints about loafers: 1) "They're too preppy"; and 2) "They remind me of Ronald Reagan." Fair enough, but if you look into the actual history of loafers, you'll realize that long before Northeastern prep schoolers got their feet on them, they were simply the best shoe for loafing around. They should be comfortable.

Works best with: Jeans and khakis; shorts in the summer, but no socks.

Tip: If you're not sold on loafers but like the idea of owning a pair of slip-ons, try a pair of boat shoes or driving moccasins, which are equally comfortable but even more casual.

RULE # 16

Buy cedar shoe trees for all your good shoes. Slipping in shoe trees every night will add years to your shoes, and this simple act of stewardship will reverberate through your life, making you more disciplined everywhere you go.

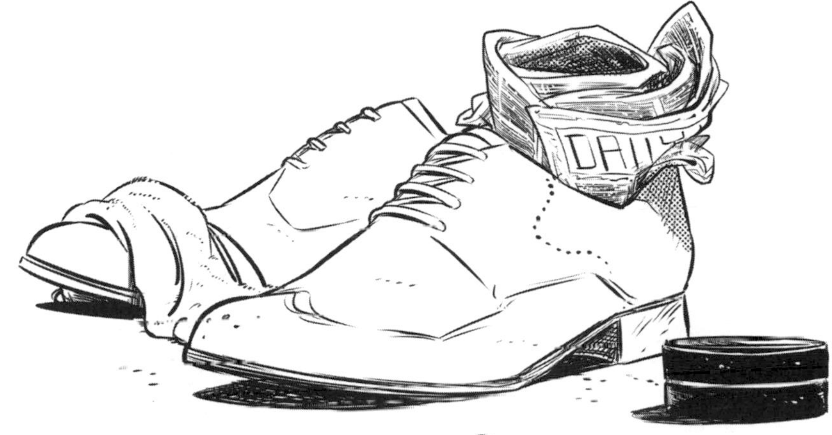

How to Resuscitate Drowned Shoes

1. **Dry.** First, wipe them off with a clean cloth. Water can ruin the leather.
2. **Stuff.** Put crumpled newspaper in them to absorb the moisture. Replace the paper when saturated. Repeat until nearly dry; insert cedar shoe trees.
3. **Condition.** Rub them down with a good leather conditioner.

Remove Stains on a White Shirt

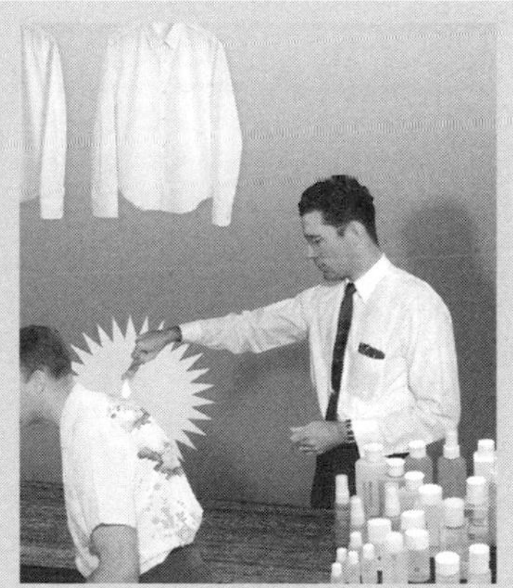

Greasy stuff (cooking oil, salad dressing, mayo, etc.): Pretreat the item with a stain remover, such as Spray 'n Wash or Shout; these use solvents to dig out big stains. Wash it in hot water, but make sure the spot is gone before drying—heat will make a temporary spot permanent.

Dye jobs (mustard, ink, grass): Pour a detergent that contains bleach on the stain and leave it for 5 minutes. Then rinse well. If that doesn't work, soak it in a bleach solution (2 ounces per gallon of water). If the stain's still there after a 15-minute soak, it's not going anywhere.

Tannin stains (wine, coffee, tea): Wash the item in a hot-water cycle with detergent. No need for pretreatment—these stains won't set unless they've been subjected to intense heat. Avoid soap, which may react with some soils to form larger compounds or bigger stains.

Saucy stains (barbecue, ketchup): Combination stains like these have grease and dyes. First, blot off excess sauce (don't rub!), using a white paper towel to avoid color bleeding. Tackle the oil with a stain-removal stick or spray, or detergent, and wash the item in hot water.

Q My girlfriend has one of those sonic face scrubbers. Should I use it?

A. On your golf balls? No. On your face? Go for it. Sonic scrubbers contain microbristles that pulsate hundreds of times a second to clean your pores, says Adnan Nasir, MD, PhD, the *Men's Health* dermatology advisor and an adjunct assistant professor of dermatology at the University of North Carolina at Chapel Hill. "They're especially great for men with oily, flaky, or clogged skin because they clean deeper than your fingers or a washcloth can, and they easily remove acne-causing grime from your skin." He likes the Clarisonic Plus ($225, clarisonic.com) because it has three speeds; that way you can vary the intensity of your scrub. Use it with a mild face wash, such as Cetaphil Gentle Skin Cleanser ($7, drugstore.com). Just two caveats: Men with sensitive skin or eczema should skip the scrubber, says Dr. Nasir, and if you share a device with your girlfriend, make sure you buy a separate brush head so you don't gunk up hers.

Banish BO

If you stink like your ninth-grade gym locker, try an antibacterial soap—body odor can be a product of bacterial growth on the skin. And skip the Indian buffet at lunch—odors from onions, garlic, curry, and spicy foods are excreted in sweat glands. Finally, do the laundry. Bacteria from sweat can cling to fabrics; the heat from your body acts like a plug-in scented warmer, but in this case it activates offending odors.

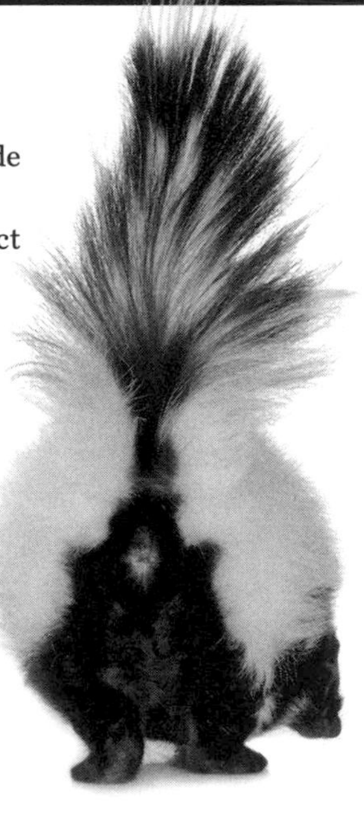

Disguise Your Gut

Those last 10 pounds have a preferred spot to settle: the area formerly known as your abs. Until you bust the bulge, memorize these sneaky style slimmers.

Embrace geometry. Look for shapes that create the illusion of an inverted triangle—broad shoulders, narrow waist. Structured blazers and shawl-collar cardigans keep balance by adding a bit of bulk to your neck and shoulders.

Ask for a regular. Rather than a relaxed or slim fit—neither of which will flatter your abdominal acreage—opt for a "regular fit" dress shirt. This style won't hug your belly or bury it in excessive fabric. Instead, it will fit uniformly, with a little room to move.

Skip the zips. Avoid wearing zip-front sweaters and cinched-waist jackets, which just draw the eye to your problem area. Buttons are much more forgiving.

Ease your belt a notch. A belt that's too tight cuts you off in an unflattering way. Buy a belt two sizes larger than your pants so you'll have more strap to tuck in a loop.

Never cinch. A cinched waist creates the illusion of bulk even when there isn't any. When you wear a sweater, opt for one without an elastic waistband and you'll still look sleek.

RULE # 17

Never wear loafers with a suit. Save them for khakis or jeans, and maybe a sports coat. A suit needs shoes with laces or buckles.

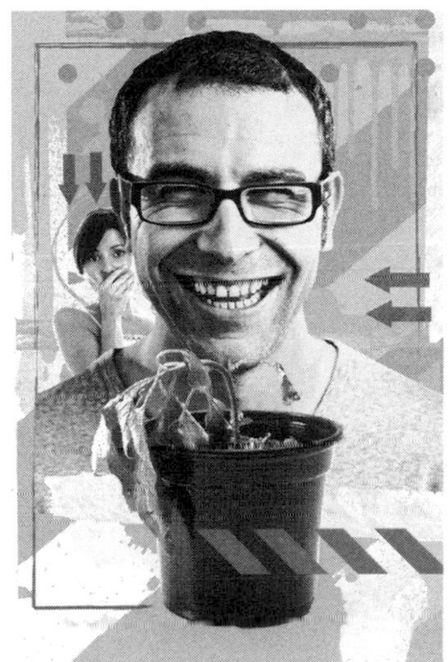

Check Your Breath

If it can peel paint, skip the mints—they only mask the stink. Use a tongue scraper to remove back-of-the-mouth bugs. How to check:

Step 1

Wash your hands with an odorless soap to remove other scents.

Step 2

Lick the back of your hand and let it dry for 5 seconds—enough time for the saliva to evaporate.

Step 3

Bad-breath bacteria's sulfur compounds will remain. Take a whiff.

Source: Harold Katz, DDS, founder of the California Breath Clinic

Clothes Remake the Man

IF YOU WEREN'T BORN WITH A MANNEQUIN'S BODY, FAKE IT!

There's no way you can add 3 inches to your height, lose 10 pounds in 10 minutes, or broaden your shoulders instantly—but you can create the illusion of having these physical upgrades and more.

Add inches. The idea: You want to create the appearance of a straight line from shoulder to toe. An easy option is a monochromatic outfit, but when you feel like branching out, try vertical stripes. They'll do more to elongate your frame than other patterns will.

Make feet sleek. "Somewhat" counterintuitively, chunky or square-toed shoes can exaggerate length. Avoid shoes with a bulbous toe; they create a clown shoe effect. Instead, stay sleek and serious with an almond-shaped toe.

Broaden narrow shoulders. If you're about 100,000 shoulder presses away from your goal, cheat the "V" look with jackets that have structured shoulders. The padding creates a sharper and stronger profile. And while a structured suit jacket creates the illusion of larger shoulders, a sweater should fit you snugly to accentuate the shoulders you already have. Contrasting body and arm colors can also add dimension.

Lengthen your legs. Maintain little or no break in your trousers to help balance your proportions. The excess fabric gathered at your ankles will only make you look like a guy who inherited his dad's pants. Try matching socks to the color of your pants to elongate even further.

Brighten pasty skin. Remember this in fall and winter: Earth tones, browns, and olive greens look soft against pale skin. Reds, oranges, and pinks bring out rosiness in your skin.

Shape the rear view. Don't hide your flat butt in relaxed-fit jeans. Choose a slimmer or tapered style that hugs your backside. Flap pockets can enhance a pancake posterior; you'll be glad they're there when you catch her checking you out from behind.

RULE #18

Change your pillowcase once a week so your freshly washed face is not resting on a buildup of your hair's oil. Use a disinfecting wipe on all your phones to reduce breakouts by your ear and jawline.

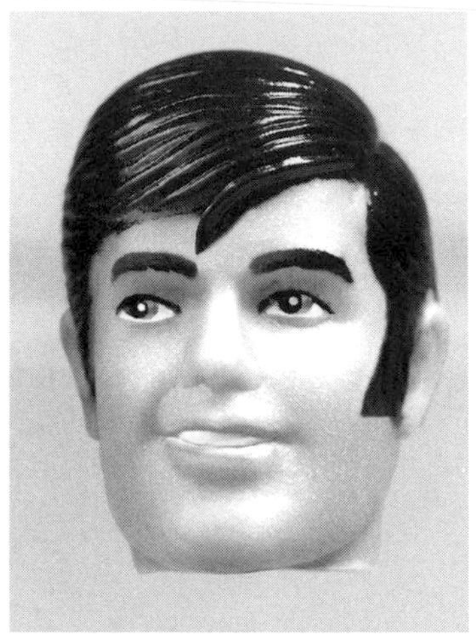

Sideburns 101

Check length. Let your face shape be your guide. If your face is round or your chin isn't very pronounced, keep 'burns at mid-ear or shorter. If you have an oblong or rectangular face, keep them a little longer—mid-ear to earlobe length.

Keep 'em narrow. Don't let them grow wider than about an inch or you'll need a sequined jumpsuit to match. Keeping them that way is easy: Buy a comb as wide as your 'burns, hold it up against them, and follow its smooth edge with a trimmer.

Avoid fluff. Watch the edges and puffiness of your sideburns. If you have shaggy hair, keep your sideburn hair short, around an eighth of an inch. Bushy 'burns push long hair away from your face, creating a mushroom effect.

Q My deodorant isn't doing a good job of controlling my BO. What should I try?

A. Hit your pits with an aluminum-fortified antiperspirant. It will block sweat, starving stench-building bacteria, says Carolyn Jacob, MD, medical director of Chicago Cosmetic Surgery and Dermatology. If your skin is sensitive, try a soothing stick, like Dove Men+Care Clinical Protection antiperspirant ($8, walgreens.com). For a clear shield when you're shirtless, go with a water-based gel, like Gillette Clinical Clear Gel antiperspirant/deodorant ($8, target.com). Still sweaty? Certain Dri Clinical Strength antiperspirant roll-on ($7, cvs.com) has the strongest sweat blocker in the highest amount available over the counter.

RULE # 19

Your socks should always match the color of your pants, not your shoes. Subtle patterns—not the Utah Jazz logo—are okay for most situations (except black tie). The pattern should pick up another color you're wearing.

How to Outgrow a Bad Haircut

Escape humiliation and grow to great lengths just by mastering the art of these grooming techniques.

Timing: Start growing out your hair in early winter, when cooler weather prevents a sweaty head. Hair grows about half an inch a month, so you'll have your new look by spring.

Trimming: If you usually go for a full-on haircut every 4 weeks, push it to every 6. But drop by the barbershop once between cuts to clean up your neck and sideburns.

Texture: Ask your barber to remove some bulk (not length) with special texturizing scissors or a razor. This allows different styling options and prevents poufing.

Touch: Keep your hair soft and pliable—and more touchable for her—by using less styling product than you would on shorter hair. And buy a hairbrush.

How to Go Long on Top

Consider your noggin shape when choosing a hair length.

SQUARE:
Length adds softness to a strong, square jawline. Stay away from a straight style or a one-length cut, either of which can overemphasize your jaw.

ROUND:
You want to add length and reduce width—your face is round enough already. Keep your hair shorter on the sides than on top. If you go especially long, keep it as straight as possible so it won't add bulk to your cheeks.

OVAL:
You're in luck. Any length can flatter this universal face shape, which is wide near the temples and narrow toward the chin. Experiment to find the style you like best.

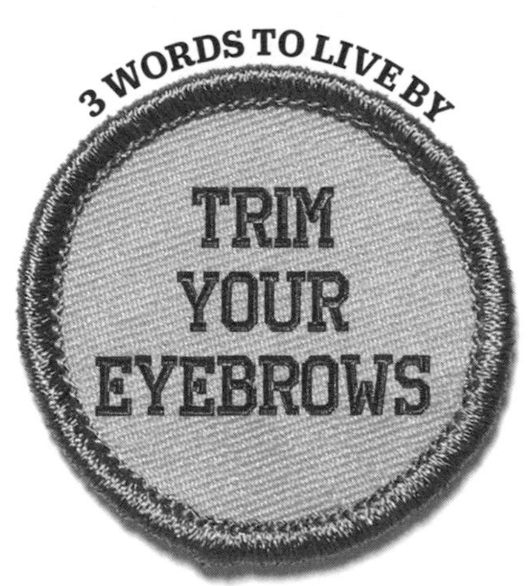
3 WORDS TO LIVE BY
TRIM
YOUR
EYEBROWS

The Four Secrets to Cleaning Up Good

More than half of women cop to judging your teeth, hair, and nails when sizing you up, a Match.com survey reveals. Here's how to ensure she likes what she sees.

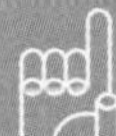

Maintain Your Mitts

First, clip each nail following its natural curve, says Angel Williams, a New York City manicurist. With a hangnail clipper, remove torn skin at the base, and then even out the edges and push back your cuticles after coating them with preshave oil. Then use a buffer to banish ugly cracks and bumps.

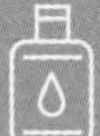

Take a Hair Holiday

Product buildup mats your mane, leaving it greasy. Skip gels and creams for a few days, and vary your shampoo routine. "Rinse vigorously daily; use a cleansing conditioner every two days and regular shampoo weekly," suggests Paul Boucher, a stylist at Floyd's 99 Barbershop in Dallas, Texas.

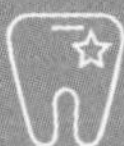

Polish Your Ivories

When considering a date, 71 percent of women scrutinize your grill, the Match.com survey found. Try this DIY whitener from Chicago dentist Jessica Emery, DMD. Make a paste of baking soda (1 tablespoon) and hydrogen peroxide (5 drops). Apply it to your front teeth, wait 15 minutes, and brush.

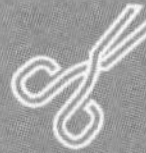

Tend to Your Brows

Work with their natural shape, says celebrity makeup artist Fabioloa Arancibia. "Brush the hairs upward and trim long pieces," she says, "but don't go crazy or it'll look spotty." We like Tweezerman's facial hair scissors; rounded tips make the job easier. *$17, tweezerman.com*

The Four Smartest Ways to Achieve a *Perfect Fit*

Even an affordable suit can look custom with just a little extra effort. Buy it a size too big and have it tailored to your body, says designer Stanley Hudson, a former *Project Runway* contestant. Zero in on these telltale details.

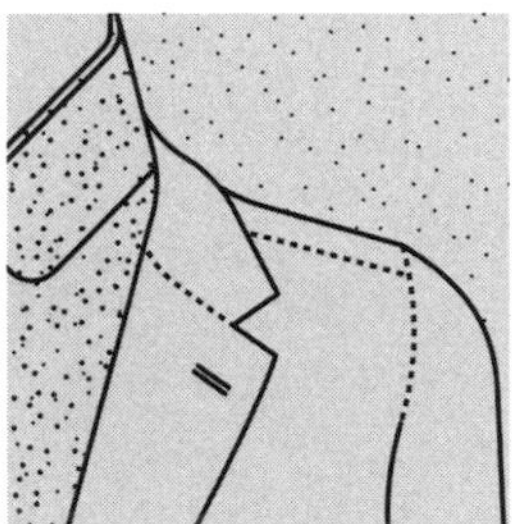

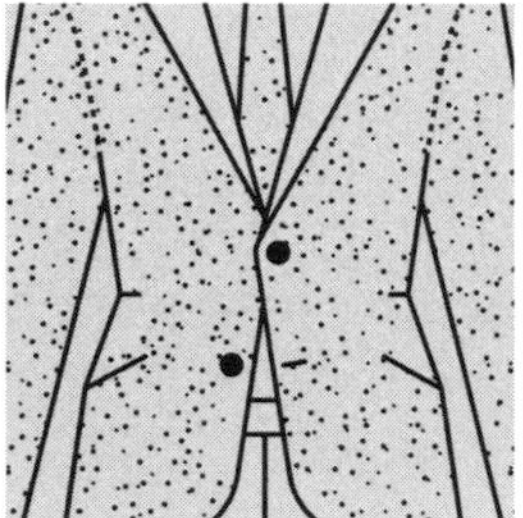

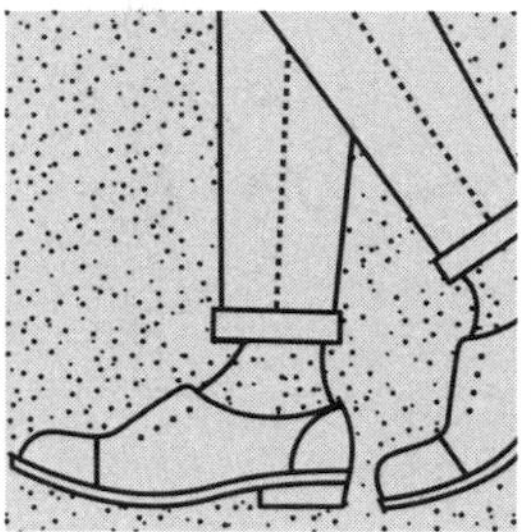

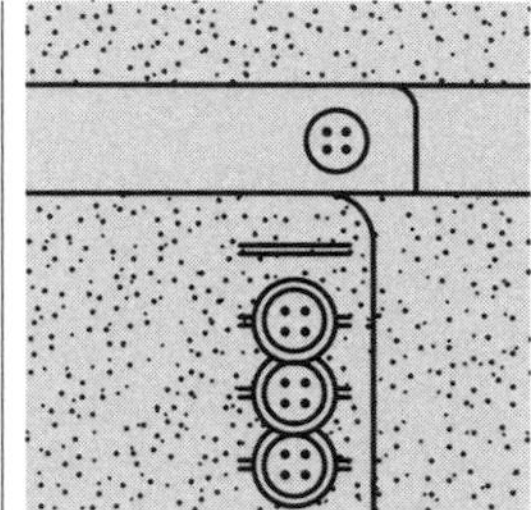

Shoulder the Burden

No matter what the jacket costs, the shoulder seams should sit directly above the edge of your shoulders, says Hudson. "Get it right while you're at the store. They're impossible to alter."

Frame Yourself

The jacket should skim your frame and be neither too loose nor too tight. Your fist should fit between the top button and your body, but you can go as snug as two fingers for a modern fit.

Slim Down

Your trousers should taper to 7 to 7½ inches seam-to-seam, Hudson says. A stockier guy can go an inch or two wider, and only really skinny guys will want an extremely slim fit.

Button It Up

Pricey suits often have functional buttons on the sleeves. "It's worth converting yours if you wear French-cuff shirts," Hudson says. Leave one or two undone and let the boss notice.

When to Change Your Razor Blade

Gillette says every five to seven uses—but the company has to sell a lot of razors to pay for the Pats' stadium. You can save some dough and extend that to 2 to 4 weeks if you soften your facial hair with hot water and lather.

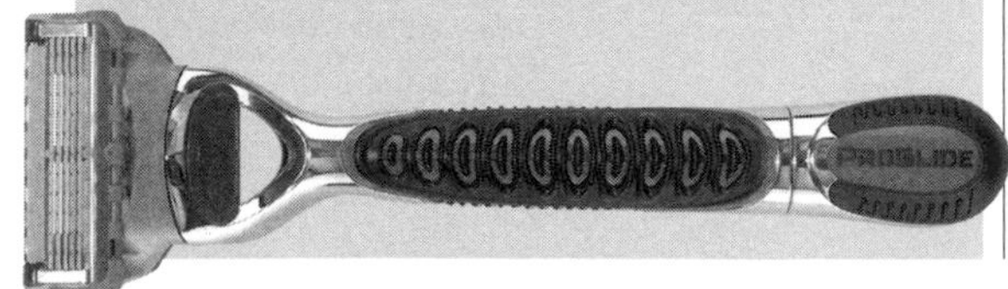

Keep Your Skin from Cracking

Women hate dry, cracked hands—on their men, too. Soften them up and you'll look instantly younger. Our skin is naturally acid to protect against bacteria, says Adnan Nasir, MD, PhD, adjunct assistant professor of dermatology at UNC Chapel Hill. Many soaps are alkaline, though, so they strip away protective oils. So look for a soap that's pH balanced or one that lists lactic acid or glycolic acid among the first half of its ingredients.

Age-Proof Your Eyes

Wrinkled, baggy, or dark skin around your eyes can make you look years older than you are. So save them now. We asked dermatologists Joel Schlessinger, MD, and Ariel Ostad, MD, for DIY solutions. Here's their advice:

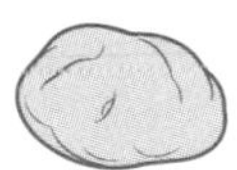

Peel a Potato

Why: Potato starch has anti-inflammatory properties, so it's good for soothing redness and irritation.

Do this: Peel and grate a raw potato, and then mash it and wrap it in a clean dishcloth. Lie down and place the pouch on your eyes for 15 minutes.

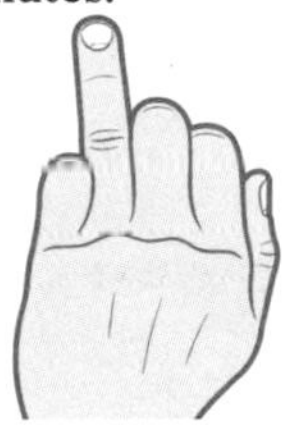

Use Your Ring Finger

Why: It's weaker than your pointer finger. Touching your eyes with your stronger finger tends to stretch the skin.

Do this: To stop an itch or apply cream, lightly tap your eye area with your ring finger.

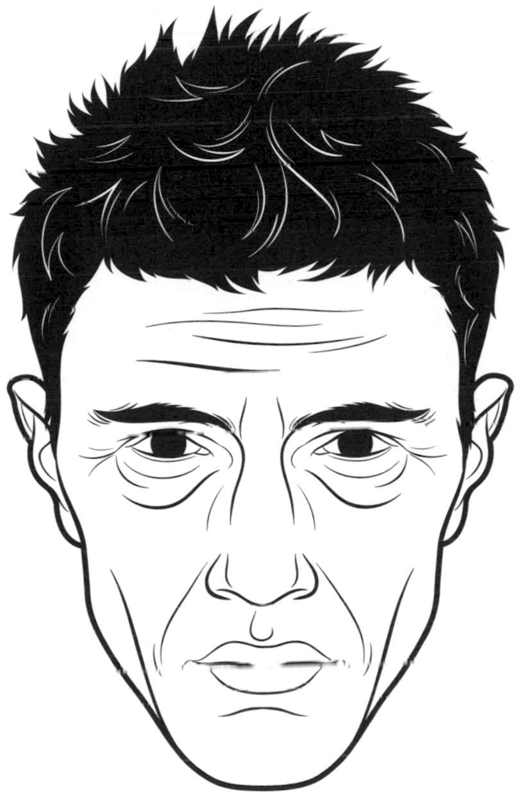

Eat Healthy Meals

Why: The more salt and booze you consume, the more fluids you retain, puffing your eyes.

Do this: Cut back on both—and sugar, too. A high-sugar diet can generate harmful molecules that damage collagen, leading to wrinkles.

Sleep on Your Back

Why: If you're on your side or stomach, the pressure of your head against the pillow for hours can cause permanent creases around your eyes.

Do this: Try sleeping faceup and add an extra pillow to prevent fluid from pooling in your face.

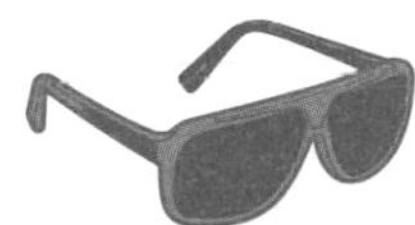

Don't Squint

Why: The skin around your eyes is up to one-thirtieth the thickness of the skin on your palms. Habitual squinting can forge deep crevices.

Do this: Wear shades outdoors. If you wear regular glasses, keep your prescription up to date.

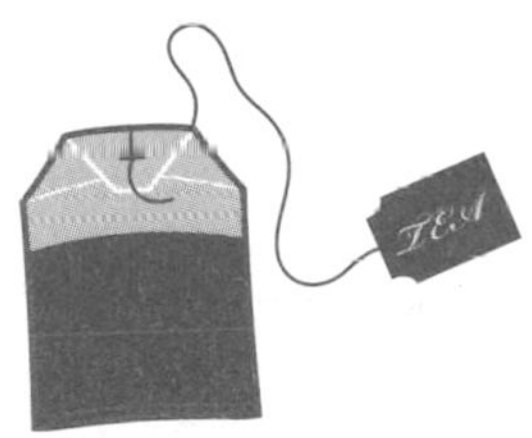

Wear Tea

Why: Green, black, and chamomile teas have astringents that constrict blood vessels and pull skin taut.

Do this: Steep two bags, let them cool, wrap each in a clean dishcloth, lie down, and place a bag over each closed eye for 5 to 15 minutes.

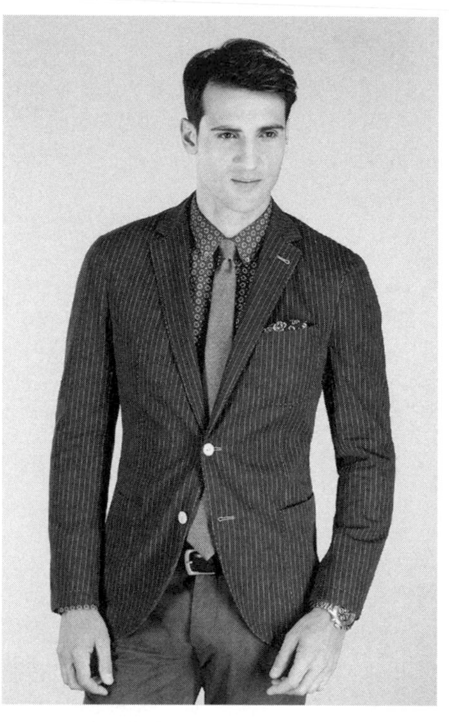

How to Play with Patterns

Most men stick to solid shirts and patterned ties, but the inverse is just as easy to pull off. The size of patterns and thickness of textures dictate how pieces should be paired. When pairing a shirt with a large pattern, choose something more subtle in your tie and vice versa.

Start with a statement pattern like a floral and repeat it on a smaller scale or subdue it by adding a solid color. For example, solid trousers or dark jeans tone down a bold striped jacket with a printed shirt. If that's too extreme, try to vary the texture of your clothes instead—like a solid-colored shirt in an unexpected fabric, such as linen or denim.

Match Your Collar

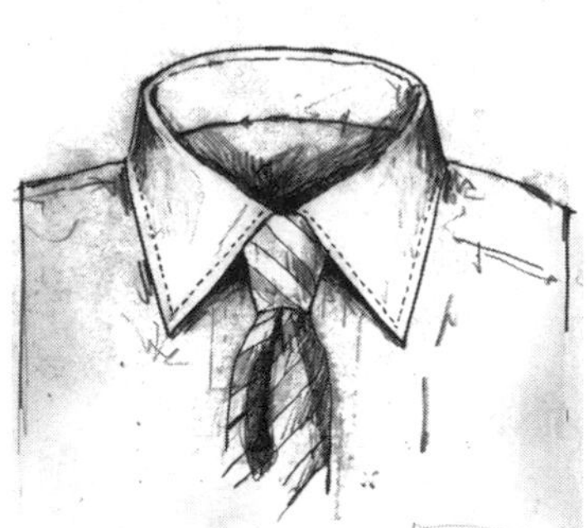

Option 1: The Point

Recommended suit

Italian two-button peak lapel with side vents

Recommended knot

Four-in-hand or half Windsor

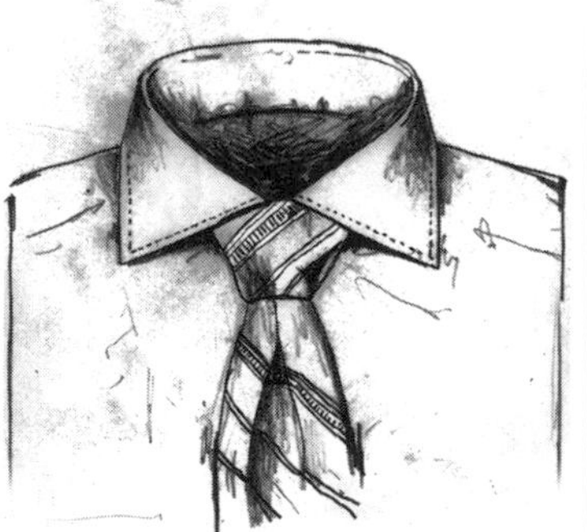

Option 2: The Spread

Recommended suit

English three-button notch-lapel suit with side vents

Recommended knot

Windsor or double Windsor

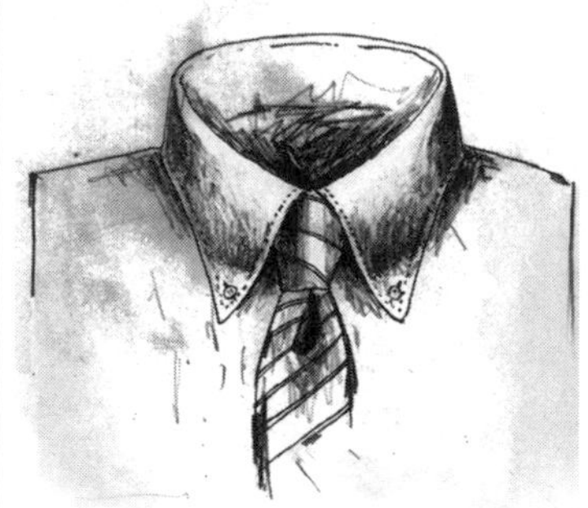

Option 3: The Button-Down

Recommended suit

Classic American two-button notch lapel with single vent

Recommended knot

half Windsor

Fast Fixes for *Style Emergencies*

Get rid of shirt nipples. You took your polo off the hanger and put it on. Now the mirror reflects what suggests you've grown perky nibs on your deltoids. Remove them by moistening your fingers and rubbing them on the protrusions until the shirt is wet. When it dries, the nipples will be gone.

Straighten a curling collar. Lost a collar stay from your shirt at work? Replace it with a large paper clip to carry you through the rest of day without a curled collar.

Uncrease your tie. Drape your tie over the closet bar in the evening to let the creases relax. Then roll it and store it in a drawer instead of using a tie rack. Gravity deforms ties.

Find your mark fast. The tip of your tie should reach just below your belt. It can be challenging to get it right every time. As a cheat, use a permanent marker to make a tiny dot on the back of the wide blade marking how low the narrow end should hang when you start tying the knot.

Get more mileage out of your jeans. They won't fade as fast if you turn the jeans inside out before washing.

Get more mileage out of your trousers. If they are wrinkled badly, have them professionally steamed. Dry-cleaning too often destroys fabric. Suit pants should be dry-cleaned only once or twice a season.

Put GQ in your shoes. If you're on a business trip and left your cedar shoe trees at home, roll up two magazines and slip them into your shoes in the evening. They'll expand to smooth out the leather and reshape while the paper will absorb the day's foot sweat.

Shine savers. Three ways to save the day if your shoes look dull and scuffed but there's no shoe shine shop or kit around: (1) Get scuff marks off shoes by applying a little toothpaste to a rag and buffing out the scuffs. (2) In an emergency, rub leather shoes with the inside of a banana peel. Then clean and buff the surface with a cloth or paper towel. (3) Spray a little Armor All leather cleaner on a soft cloth. Now pretend you're wearing Pirellis on your feet and quickly buff those Italians to a high shine.

Shave with olive oil. Out of shaving cream? Massage a glug of olive oil into your beard. You may never go back.

The Rules of Pairing Shirts and Ties

Nothing freaks a guy out more in the morning than selecting a tie to go with his shirt. But different patterns and textures can look stylish—if you follow this guide.

Sophisticated Look

WHY IT WORKS: The dominant colors in both shirt and tie are the same tone, but not a perfect match. The flecked texture of the wool tie provides a contrast with the shirt's classic windowpane.

Conservative Look

WHY IT WORKS: Stripes and checks can work when the shirt and tie share a common color. Make sure one of the two is bolder than the other.

Casual Look

WHY IT WORKS: The bigger the checks, the more casual the shirt. Match that feeling with a textured tie in a loose knot. To make it more formal, switch the tie for a silk one and tighten the knot.

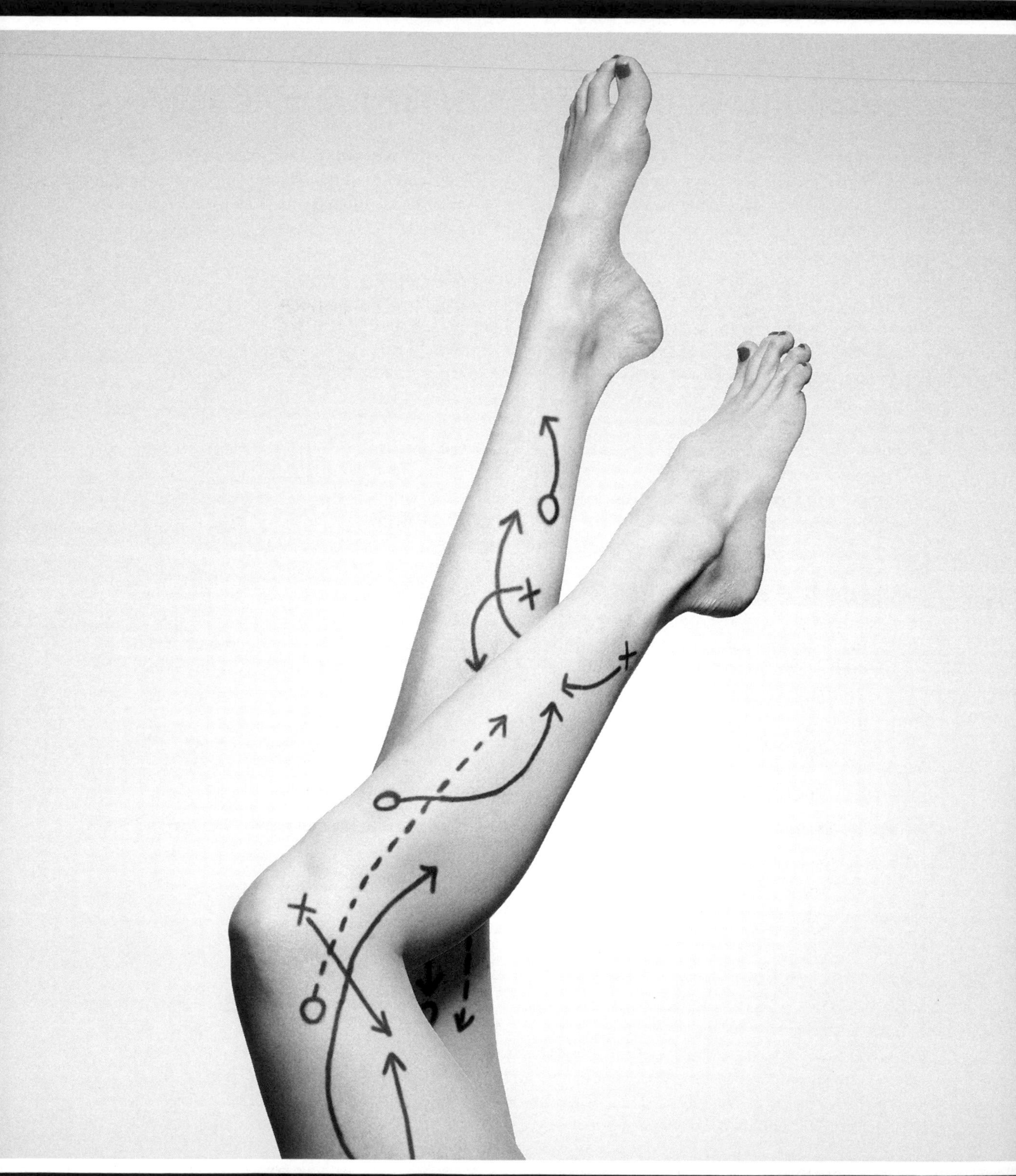

Women

More Useful Than Your Good-Looking Friend's Little Black Book, This is Your Manual to the Female Species

So much is made of trying to find, attract, and understand women—and for good reason. Of all a man's adventures, identifying the right female and wooing her can be one of life's most challenging and exciting. For an apt analogy, consider upland bird hunting for woodcock. Even better, the ruffed grouse. The ruffed grouse is the most wary and cunning of all land game birds found in the northern United States. It's wild and shy, rising and fleeing swiftly usually long before the hunter is in range, often taking refuge in the ladies' room—*er,* the branches of a tree. Success with the ruffed grouse requires much practice and skill on the part of its pursuer, but at least the grouse hunter has an advantage—his trusty pointers and setters. When it comes to pursuing women, you can try using your friends to flush 'em. But you're mostly on your own. Fortunately, *Men's Health* has been helping readers find, attract, and understand women for more than 25 years. That's a lot of wisdom to help you try to answer that elusive question—*What Do Women Want?*—and much of it can be found on the following pages.

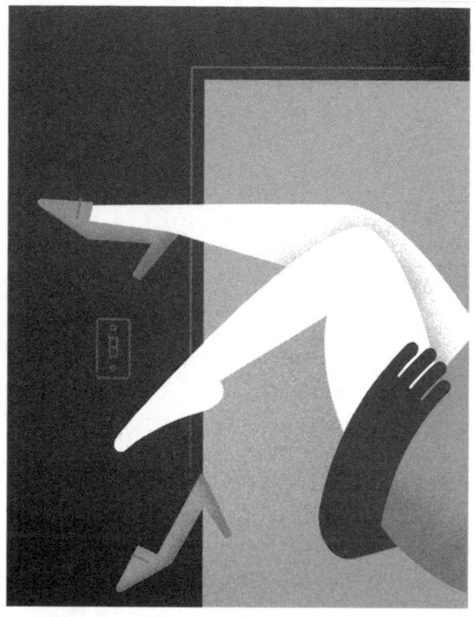

How to Pick Up Women

(WITH YOUR DIGNITY AND YOUR LUMBAR DISCS INTACT)

Prepare for Liftoff

If you're right-handed, approach your gal's left side. (Reverse these directions if you're a lefty.) Place your right arm across the middle of her back. Now push your hips back as you bend at your knees. Place your left arm across the back of her knees. Have her position her left hand on your right shoulder to help with stabilization.

Secure Your Core

Tighten your abs as much as you can—as if someone were going to punch you in the stomach. (This stabilizes your torso, which keeps your back safe.) In one motion, lift your bride: Push your hips forward and straighten your knees while maintaining a straight back. As with lifting any heavy object, your legs do the work.

Let Her Down Easy

Standing straight with tightened abs, walk across the threshold. To bring her back down to earth, reverse the lifting motion. Keep your back straight as you push your hips back, bend your knees, and guide her feet to the floor. Make sure to support her torso with your right hand so she doesn't fall.

RULE #1

You're 227 percent more likely to meet a potential girlfriend through a friend or family member rather than in a bar, at the gym, or on the street.

3 WORDS TO LIVE BY
HOLD
THE
DOOR

RULE #2

Look up. The direction of a woman's gaze could reveal her intentions, a study in *Psychological Science* shows. Using photographs and eye-tracking devices, researchers found that someone who's romantically interested in a stranger fixates more on the face. If it's pure lust, the eyes tend to target the body. These eye patterns—in men and women alike—were perceptible within a second and a half.

How to Date
Out of Your League

The secret lies in the two Cs: confidence and compliment, says Barton Goldsmith, PhD, author of *100 Ways to Boost Your Self-Confidence.*

Pump Yourself Up

You're nervous because you think she can see your faults. Guess what? She'll see them only if you show them to her. So before you approach her, take a minute or two to boost your own confidence. Remind yourself why you rock and then visualize those traits front and center as you interact with her. Do you have an amazing sense of humor? Visualize her laughing, and that talent may be more likely to break through. Dashing blue eyes? See her staring into them.

Ease into Conversation

Wait for an opportune time to approach her one-on-one (when her friend goes to the bathroom, or she steps up to the jukebox alone). You don't want to interrupt or surprise her; that'll put her on the defensive. As you initiate conversation, keep your shoulders back and hands at your sides—a warm, welcoming stance. Open with a polite "Excuse me . . ." instead of an intrusive "Hey" or "What's up?"

Say Something Nice

A pickup artist might tell you that a backhanded compliment will pique a woman's interest because she's already heard all the nice compliments. Don't believe it: You just have to use the right compliment. Instead of commenting on a physical trait, like her eyes, ask her about that funky piece of jewelry or cool T-shirt. This diverts the conversation from her, which she'll appreciate, and her answer will provide jumping-off points for more topics.

Seal the Deal

Because you approached her, it's your responsibility to proffer your number first. Give her a reason for contacting her: "If you really want to catch that new Wes Anderson movie, why don't I text you next weekend when it's out?" You'll reinforce the fact that you're interested in her while keeping the talk cool, confident, and casual.

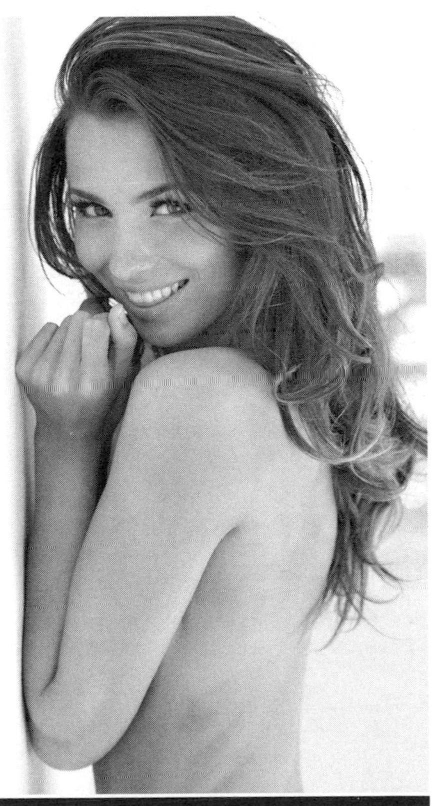

What Her Past Says

Women who have low intimacy levels in college may be more likely to divorce later in life, according to a study in *Personal Relationships*. When researchers at the University of Massachusetts at Amherst tracked down 167 people who had taken a psychological test 34 years earlier, they found the correlation—only among women. Women tend to take a more active role than men in maintaining a couple's closeness, so a relationship in which the woman shows less intimacy may be more likely to falter, says study author Mark Weinberger, PhD.

What to Do When Her Name Slips Your Mind

Is that you, Mulva? Forgetting happens. Instead of asking again, coax her to tell you a story, says Josh Piven, coauthor of *The Worst-Case Scenario Survival Handbook: Dating and Sex*. What was her childhood nickname? Was she named after anyone? If the answer doesn't shed light, be creative. Make up a nickname for her or think of something cool you read recently and tell her about it. Then offer to e-mail it to her. Her address will probably contain a clue to her name.

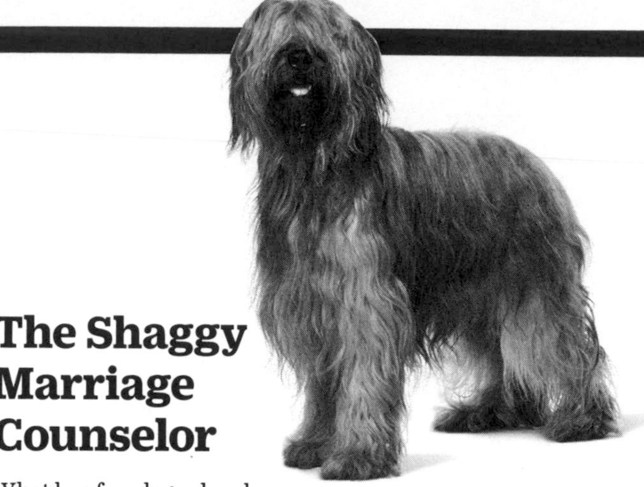

The Shaggy Marriage Counselor

What has four legs, drools, and lowers blood pressure? A dog, according to a study in the *Journal of Psychosomatic Medicine*. Researchers analyzed 240 couples, half of whom owned a pet. In times of stress, couples who were pet owners had lower blood pressures and heart rates than petless couples, the researchers say, suggesting that pets have a calming effect on couples.

Will She Go Home with You?

Tough to predict when her husband keeps interrupting, but there are ways to know what she's really thinking. Some clues from Tonya Reiman, author of The *Body Language of Dating*.

You Think the Girl at the Bar Is Interested

Do this: Glance at her feet. People subconsciously move toward their desires. Her upper body might not be turned toward you, but if her feet are pointed at you, she's subconsciously positioned herself in your direction. Go on, say "hi."

It Looks like She Wants to Kiss, but You're Not Sure

Do this: Take a look at her lips. She'll touch and lick them more than usual. And if she's into you, it's perfectly okay to stare—just make sure you're staring at her eyes, not just her lips. Now, quick, seize the opportunity!

She Says She's Not Mad, but You Suspect Otherwise

Do this: Watch her jawline. She'll instinctively close her mouth and tighten her jaw when she's angry. If she's perfected her poker face, check her hands. If she's clutching her knuckles or something else, let her cool off.

You're Not Sure She Loves Your Gift

Do this: Look where she puts the goods. If she really likes the gift, she'll spend time with it. If she removes it from sight, don't act apologetic. Mention why you bought it for her, which will emphasize your thoughtfulness.

Buy the Perfect Gift EVERY TIME

Streamline your shopping by asking yourself these four questions first.

1 "What did we talk about last?"
"People are always dropping ideas," says Lash Fary, who creates gift baskets for Hollywood events. Her train commute sucks? Buy her an iTunes gift card. She just signed up for a yoga class? Buy her a mat for home.

2 "Can I tie in a personal experience?"
You know what's better than that iTunes gift card? One to a restaurant you've been to together. "Use nostalgia to your advantage," says Fary. "The thoughtfulness behind it will make a small gift seem bigger."

3 "What does he or she do regularly?"
Can't think of anything? Then you're not trying hard enough, says Fary. Think about it: Your wife brews coffee every morning. Your brother hikes every week. Your buddy has two dogs. Your list writes itself!

4 "What's the purpose of this gift?"
If you can't answer this question, keep shopping. "Ultimately," says Fary, "gifts should be a reflection of how well you know the needs of the person you're buying them for."

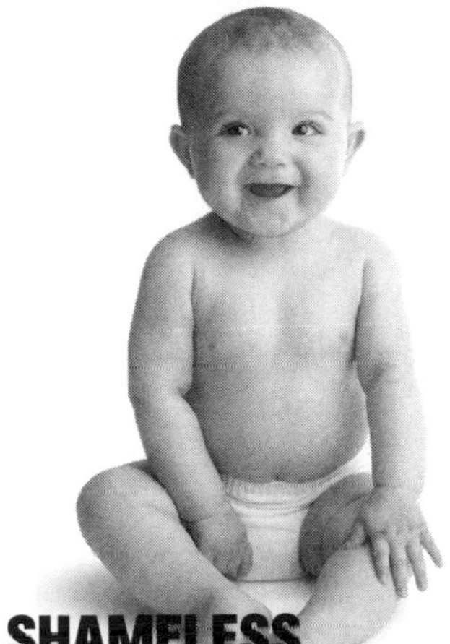

SHAMELESS PICKUP TRICK

BE A BABY MAGNET

She may go gaga over you if you try some baby talk—that is, when directed at an actual baby, not the babe. Women in a French study were 28 percent more likely to give their number to a guy if he cooed over someone's infant.

Try Group Play

Think she might turn down that date? Offer to bring friends. According to a DatingAdvice.com survey of more than 1,000 people, over a quarter of single ladies prefer their first dates to be in groups.

***Bonus:* You just fixed up your friends.**

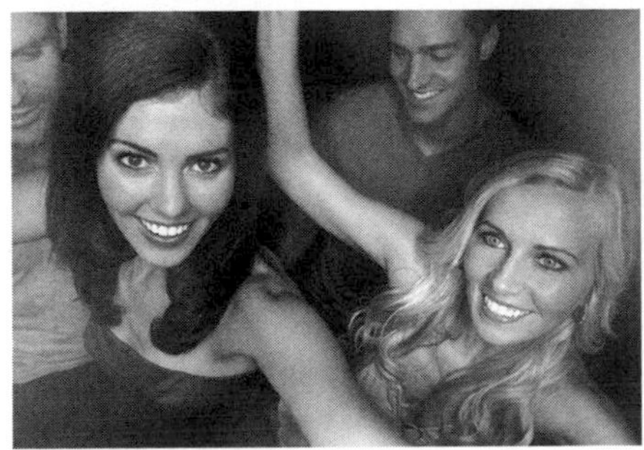

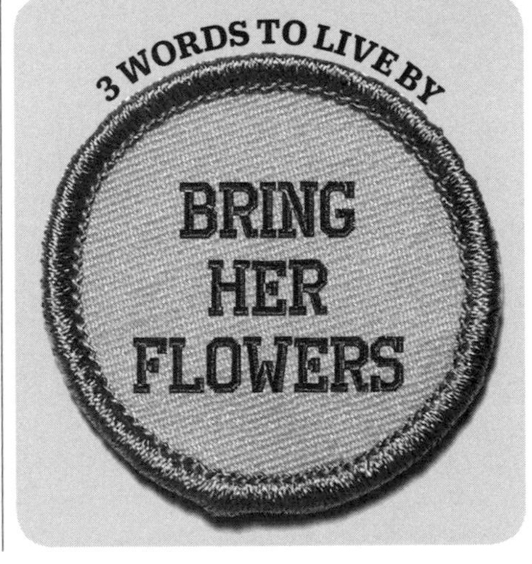
3 WORDS TO LIVE BY
BRING
HER
FLOWERS

Help a Lady with Her Coat

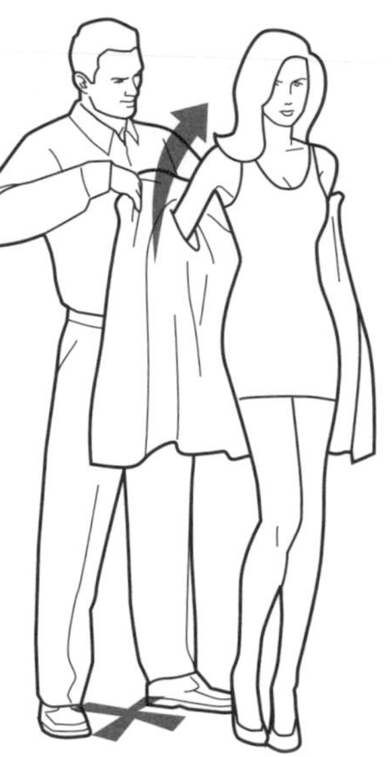

PREP

To avoid an elbow to the face, first ask, "May I help you with your coat?"

PUTTING IT ON

STEP 1

Stand about a foot behind her, and slightly to her right if she's right-handed. Hold her coat open just above her waist—any higher and she'll have to perform armhole acrobatics. Spread your arms wide, opening the jacket.

STEP 2

After her arms slip in, pull the right side of the coat toward her shoulder and then extend the left side out around waist height. Pull the left side over her shoulder.

STEP 3

Give her a quick squeeze on the shoulders to show affection. Now back away and let her pull her hair out from under the collar herself. Messing with a woman's hairstyle is dangerous.

TAKING IT OFF

STEP 1

As she shrugs off her coat, stand behind her to catch it as it slides from her shoulders. If you pull it off, you'll also pull her arms back. Not helpful.

STEP 2

Tuck her scarf halfway into one of her coat sleeves before handing the coat to the attendant so it's there for her return.

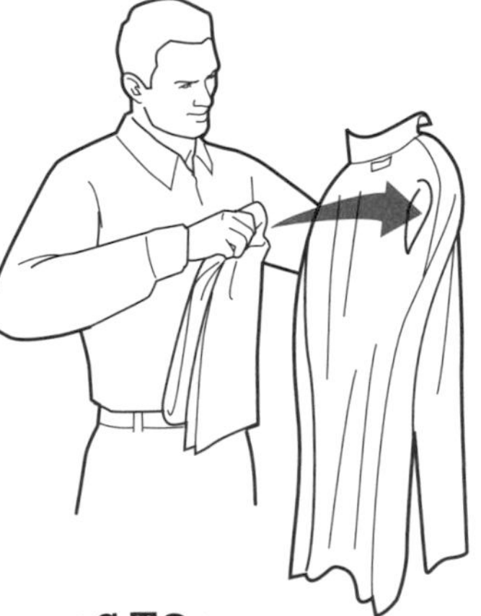

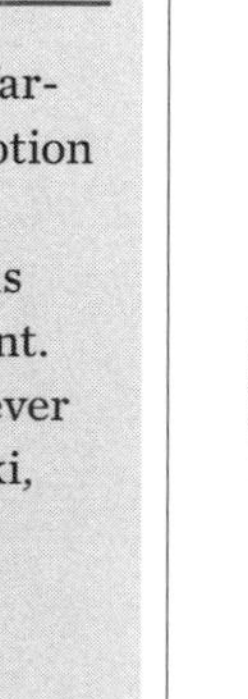

Q Is there any science backing up pheromones and how they attract women?

A. Sorry, fellas, but a shower and a smile will go a lot farther with the ladies than your sweaty armpits. The notion of sex-attracting pheromones was first propounded 50 years ago, when a scientist noticed that male moths stayed upwind to attract female moths with their scent. This is true for moths, but no such phenomenon has ever been shown to apply to humans, says Charles Wysocki, PhD, a neuroscientist at the Monell Chemical Senses Center in Philadelphia.

"There is no biomedical literature to support the claim that humans use attraction pheromones," he says.

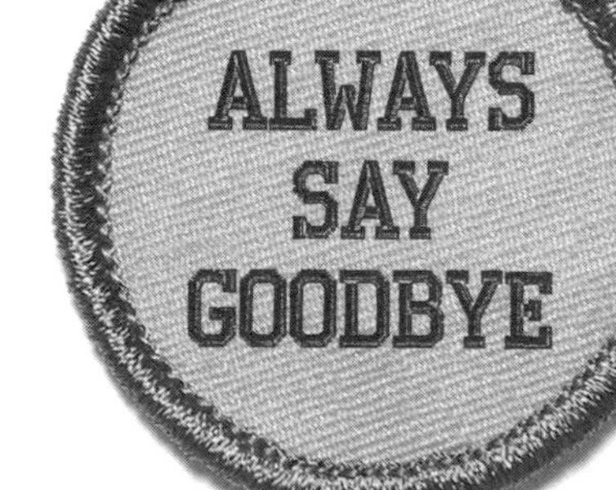
3 WORDS TO LIVE BY
ALWAYS
SAY
GOODBYE

The Monet Shot

Forearms are packed with pleasure nerves that respond best to a touch traveling between 1 and 10 centimeters per second, scientists report in the journal *Nature Neuroscience*. These "C-tactile" nerve fibers (also found on the legs and face) send signals to the limbic system, an area of the brain associated with trust and affection. For best results—whether with your wife of 10 years or a first date—gain her attention with a brief stroke, using the force of an artist's brush.

Fact:

Only 18 percent of women are able to recognize when a man is flirting with them.

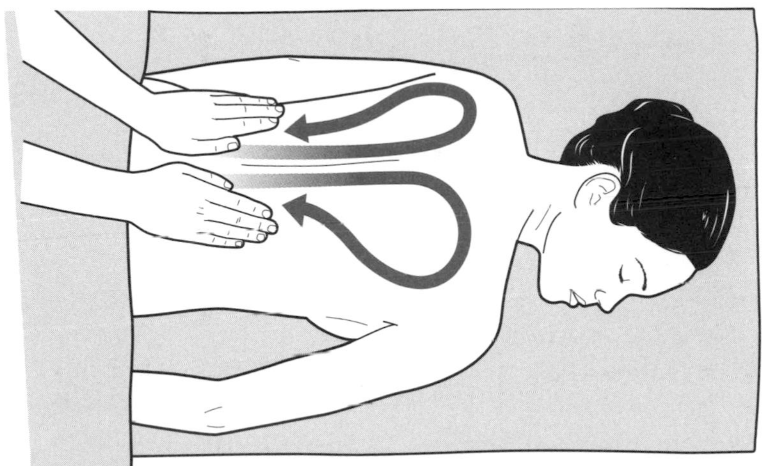

Give Her a Great Back Massage

Like great sex, a great massage requires a warmup, varying intensities, and a cooldown. Ready to start? Here are your moves.

Move 1: The Circle Back

Make circles in opposite directions with both palms, slowly moving all over her back and shoulders. Vary the size of the circles and the pressure you apply as you move up and down her back. Periodically switch the direction of your circles. Because this move is less intense, it's a good one for starting and ending the massage.

Move 2: The Heart Warmer

Place your hands on each side of her lower back about half an inch from her spine, and gently lean into your palms. Applying pressure, glide your hands up her back to her neck and then outward along her shoulder blades. Continuing the motion, bring your hands to the start position, completing a heart-shaped route.

Move 3: The Spine Tingler

Starting at her lower back, place your thumbs on each side of her spine and slowly rub your thumbs into the muscles, avoiding direct contact with her spine. Alternate hands, spending a few seconds in each spot before moving your thumbs up an inch. Work to her nape and then back down. Repeat the movement several times.

Move 4: Bring It Home

Aim for a 15-minute session. She'll be plenty relaxed—and you won't develop muscle cramps. To bring the massage to a gentle conclusion, place your hands in the center of her back and hold them there for 10 seconds. Then leave the room for a minute or two so she can come back to reality. Accept her high praises.

Pass Her Google Exam

The readers of *Women's Health* clue us in to search-result gaffes.

A Barren LinkedIn

Of the women surveyed 41 percent would scan your profile. Evolution has wired them to seek competent males, say Helen Fisher, PhD, so play up your career successes.

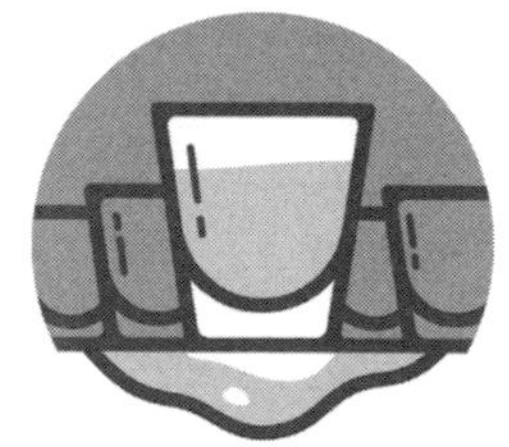

Friday Night Pics

Some 62 percent dislike partying photos. Sure, tag pictures with friends, but brewing the beer, not doing keg stands, says flirting expert Jeffrey Hall, PhD.

Lame One-Liners

Being truly funny can enhance your attractiveness online, the survey revealed. But make sure your jokes don't all start with "I" or criticize other people, Hall says.

An Outdated Blog

Delete any potentially embarrassing content, hopefully before she sees it. Then look up "Google removal tool" for details on scrubbing those search results.

61

Percentage of women who say they wish their partner was more spontaneous

PICKUP TRICKS: GO LOW

Drop your voice and she may drop her inhibitions. Women perceive men with deep voices as more attractive, according to a study in the journal *Personality and Individual Differences*. (Sorry, you won't find that one at Barnes & Noble.)

RULE #3

Simplest way to be romantic: Shave on the weekend.

How to Write a LOVE LETTER

Nothing stirs passion like pen on paper—as long as you don't try to sound like Lionel Richie. She wants to hear you, so write like you talk—goofy voice and all, says Samara O'Shea, author of *For the Love of Letters*. Tell her why you're writing ("I've been thinking about us a lot") and touch on a couple of great memories. Then transition to the present: ("Six years later I'm still crazy about you.") List a few things you love about her, tease her gently about something that drives you nuts ("There's no one's shoes I'd rather trip over") and close with a sign-off ("love, Joe"). Place the note somewhere surprising like a coat pocket or, if you live together, your own mailbox. Then stand by for some enthusiastically requited affection.

Pick Flowers She'll Love

When dealing with women, flowers are your best buds. We asked more than 350 women which flowers they'd want for different occasions. Then we checked in with Kate Law, head floral designer at ProFlowers, for some creative upgrades.

Come Up Roses

When women are looking for romance—for Valentine's Day, say—red roses win every time. But that's not to say you can't still surprise her.
Upgrade: Instead of cheap-looking baby's breath, supplement her bouquet with green Fuji mums, and choose pink roses over expected red.

Slip Her the 'Lips

Women we polled said they'd like to receive tulips for an accomplishment, such as a promotion. Tulips are simple but thoughtful, says Law.
Upgrade: Tulips are elegant. Law suggests showcasing them in a glass vase, with the stems cut so the flowers rest just above the lip.

Seek Out Lily

Lilies ranked high on birthday lists. They're celebratory blooms.
Upgrade: For a classic look, go with a solid bouquet of one color—and ask for tango lilies. They have bursts of color throughout their petals, which give them a unique, sophisticated appeal.

Wait a While

There's one time when a woman probably doesn't want you to give her flowers: the first date. While you may think the offer is thoughtful and surprising, most women will think you're just trying too hard. The vast majority of women we asked advised arriving without a bouquet.

Plan the Perfect V-Day

Charm your partner's heart or transform a new fling into more by way of Cupid's arrow. Try these Valentine's Day dates for any, and every, part of your relationship.

A New Couple

Skip the predictable dinner in favor of low-pressure fun like indoor mini golf. Let her kick your ass and then schedule a rematch to keep the momentum.

A Few Months In

Build your bond by giving back—cleaning up a local park, say. Finish the day and keep the teamwork going by cooking at home. Don't forget a bottle of red.

Nearly Engaged

Re-create your first date. Add thoughtful details, like wearing the same shirt you had on that day. You might just inspire her to revisit the lingerie drawer.

Married

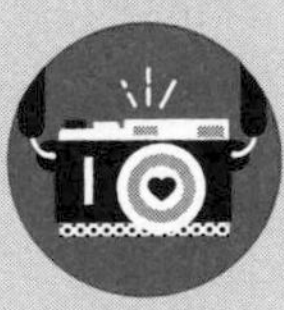

Be a tourist in your own city. Yes, that means you'll need to take that double-decker bus ride. You'll see your town—and your mate—in a brand-new light.

How to Buy *Lingerie*
WITHOUT EMBARRASSING YOURSELF

We've all been there: dawdling amid the teddies and garter belts, eyeing what other women are buying. Here's a less creepy way to shop for sexy bits for a woman, according to Jennifer Carroll, author of *Underneath It All.*

Be a Bra Detective

Avoid the hand-cupping and "they're about this big" descriptions by noting a few of her bra and panty sizes. In doubt? Ask her! There's no bigger buzzkill than a sexy gift she can't slip into 5 minutes later.

Consider Her Shape

In the right outfit, she can go from lovely to stunning. Think about her best attributes and use the guide below to choose the best style for her body type.

Recruit Help

Head for the oldest employee—she'll be more sensitive to specifics like a paunch or small breasts. Tell her your gal's size and style, and she'll help narrow the search.

Emphasize Her Assets

HER KEY ASSETS	IDEAL STYLES
Long legs	Baby doll, short nightie, bra-and-panties set. A thigh-skimming style adds emphasis to legs.
Big chest	Sheer bra, chemise with built-in cups and underwire. A sheer bra flaunts her assets; built-in cups support her bust.
Petite breasts	Sheer camisole-and-panties set; lacy bra (no underwire). A- or B-size breasts don't need the support of underwires.
Flat stomach	Three-piece bra, panties, and garter set. This sexy trio draws attention to her trimmed tummy.
Great butt	Lacy tanga panties or boy shorts. Peekaboo cut accentuates her curves more than a G-string.

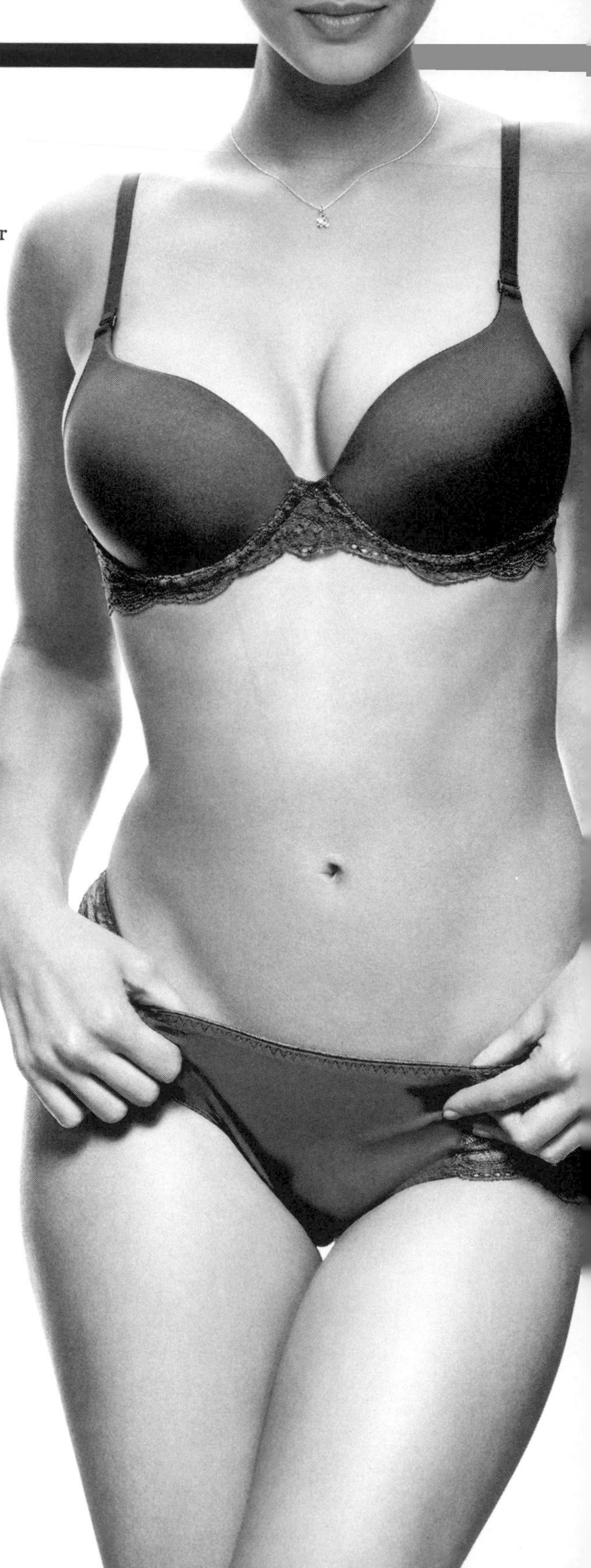

Buy a Bra She'll Wear

1. Size Her Up

What is Victoria's secret? "The brand tends to undersize its bras," says plastic surgeon Bradley Bengtson, MD. This can create confusion for you, the guy buying his GF a bra. "Write down the sizes of three bras you see her wear a lot," says Alexis Isadora, owner of Brooklyn Fox, a lingerie shop. "Go with the middle size."

2. Choose a Cut

The most popular bra style among women: full coverage. Step out of that comfort zone: For an A or B cup, try a demi style. For C or larger, choose a more supportive three-quarter cup. One rule: Resist padded push-up bras. "These are Barbie-doll culture," says Isadora. "The point is to feel sexy, not to fit a stereotype."

3. Pay Attention to the Details

Clueless about color? "Black is always a safe bet," says Isadora. "I also love the 'sweet' look—a beautiful white lace or cotton bra." Venture into red, leopard, or neon only if you see similarly wild styles in her drawer. If you're going lacy, spring for high-quality semisheer French lingerie, like Aubade.

Flirt like a Pro

Seduce with stimulating conversation and these tips from Daniel Menaker, author of *My Mistake* and *A Good Talk: The Story and Skill of Conversation.*

Take Your Cue

First, find out if she even wants to flirt. Is she giving you eye contact? A smile? Teasing you? Do the same back at her. But don't poke fun at her hair, height, or physical traits. Her outfit is a safer target. ("A Jets hat? So you're into losers, huh?")

Make a Connection

If you feel you're on a repartee roll, shift the talk. Ask what she thinks of the bartender's haircut, or crack a joke about the rowdy fan a few rows down—any other "third thing" that takes the pressure off the two of you. Plus, you'll have an inside joke to use later. Speaking of which . . .

Close the Deal

If she's into you, she'll be asking you questions and following up with more personal answers. Ask for her number. Give her a reason for staying in touch: "I'd like to try that Thai place you mentioned. Why don't I text you next weekend?"

4 THINGS TO NEVER SAY TO A NAKED WOMAN

"There's something really weird I want to try with you."

"That orgasm seemed as phony as Cheez Whiz."

"Not now, thanks. This book is really getting good."

"Is that supposed to feel good?"

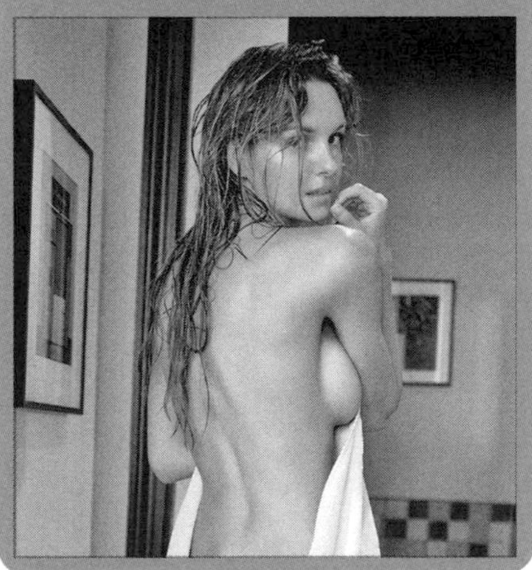

Deliver a Hot French Kiss

Make her say "ooh la la!" with these three simple steps from Justin R. Garcia, PhD, a researcher at the Kinsey Institute for Research in Sex, Gender, and Reproduction, and William Cane, author of *The Art of Kissing*.

Lead Her On

Don't go in all tongue wagging. In fact, don't start the kiss by kissing at all. Stimulate her secondary erogenous zones by using your hands to softly touch her neck, jawline, or hair. This prolongs the anticipation.

Build the Mood

Hot kisses start slowly and intensify. Begin by kissing her lower lip softly. She can breathe easier when you do this, which means she can control the kiss. When you feel her excitement building, lightly touch the tip of her tongue with yours. The tip has more nerve endings than almost any other part of the body.

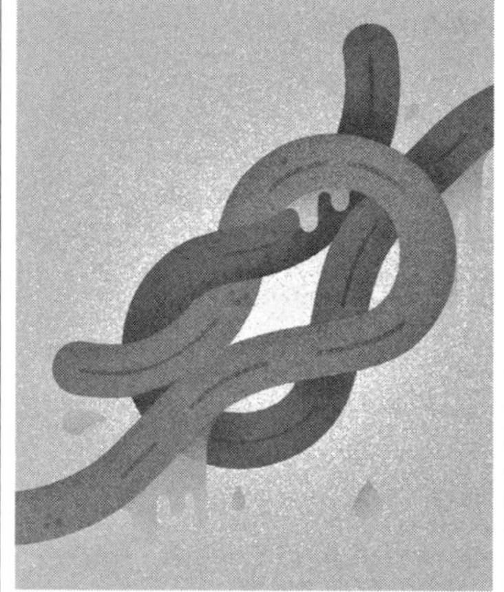

Put Your Body into It

As the kiss heats up, step toward her to where she can rub your back and pull you even closer. To heat things up, open your mouth wider to let her involve her tongue more. Gradually add quicker soft-tongue movements. Don't forget about your mouth's other power: giving her compliments. You can extend and intensify the kiss by pausing to whisper endearments in her ear, after which you can segue into neck kisses.

Marriage, with Benefits

If you're susceptible to vice, find a wife. She'll save you from yourself—and improve your life—in a variety of ways. Notably, she'll . . .

1. Increase Your Pay

A Virginia Commonwealth University study found that married men earn 22 percent more than their similarly experienced but single colleagues.

2. Speed Up Your Next Promotion

Married men receive higher performance ratings and faster promotions than bachelors, a study of U.S. Navy officers reported.

3. Keep You Out of Trouble

According to a U.S. Department of Justice report, male victims of violent crime are nearly four times more likely to be single than married. And of course, single guys wind up in jail much more often.

4. Help You Beat Cancer

In a Norwegian study, divorced and never-married male cancer patients had 11 and 16 percent higher mortality rates, respectively, than married men.

5. Help You Live Longer

A UCLA study found that people in generally excellent health were 88 percent more likely to die over the 8-year study period if they were single.

RULE # 4 **Good kissing trumps personality and looks for women considering a long-term relationship, according to a study in the journal *Evolutionary Psychology.***

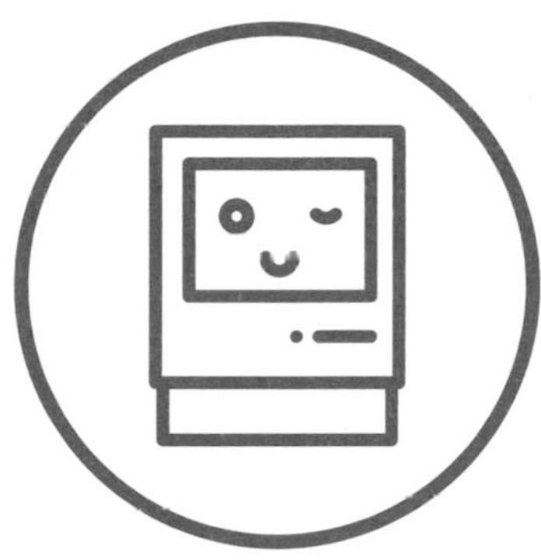

MAKE THE FIRST MOVE

Don't be shy online. Your chances of landing a looker on a dating site increase if you initiate contact instead of waiting to be chosen, according to a report in the *Journal of Marriage and Family*. Why? Everybody takes a shot at someone hotter. So if she reaches out to you, you're likely to be the more attractive partner, and vice versa, says lead study author Derek Kreager, PhD. About 80 percent of men's messages go unanswered, probably because everyone's after the same people. So try your luck with that stunner, but also contact women with less dazzle—and more space in their in-boxes.

Vacations That Turn Her On

1. Tropical beach
2. European tour
3. Bed-and-breakfast in the country
4. Trip to wine country
5. Cruise

Vacations That Turn Her Off

1. Safari
2. Gambling trip
3. Charity work
4. Wedding
5. Theme park

Source: Poll of 327 women by TripAdvisor

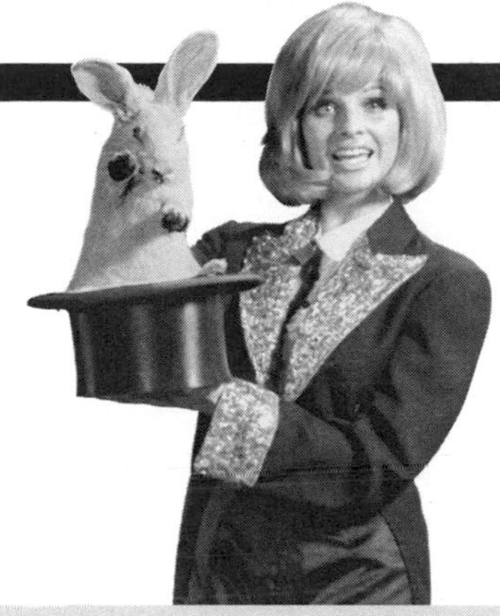

Get Her Number with Magic

The principle: Magicians know that audiences "see" the same things differently. "That's because there are no absolutes for the brain," says neuroscientist Susana Martiez-Conde, PhD. Your mind perceives things based on context, either actual or implied. This is the basis for many illusions. You just need to create the right context, says magician Francis Menotti.

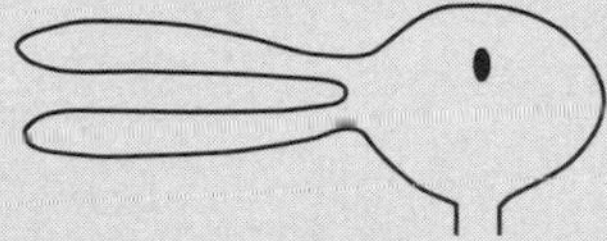

How to use it: Try this trick the next time you're at a bar and want to break the ice with a woman. Sketch the image above on a piece of paper and ask what she sees. It can be viewed as either a duck or a rabbit, but people usually see one, not the other. If she sees a rabbit, tell her you can transform the picture—without touching it—before her very eyes. Then say two magic words: "quack, quack," and she'll see the duck. "You can influence people with psychological subtleties," says Menotti. And if she sees the duck? Say "Bugs Bunny." Presto! You've made her smile.

Four Dates You Should Never Forget

Therapist Rober Taibbi, LCSW, suggests a few subtle celebrations to earmark.

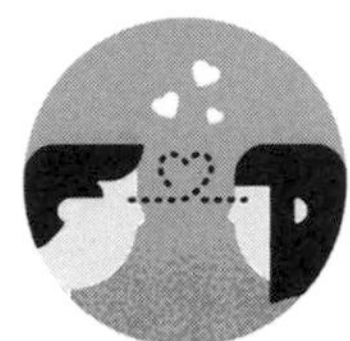

When You Meet

Pull up a stool at the pizza joint where you first flirted, says Taibbi. Or do one better: Make the pie at home and skip dealing with the grouchy counter guy.

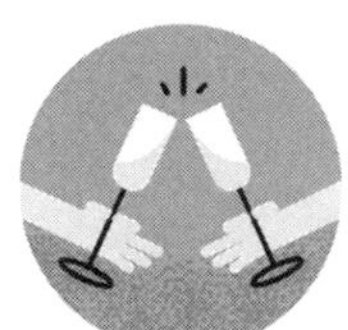

Her Big Promotion

She killed it, so raise a glass, says Taibbi. Try: "I knew this would be a big change and hard work, but it's paid off. I'm proud of you." Now pop that bubbly.

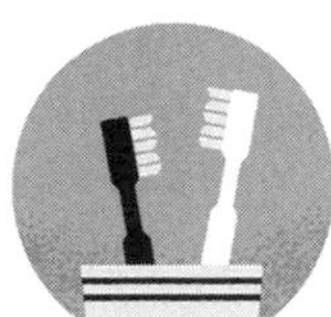

When You Moved In

Surprise her with an upgrade to your abode: Plant a tree in the yard, buy that piece of art she's had her eye on, or spring for luxury sheets. (Then test 'em out!)

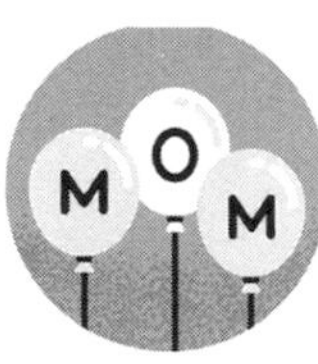

Her Mom's Birthday

Cute, right? But seriously: Help her mom kick back, and maybe toss in that new book she wants, and you could earn a powerful ally.

How to Argue and Win

What's the argument about?

A. The In-Laws

SAY THIS: "Let's go outside for a few minutes."
WHY THIS WORKS: Taking a walk with her or snuggling up on a lawn chair will remind her that, at the end of the day, it's just the two of you. Worry about what works for you—not for your parents.

B. Trivial Matters

SAY THIS:"I know you're upset about [whatever], but it feels like there's something else going on. Let's talk about the other stuff."
WHY THIS WORKS: If you think she's overreacting, a larger issue is probably fueling her rage. That's what you need to know about—and calmly address.

C. Parenting

SAY THIS: "We need to find a balance between being strict and flexible. When do you think we should be flexible?"
WHY THIS WORKS: Firm and flexible parenting styles can coexist—as long as you act together as a team. No one should always be the bad guy.

D. Hell if I Know . . .

SAY THIS: "Okay, let's focus. What are a few things we could do differently here?"
WHY THIS WORKS: Sometimes she just needs to vent general dissatisfaction. Directing your energy toward action, not anger, can soothe her nerves.

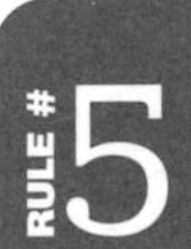

Wash your sheets. The average guy changes his linens four times a year, but 65 percent of women say they're more likely to have sex with their partner if the sheets are clean, report two UK surveys. That's wash, rumple, repeat.

What's the State of Your Union?

The sex and benefits of coupledom are pretty awesome, but maintenance is a must. Are you keeping up your end? Use this flowchart to troubleshoot key problem areas, and deploy the power tools that just might rescue your relationship.

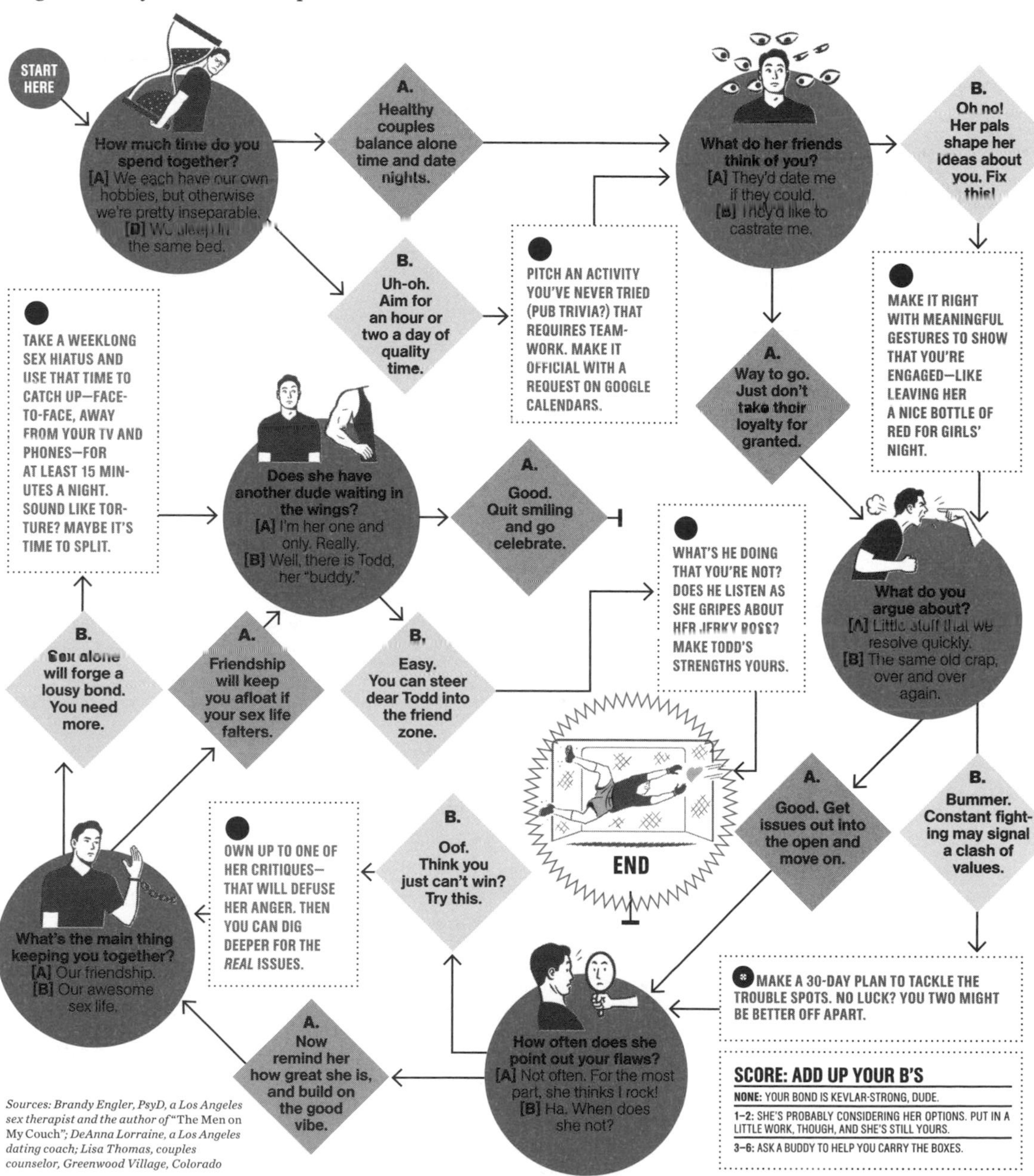

START HERE
How much time do you spend together?
[A] We each have our own hobbies, but otherwise we're pretty inseparable.
[B] We sleep in the same bed.
A. Healthy couples balance alone time and date nights.
B. Uh-oh. Aim for an hour or two a day of quality time.
PITCH AN ACTIVITY YOU'VE NEVER TRIED (PUB TRIVIA?) THAT REQUIRES TEAMWORK. MAKE IT OFFICIAL WITH A REQUEST ON GOOGLE CALENDARS.
What do her friends think of you?
[A] They'd date me if they could.
[B] They'd like to castrate me.
B. Oh no! Her pals shape her ideas about you. Fix this!
MAKE IT RIGHT WITH MEANINGFUL GESTURES TO SHOW THAT YOU'RE ENGAGED—LIKE LEAVING HER A NICE BOTTLE OF RED FOR GIRLS' NIGHT.
A. Way to go. Just don't take their loyalty for granted.
TAKE A WEEKLONG SEX HIATUS AND USE THAT TIME TO CATCH UP—FACE-TO-FACE, AWAY FROM YOUR TV AND PHONES—FOR AT LEAST 15 MINUTES A NIGHT. SOUND LIKE TORTURE? MAYBE IT'S TIME TO SPLIT.
Does she have another dude waiting in the wings?
[A] I'm her one and only. Really.
[B] Well, there is Todd, her "buddy."
A. Good. Quit smiling and go celebrate.
WHAT'S HE DOING THAT YOU'RE NOT? DOES HE LISTEN AS SHE GRIPES ABOUT HER JERKY BOSS? MAKE TODD'S STRENGTHS YOURS.
What do you argue about?
[A] Little stuff that we resolve quickly.
[B] The same old crap, over and over again.
B. Sex alone will forge a lousy bond. You need more.
A. Friendship will keep you afloat if your sex life falters.
B. Easy. You can steer dear Todd into the friend zone.
END
A. Good. Get issues out into the open and move on.
B. Bummer. Constant fighting may signal a clash of values.
What's the main thing keeping you together?
[A] Our friendship.
[B] Our awesome sex life.
OWN UP TO ONE OF HER CRITIQUES—THAT WILL DEFUSE HER ANGER. THEN YOU CAN DIG DEEPER FOR THE REAL ISSUES.
B. Oof. Think you just can't win? Try this.
MAKE A 30-DAY PLAN TO TACKLE THE TROUBLE SPOTS. NO LUCK? YOU TWO MIGHT BE BETTER OFF APART.
How often does she point out your flaws?
[A] Not often. For the most part, she thinks I rock!
[B] Ha. When does she not?
A. Now remind her how great she is, and build on the good vibe.
SCORE: ADD UP YOUR B'S
NONE: YOUR BOND IS KEVLAR-STRONG, DUDE.
1–2: SHE'S PROBABLY CONSIDERING HER OPTIONS. PUT IN A LITTLE WORK, THOUGH, AND SHE'S STILL YOURS.
3–6: ASK A BUDDY TO HELP YOU CARRY THE BOXES.

Sources: Brandy Engler, PsyD, a Los Angeles sex therapist and the author of "The Men on My Couch"; *DeAnna Lorraine, a Los Angeles dating coach; Lisa Thomas, couples counselor, Greenwood Village, Colorado*

Give Her the Universe

Summer is the perfect time to offer up some celestial razzle-dazzle, says astronomer Geoff Chester of the U.S. Naval Observatory in Washington, DC. So find the darkest skies you can, lie down on a blanket with her, and start exploring. (The sky, that is.)

PLAY MIND TRICKS

It takes 30 minutes for your eyes to fully adapt to darkness. Use that time to have a satellite-spotting contest: Scan the sky for what appear to be fast-moving stars. When the half hour is up, you'll be able to see thousands more stars than when you first came out.

ZOOM IN

Take turns scanning the sky with binoculars. (Use at least a 50-mm aperture. We like Celestron's SkyMasters 9x63, ($220, celestron.com). Don't worry about finding anything—just enjoy the view. You'll quickly stumble across star clusters and

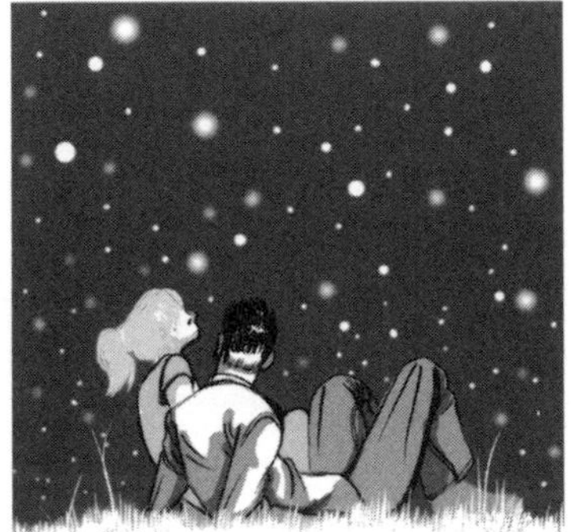

nebulae. Here's an easy grab, though: the Andromeda galaxy, which sits low in the east. (It's the width of five full moons.) If you start wondering what you're looking at, download Star Chart to your iPhone ($3) or the free Sky Map to your Android. Hold the phone up to the sky to ID celestial objects.

GO FOR A MOONWALK

Stroll a moonlit beach. "This is most fun during the full moon, when many shore critters, such as ghost crabs, aka sand crabs, are very active," Chester says. Then conduct some lunar science. If the moon is near the horizon and seems huge, prove to her that it's the same size no matter where it is in the sky. Hold an aspirin tablet at arm's length up by the moon—they'll be the same size. Repeat this later in the night, when the moon is higher, to prove the "summer moon illusion" is just that—an illusion.

Turn Sunscreen into Massage Oil

STEP 1

Pick a sunscreen that contains grapeseed extract. Its emollient qualities make it a common choice for massage oils.

STEP 2

Have her sit on the sand, and kneel behind her. This way she's grounded and won't squirm when you start applying pressure.

STEP 3

Squirt a dollop into your hand. With your wrists together, wrap your hands around the back of her neck; slide back and forth to spread the lotion.

STEP 4

Form a soft fist and put sunscreen on your knuckles. Use them to massage from the base of her neck down both sides of her spine.

STEP 5

With sunscreen on your open palms, graze your hands down her rib cage on both sides. Move slowly so it doesn't tickle.

STEP 6

Apply pressure with your thumb to her lower back and then on her neck. Move in small, slow circles all the way up and down the sides of her spine.

Source: Robert Wolf, LMT, a massage/wellness expert based in NYC

The Dance Move Hall of Lame

You should be dancing, yeah—but like JT, not like this goofball (shown below). Justin Timberlake's chief choreographer, Marty Kudelka, says "Showing confidence—even if you're faking it—is more impressive than trying too hard."

Less is more: "Stick to a simple one-two step: left to right, right to left," he says. Men who use their upper body are seen as better dancers and therefore more attractive, a German study found—and JT proves it.

"If you watch Timbaland and Justin in the studio, as soon as the beat drops, they lean back together," says Kudelka. "If you lean forward, it just looks goofy. But when you lean back, your whole upper body gets involved—your shoulders are going with you."

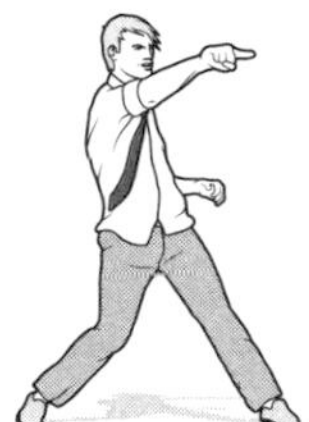

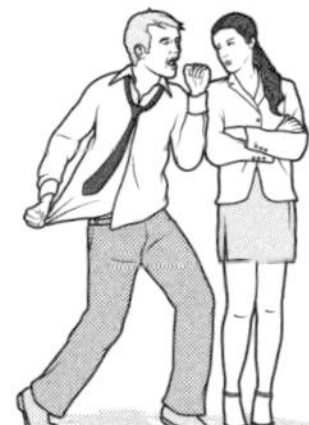

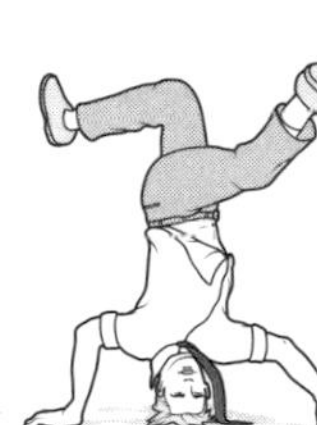

The Point
"That's just awkward," Kudelka says. "Women may laugh, but they don't actually think it's funny."

In-Her-Face Lip Syncing
"It's probably a crutch, but it's a bad one. Even if you feel like it's helping you relax, it's corny."

Break Dancing
"Who wants her man flopping around on the floor?"

Neck Nibble While Grinding
"You need to go home at this point. Get a cab."

SCORE WITH SCRUFF

Show your potential for serious growth—starting with your mug. Women perceive a man sporting a 10-day beard as more attractive than a clean-shaven guy, according to a 2013 study in *Evolution and Human Behavior.* Keep the fuzz between $\frac{1}{4}$ and $\frac{1}{2}$ inch with the help of an electric trimmer. And soften your whiskers with a few drops of beard oil three times a week or so to keep those bristles from leaving rug burns.

SHAMELESS PICKUP TRICK

BE MORE GIVING

Volunteer at a local triathlon. It's a one-day commitment and an easy way to meet (and impress) beautiful, athletic women. In a Cornell University study women favored altruistic men in both relationships and one-night stands.

Q Do women really want men to show their vulnerable, sensitive sides?

A. No. Start weeping and she'll start worrying. "She was attracted to your strength. She needs you to be strong," says Scott Haltzman, MD, psychiatrist and author of *The Secrets of Happily Married Men.* But between the tears and stoicism, there's a happy medium. She wants to see some emotion to show that you have some depth and a range of reactions. "They want to know that you care about something," says Dr. Haltzman.

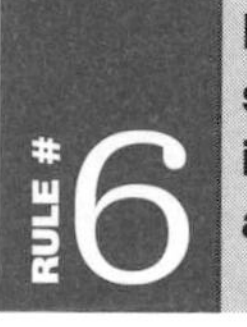

Be more spontaneous in the bedroom and out.

Make Her Your Centerfold

You have an awesome new camera. She's shy. We'll help.

Encourage Her

Even models who are paid for sexy photo shoots perform better when photographers say they're gorgeous. Talk her up, telling her how great she looks. And keep things light—if you joke around, she'll be more relaxed.

Choose Poses

Don't expect her to go all Bettie Page as soon as you start snapping. Instead, help her pick some poses that make her feel sexy. Start with these classics, which work whether she's naked or in a nightie.

1. Sitting at the edge of the bed with her legs drawn up, her head resting on her knees, and her chest against her thighs. Take a shot from the side.
2. Lying on her back diagonally across the bed with her head at the bottom corner. Have her raise her arms above her head and look back toward you. Tell her to arch her back and point her toes. (Her waist will look thinner and her legs longer.)

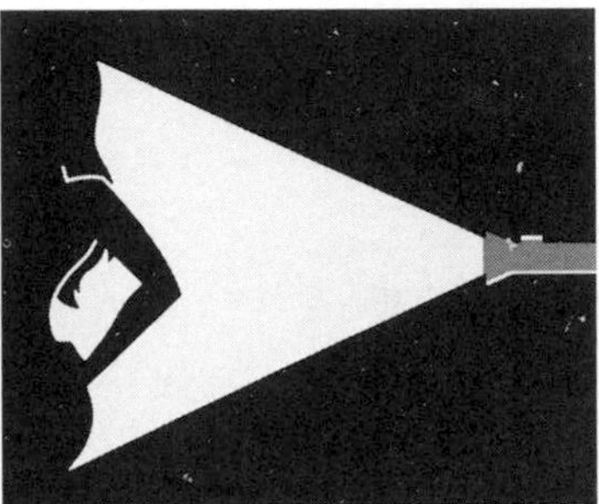

Play with Lighting

Automatic flashes aren't flattering. For a softer effect use flashlights or position two lamps, with shades, on each side of her. Or open the drapes and use natural light.

Set Your Camera

Switch to aperture (A or AV) mode. An aperture of 16 and a shutter speed of 1/30th of a second should work well in low light. For the best color, set your white balance to "tungsten" if you're using lamps. Then set your ISO: In low light, 400 to 1600 will work, with 400 giving you the smoothest result. (Experiment beforehand so you don't kill the mood with your camera fiddling.)

Don't Let Her Peek

You'll ruin the momentum if you let her look at every shot. Promise that you'll show her all of them—later, when you're both in bed.

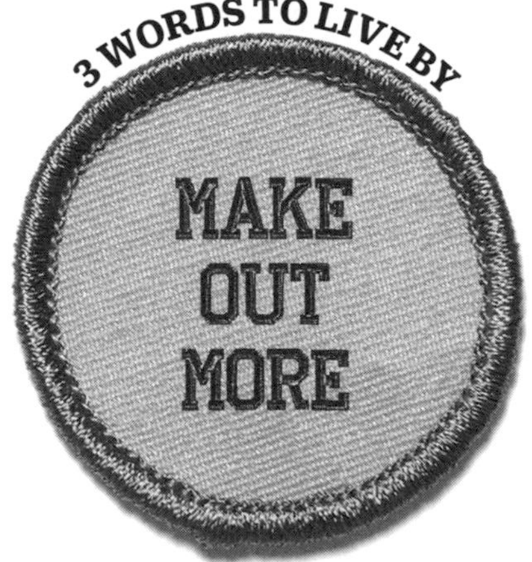
3 WORDS TO LIVE BY
MAKE
OUT
MORE

SHAMELESS PICKUP TRICK

FLY SOLO AT A WEDDING

The romantic setting primes the bride's single gal pals for pairing off. And as a friend of the couple, you've been prescreened. And there's dancing. And booze. Wear your best tailored suit. Men in perfectly fitting suits are more successful and confident than guys in ill-fitting off-the-rack attire, a British study shows.

SHAMELESS PICKUP TRICK

WORSHIP THE SUN

Sunshine casts you in a better light: Women are more likely to give a man their digits on a sunny day than on a cloudy one, according to a French study. Your line: "Don't you love the sun?" It can feel like you're celebrating together, so it's a perfect pickup tactic at the park. At the beach, invite her and her friends to play volleyball. Women feel vulnerable in beach situations when they're in minimal clothing. If your approach is social, she's more likely to say yes.

Show Her— YOUR PADDLE!

Sexual attraction really is primitive: Tackling "caveman challenges," like handling fire or swimming in moving water, is more alluring to women than taking modern risks like riding a motorcycle without a helmet, a University of Alaska study finds. Primal physical danger lets you flaunt your evolutionary fitness, the researchers say, but 21st-century risks only advertise poor character or lack of good judgment. Take your pick: rock climbing, whitewater kayaking, or deep-sea diving—the women in the study found them all sexy.

RULE # 7 **Among her favorite sex toys is the one at the end of your arm.**

Seduce Her WITH TWITTER

Laurie Davis, online dating coach and founder of eflirtexpert.com, explains how to tweet your way to a date.

STEP 1
THE PERFECT PROFILE

Twitter pics are tiny, so use a head shot in which your face and shoulders fill most of the frame. Keep your bio simple but specific.

STEP 2
FIND YOUR SCENE

To avoid awkward "I'm married" moments, follow @LuvatFirstTweet. Build your profile by answering questions that pop up in your Twitter feed. They'll match you with like-minded tweeters.

STEP 3
CHAT HER UP

Catch her eye by commenting on a conversation she's having or by delivering snappy one-liners about her love for the Yankees. The key to connecting is skipping bar talk ("What do you do for a living?") and talking about things as they happen.

STEP 4
TAKE IT BEHIND THE SCENES

If she seems responsive, DM her to amp things up. Now you can get a little flirty. Instant reply is part of Twitter's charm, so ditch the old "don't seem too eager" rule. Message to your heart's content, as long as she's into it.

STEP 5
MOVE OFFLINE

If the ultimate goal is to meet up, suggest a phone call or Skype session. If you're still not sure, suggest you meet her at a tweetup—a Twitter version of bar night in cities nationwide.

RULE # 8

"People who love each other and have a good relationship are best friends, and best friends are basically good to each other."—Michael McKee, PhD, a psychologist at the Cleveland Clinic

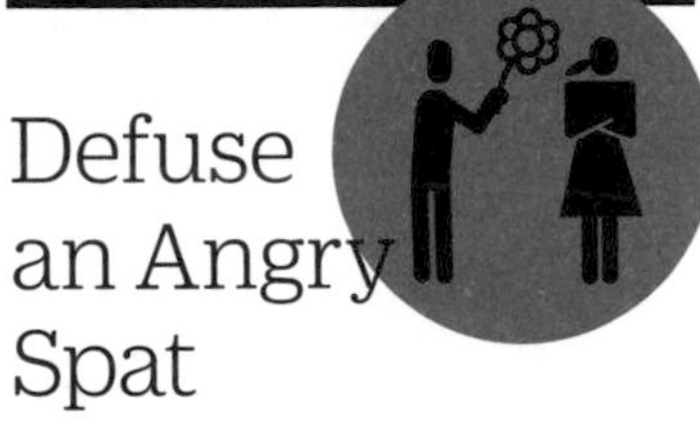

Defuse an Angry Spat

Therapist Don Cole helps you make peace at warp speed.

Call a Code Blue

... or any other predesigned safe word to signal a 30-minute time-out. The first step is getting both of you to a calmer place.

Snuff Your Fuse

Set your phone alarm for 25 minutes and use that time to distract yourself with something you enjoy doing, like shooting some hoops.

Be the Bigger Man

Spend 5 minutes of your time thinking about how you can be the first to take a *little* responsibility. Now it's her turn.

Survive the Spoon

She loves it, but you can't wait to liberate your arm and roll over for some real sleep. Give her the snuggle she craves—and then give yourself some space . . .

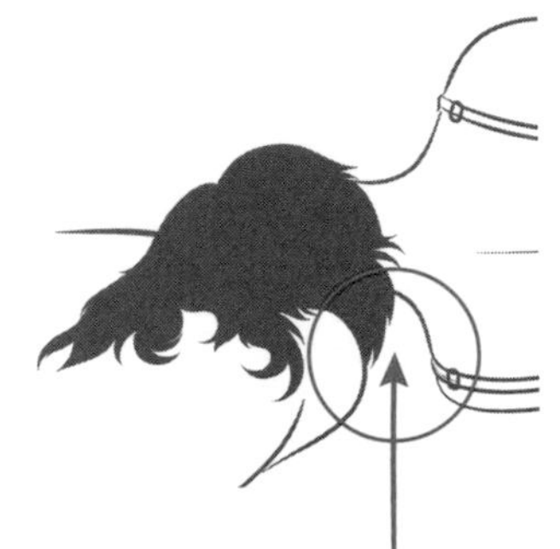

1 Make Room

Move both pillows about a foot down from the headboard. This provides room for your arms to extend above your head if that proves more comfortable.

2 Defeat "Dead Arm"

Assume a standard spooning position, but have her lie so just her head (not her neck) rests on the pillow. See that gap between her neck and the bed in the photo at the top? Instead of wedging your arm under her torso, thread it through the gap so it extends out in front of her body. Your other arm is free to wrap around her.

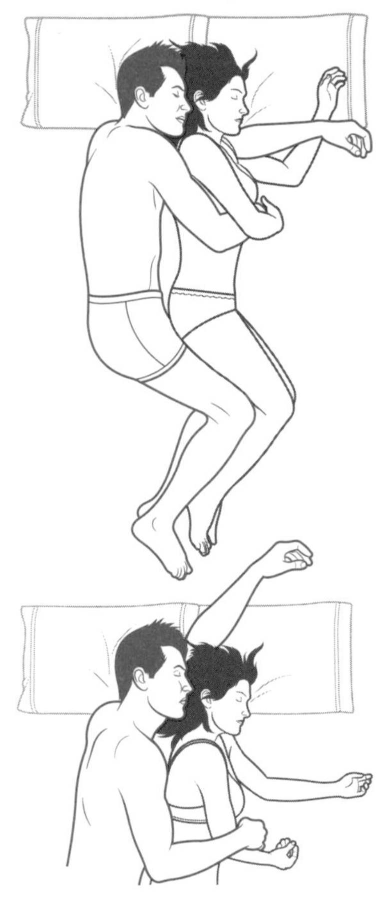

3 Withdraw Stealthily

Is she asleep? Slip your arm out from under her neck—the pillow will support her head. Now you can extend that arm overhead, Superman-style, toward the headboard, or tuck it between your body and hers. Now fall asleep—or roll over.

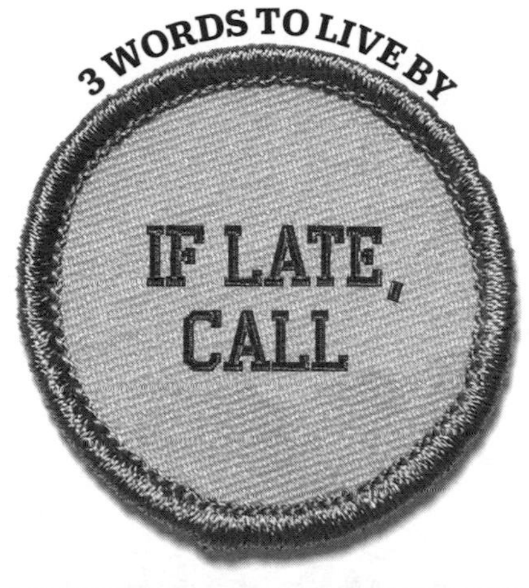
3 WORDS TO LIVE BY
IF LATE, CALL

Q Is it true that scary movies can actually turn women on?

A. Like a light. "Being scared is physiologically arousing, and in the right company, it may eventually carry over to sexual arousal," says Joanne Cantor, PhD, a professor emerita of communications at the University of Wisconsin, who studies the ways people are affected by media.

After the movie, your date may find your glances more erotically charged and your touches more stimulating. But watch out—trying to scare her into your arms could backfire. "If the movie turns out to be too much for her, she may start wondering why you brought her to see it, and her physiological reaction will just intensify that confusion," Cantor says. So if she isn't into over-the-top terror, à la *Saw VI,* watch a classic thriller instead, like *The Silence of the Lambs.*

READ HER SIGNALS

How often do you feel the heat? Frequency of touch is a primary predictor of relationship happiness among men, a Kinsey Institute study reveals. "Touch is inherently reciprocal. You can't touch without being touched," says Matthew Hertenstein, PhD, of DePauw University's touch and emotion lab. "And it's a very specific language—touch relays distinct emotions, not just 'bad' or 'good.'" One problem: Some men aren't good at perceiving women's skin-to-skin signals, he says. Use this chart to decode her touch—and never mistake her sad snuggle for her sexy cuddle again.

	WHERE SHE'LL MAKE CONTACT	HOW SHE'LL DO IT
anger	Shoulder, arm	Push, shake, hit, squeeze, slap
fear	Arm, face, shoulder, hand	Press, light touch, shake, squeeze
happiness	Arm, hand	Swing, shake, squeeze, high-five
sadness	Hand, shoulder	Nuzzle, light touch, stroke, rub
disgust	Arm, hand	Push, slap
love	Shoulder, hand	Hug, light touch, stroke

Fact: 97 Percentage of women who say a man's sense of humor is as important as his physical attractiveness

Source: Match's Singles in America study, 2015

Rescue a Woman from a PARTY BORE

She's been cornered by some blowhard. Your mission: Save her! Here's how, according to UCLA psychologist Gerald Goodman, PhD.

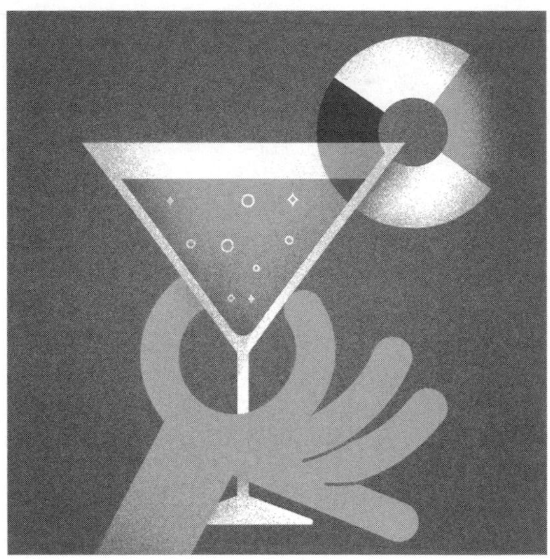

Do Some Reconnaissance

Make sure she actually wants to be rescued. Are her arms crossed? Is she checking her phone a lot? Has she locked eyes with you across the room? Is she mouthing the word "help" every time he turns away? Yep, those are pretty unmistakable signal flares.

Create a Diversion

When you sense a lull in their "conversation," casually approach and introduce yourself to both of them. Find the common ground. Go with something like, "So, how do you two know our host?" Or ask if they've tried the killer martinis. Once you're in, focus more on him. When you show him respect, he feels less threatened by you.

Be the Bore Antidote

Do the exact opposite of what he's doing; she doesn't need two gasbags to deal with. You'll come across as the more appealing guy. Analyze his movements. Is he talking her ear off and obnoxiously laughing at his own jokes? Then avoid cheap humor and let her lead the conversation. Is he hitting on her yet staring at every pair of breasts that pass by? Then it's your job to keep your gaze on her.

Shift Your Interest

Once his guard is down—he's talking more slowly, his shoulders are relaxed—switch your focus to her. Ask questions that prompt thoughtful responses. ("What else would you be doing tonight if you weren't here?") Keep your eyes solely on her and follow up on her responses. This helps transition the three-way chat into something a bit more exclusive. If he tries to steal the spotlight, shift your body so you're facing only her. Then proceed with your conversation.

Spirit Her Away

At the next lull, say it's been a pleasure and tell him you'll see him around. Mention to her that you're off to grab another drink and casually invite her along. By doing this, you're not only bypassing confrontation but also making it clear to the schmo that he's uninvited. Plus, if she follows, it reassures you that she was interested in you in the first place.

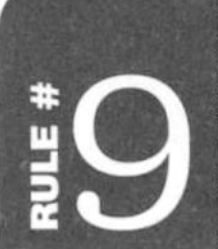

Mastering the fine art of etiquette could make the difference between a date and a blow-off. Use your manners always and as naturally as possible even if you think women are nowhere near. They are or will be as soon as you slack off. Women notice men who display class.

Keep It in Your Pants

Your wad of Benjamins, that is. Women are more attracted to men who save money, a University of Michigan study reveals. Dating profiles of people who stated that they'd save most of a financial windfall were deemed 36 percent more desirable than profiles of those who'd spend it. Saving shows self-control, says study author Scott Rick, PhD, but spending can signal rash behaviors like belligerence or even cheating. So don't be a tightwad, but do point out your smart-money ways.

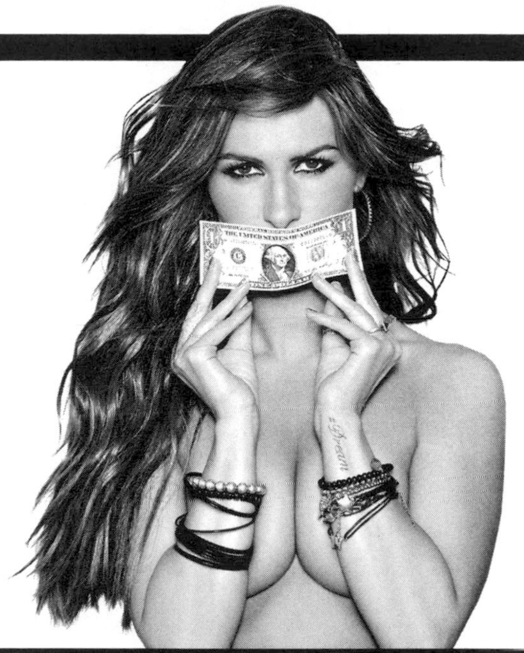

Fact:

14+ inches: Female hip width correlated with a greater likelihood of agreeing to a one-night stand, according to a study in the *Archives of Sexual Behavior.*

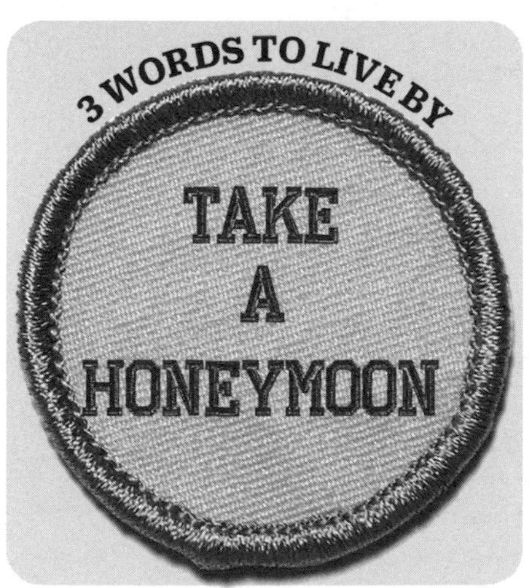
3 WORDS TO LIVE BY
TAKE
A
HONEYMOON

Slow Dance with Her

Find the Beat

Try tapping your foot to the beat. Listen for a "quick, quick, slow" rhythm or a moment when your foot can pause.

Lead Firmly

Imagine your stomach guiding you in each step's direction—this will give you a stronger lead.

Make a Box

Step forward slowly with your left foot; take two beats to do it. Bring your right foot forward and to the right (quick: in one beat) and place your left foot beside it (quick). Step backward on your right foot (slow) and take a side step with your left foot (quick), bringing in your right foot (quick). Repeat.

Fact:

44 **Percentage of men who prefer a woman to be totally bare down there.**

4 Gifts She'll Want to Unwrap

We polled the readers *of Women's Health* to find out which types of gifts they prefer most. Here are the top picks, plus the smartest, easiest ways to buy them.

Event Tickets

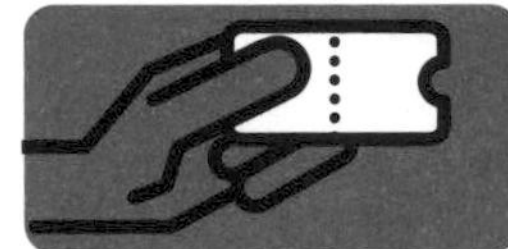

Go to eventful.com to find out which concerts, festivals, comedians, and plays are coming to your town. Just remember, this is for her, not you.

Jewelry

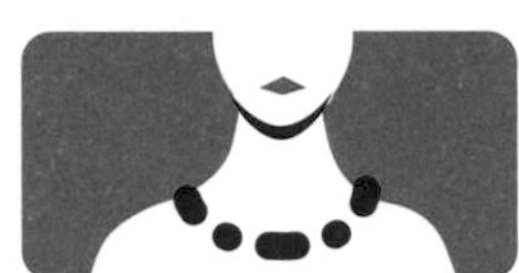

Red Envelope lets you engrave a personal message. But skip the rings unless you're proposing, says Tracy Steinberg, author of *Flirt for Fun & Meet the One.*

Spa Treatment

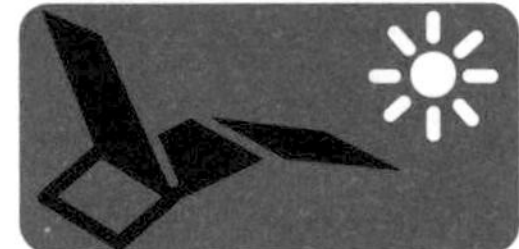

Many spas sell package deals that let her choose from a menu of services, says Steinberg. So don't try to guess what she wants; give her options.

Fitness Gear

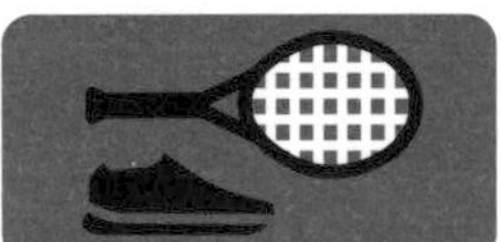

Sign up for The Clymb, a site that offers deals up to 70 percent off retail. Once you've purchased her gift, you can cancel the daily e-mails.

Feeling Light-Headed?

It takes about 3 ounces of blood to make your penis erect.

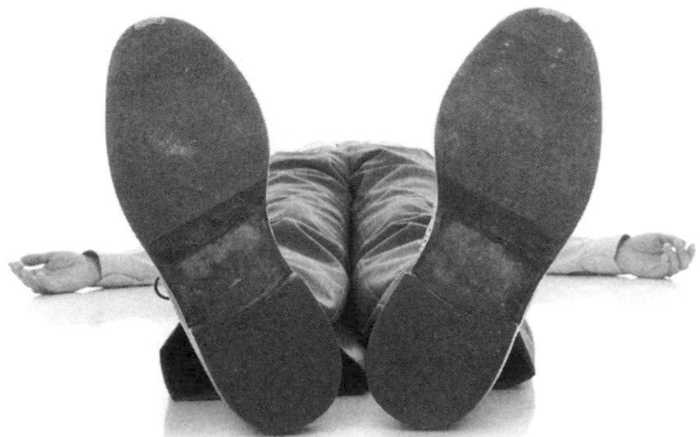

Speak Her Language

CAN'T TELL WHAT SHE MEANS? HERE'S A CHEAT SHEET.

- WHAT SHE SAYS
- **WHAT SHE MEANS**

"Are you hungry?"

I'm starving. Feed me.

"You g-chat with my best friend?"

That's weird. Find your own friends.

"Are you coming to my family's party?"

You're coming to my family's party.

"We can do whatever you want to do tonight."

Please, please, please let's do what I want to do.

"I'm fine."

I'm totally not fine. And if you'd paid attention to that tiny change in my voice, you'd know something's up and address it.

"How dressy is this event we're attending together?"

Tell me everything you know about it, including its location, who's invited, what you'll be wearing, if there will be dancing, and whether the other women there will be wearing heels.

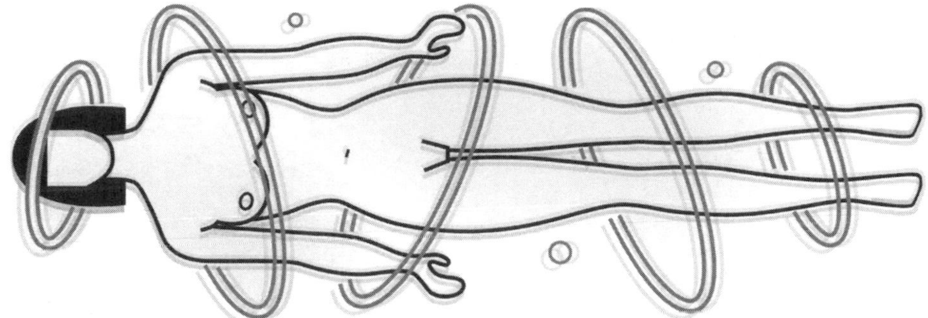

How Hormones Make Women Act Wacky

She's suddenly furious.

The cause: Low progesterone

Next time she tears your head off over nothing, it may be because her progesterone level plummeted. This hormone controls the junctions where neurons exchange messages. In days prior to a woman's period, her progesterone drops, making those synapses extra-excitable.

Best defense: Wait it out. "Don't even ask her what she wants for dinner—just make something," suggests Louann Brizendine, MD, a neuropsychiatrist and author of *The Female Brain*.

She bawls uncontrollably.

The cause: Too much cortisol

The dial that determines how intensely people feel emotion is located in the amygdala, the part of the brain that processes memory and feelings. Those emotions are balanced by the calm, rational part of the brain, the prefrontal cortex. A surge in the stress hormone cortisol can crowd out signals from the prefrontal cortex, letting the amygdala run amok.

Best defense: Hold her. Trying to solve the problem will only make things worse. Physical contact boosts levels of oxytocin, which should counterbalance the cortisol.

She's Martha Stewart on acid.

The cause: High estrogen and oxytocin

These two hormones bring out her innate (and often annoying) mothering instincts. "This usually happens the week after her period ends," says Dr. Brizendine.

Best defense: Clean the house without being asked and she may show her appreciation by helping you buff the dining-room floor, together.

The Kama Sutra of Cuddling

Snuggling doesn't necessarily conclude with blue balls. One in three people in a University of Michigan study said that snuggling usually leads to sex. Study author Sari van Anders, PhD says, "People who enjoy and frequently engage in cuddling are often the same people who frequently engage in sex." Some useful statcs that may help ensure that your spooning ends with forking (percentages may not add up to 100 percent if more than one response was given):

Activities While Cuddling:

66% Movies/TV
18% Sleep/rest
3% Eating
28% Talking
14% Reading
2% Games
24% Massage
5% Music

Coverage While Cuddling:

15% Nude
64% Partially clothed
21% Clothed

Why People Snuggle:

7% Sex
17% Feeling safe
20% Affection
15% Feels good
20% Relaxation
24% Intimacy

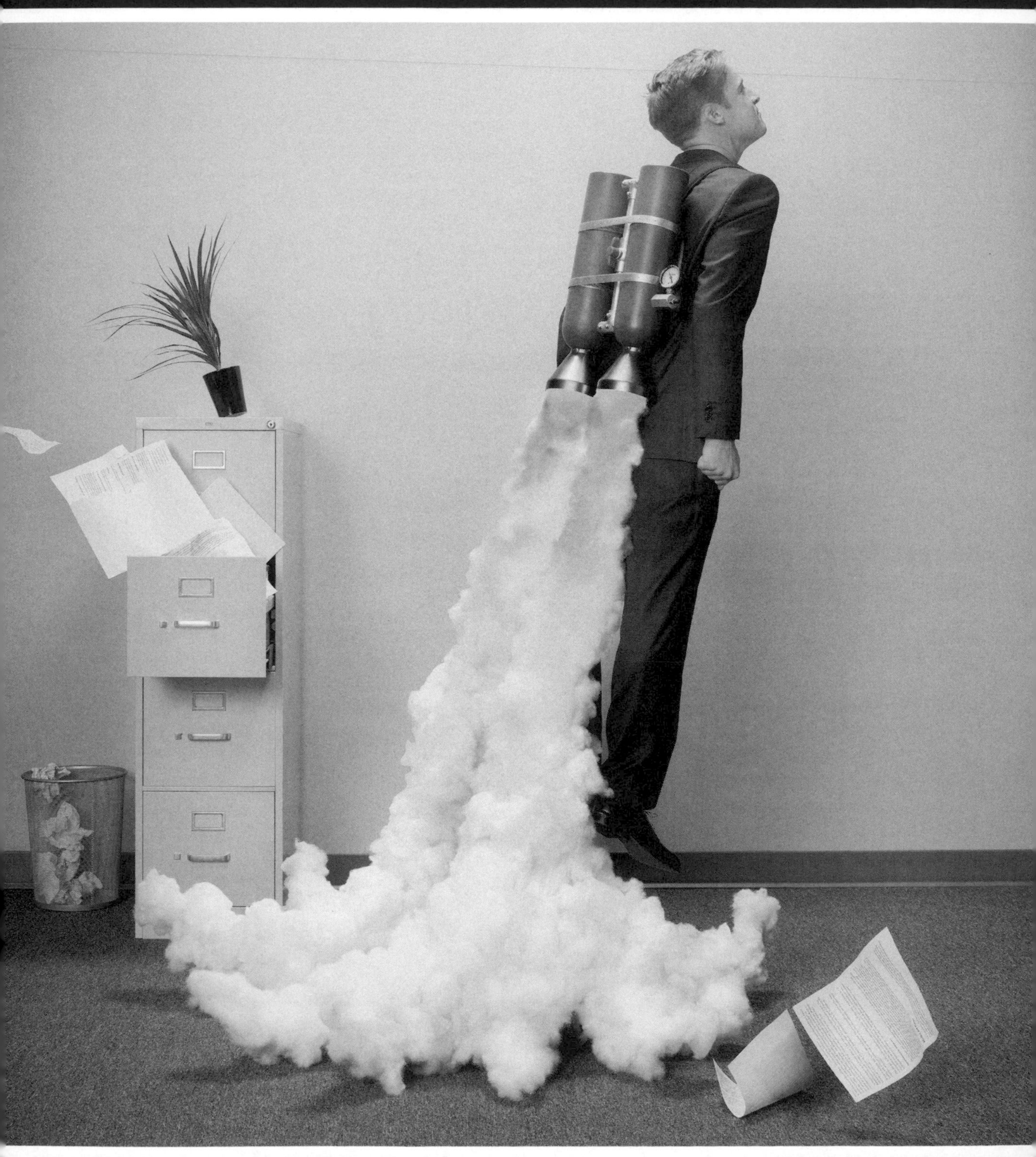

Work

Survival Strategies for the Daily Grind and Those Times When You Must Travel for Business

Remember the good ol' days of secure employment when budgets were flush, pompous senior management didn't exist, mergers and acquisitions and layoffs never ruined your day, and you could always count on raises and even bonuses? Of course you don't, because those days never happened, or if they did, you were still in high school.

Nope. Work is tough, just like it always has been, and now, thanks to required sensitivity training seminars, it may even suck more. When it comes to working, we are huge advocates of finding a good mentor and cultivating that relationship. Why? Because a guy or gal who's been through it all can dispense useful advice that'll help you avoid the potholes of postmodern office politics and manage today's Machiavellian managers. They will energize your work and help you to succeed. They also usually have a bottle of good bourbon close at hand.

If you can't secure a mentor before your next performance review, then sit down, son, and read through the workaday wisdom on the next few pages. It'll be a good start, and there will be time for mentors. After all, you're going to be working for a long, long time.

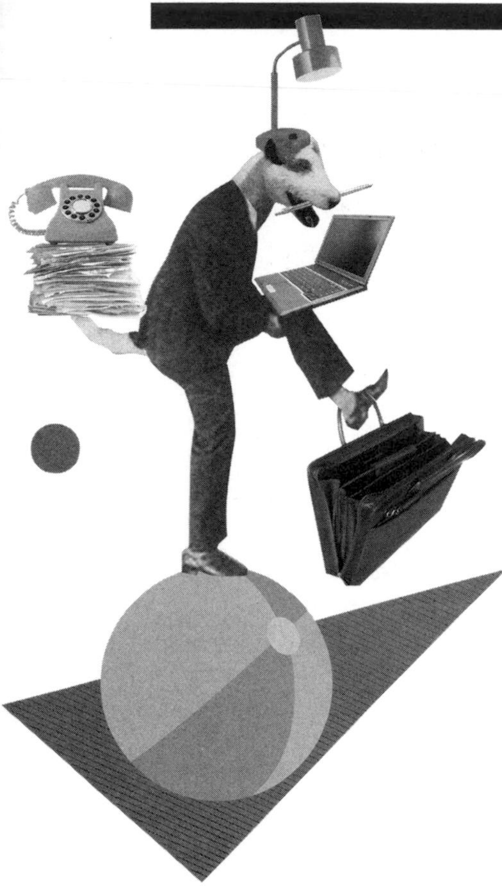

How to Train Your Boss *Like a Dog*

HE MAY LEAD, BUT YOU CAN BE HIS MASTER.

He's Shouting at You

Your move: When he's angry about something, don't give him any guff. Wait for him to calm down, and then offer a bit of good news to please him.

Why it works: Dog trainers call this the "least reinforcing scenario." Like dogs, people feed off reactions. Bossy dogs stop barking if you ignore the noise and instead focus on rewarding them for keeping quiet. So will bossy bosses.

He's Dumping Bottom-Barrel Work on You

Your move: Stay busy, limit chitchat, and trumpet your new projects.

Why it works: When a dog wishes to disengage from another dog's advances, it often sniffs the ground as if terribly engrossed in a scent—a cutoff signal. Similarly, your boss is less likely to interrupt you with a trivial assignment when he senses you're already busy.

You Can't Keep His Attention

Your move: Improve your body language so he'll focus on you. Use assertive hand gestures. Make eye contact, smile, and be animated. If your boss is walking, fall into step and match his gait.

Why it works: Dogs stand tall when they're being assertive. They move with purpose. If you do the same, your boss will respond instinctively.

RULE # 1

Never tell anyone "Welcome aboard!" unless you're on an actual boat.

What's the Safest Stall in the Men's Room?

The closest one to the men's room door. It has the fewest germs and the most toilet paper, because everyone walks past it.

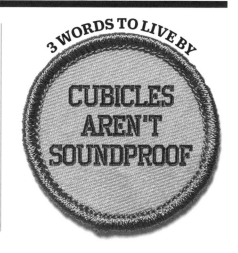

3 WORDS TO LIVE BY
CUBICLES
AREN'T
SOUNDPROOF

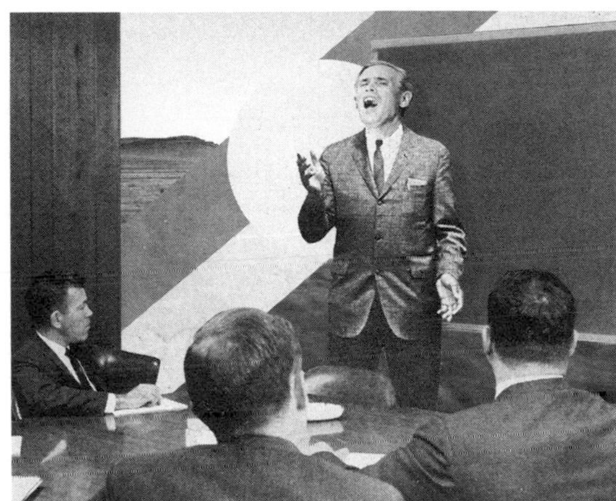

Give an Award-Winning Presentation

Using PowerPoint to make your point is like asking a woman for a date via e-mail. Got something to say? Then lose the pointer and keep your listeners tuned in with this professional-tested attack plan. Think about it: When was the last time you saw Barack Obama run a slideshow?

Amp It Up

Use exaggerated hand movements. It may feel over the top, so practice in front of a mirror until the actions look natural.

Use Catchphrases

An attorney trying to win over a jury might say a defendant put "profits over people." Such phrases can make a speech forceful.

Add Reference

If you're talking about a product, hold one up along with a competitor's to show differences. Props kill monotony.

Ask Questions

Pose some of your own to spark a conversation. Your audience will be more enthusiastic—and you'll avoid awkward silence if nobody raises a hand.

5 Things to Lose When You Graduate and Get a Job

1. Futons

As an adult earning a paycheck, your bed and couch should be two separate things, not a single piece of furniture that hurts both your spinal cord and your dignity.

2. Ramen Noodles

When you are earning a paycheck, the criteria for a meal shouldn't be whether it costs less than a quarter.

3. Dirty Bathrooms

Penn State University researchers did a study of almost 500 bathroom sink drains in 131 buildings around the country and discovered a high frequency of fusarium, a fungus known to cause ringworm and potentially blinding corneal infections. Can you afford Clorox?

4. Novelty Condoms

Safe sex isn't something that gets less relevant as you get older. But a penis with the smirking face of Gene Simmons isn't a good look on somebody who files a tax return.

5. Creative Facial Hair

Sure, facial hair can be a great way to create a new identity with very little effort or expense. But unless you work for the New Jersey Department of Transportation, you shouldn't need a Fu Manchu or a handlebar to announce to the world, "Hey, look at me! I'm unique and interesting!"

Survive the Office *Secret Santa*

A poll of almost 400 *Men's Health* readers turned up these top three Secret Santa gifts they'd most like to receive from a coworker. Buy one and you're in the clear.

1. Six-pack of craft beer
2. Local restaurant gift certificate
3. iTunes gift certificate

Don't spend more than $20. Most guys we polled say that's the amount they would spend.

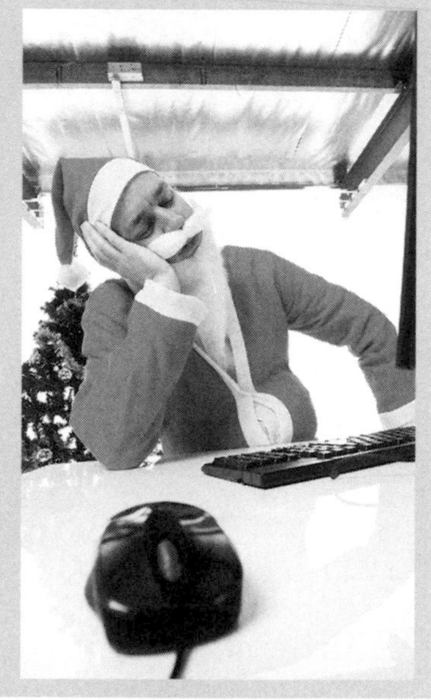

Plan a Great Holiday Party

To estimate the number of invitations, follow this formula. Number of people you want to attend X 0.6 = Y number of people to invite

How it works: Thirty percent of the people you invite to a holiday party will RSVP to decline, and 15 percent of people who say yes won't show up, according to Lara Shriftman, coauthor of *Party Confidential*. This formula, from the UCLA math department, factors in both.

How to Ask for a Raise

In a perfect world the boss would drop a stack of Benjamins on your desk and hand you a bottle of Johnnie Walker Blue every quarter along with a slap on the back. That ain't happenin'. If you want something, you have to ask for it. Especially money and promotions. Here's how to do it:

1. Timing Is Everything

You can't just barge into your boss's office unannounced, demanding a handsome reward—you'll have to be a bit more methodical. Wait until you and your team nail a big project to bring up a raise. Chances are the success will prompt a congratulatory note from your boss, which is your cue to schedule a meeting, says Jim Hopkinson, author of the book *Salary Tutor: Learn the Salary Negotiation Secrets No One Ever Taught You.* Ask to sit down and discuss your accomplishments several months before your annual performance review—which is when your boss might automatically grant a smaller salary bump than you're looking for. "If you walk in to your review and they've already given you a 4-percent raise, there's not a lot of room to play off of that," says Hopkinson.

2. Sell Yourself

Once you've scheduled a face-to-face meeting, do your homework. Find the current market rate for your position on sites like PayScale.com, Salary.com, and Glassdoor.com, and bring it with you to the meeting. Combine the report with a personal portfolio as if you were on a job interview, and emphasize your accomplishments. Say something like, "These were the three goals you outlined at the kickoff meeting this year, and here's how I accomplished all of them." "It's all about the bottom line," says Hopkinson. Your three selling points: "Here's what I'm doing, here are the skills I'm bringing to the table, and here's what the marketplace is like." It's hard to argue with results, after all.

3. Silence Is Golden

Sometimes the best thing to say during a negotiation is nothing

Master the Art of Small Talk

Chitchat your way out of three potentially uncomfortable conversations. Heck, you might even befriend the boss.

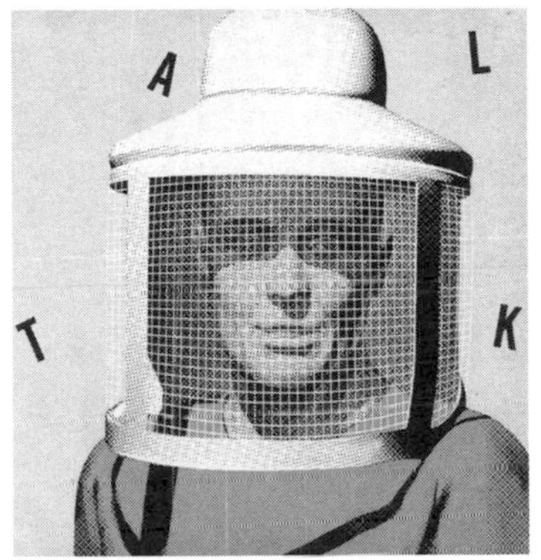

Your boss in the elevator

Resist the urge to pitch an idea. Instead, use the opportunity as a setup to pitch. Talk about a shared interest—Thai food, baseball. Then, after some banter, close with, "Glad I caught you, actually. Do you have a minute this week to discuss a new idea I have?"

Random dude running an errand

Look, he's being nice. So when he comments on envelope prices at the post office, counter with a joke. ("Yeah, and they don't taste any better either.") You're showing lighthearted goodwill. Consider it practice for when a gorgeous woman chats you up.

You're not knowledgeable about the topic

Ask a question that throws the ball back into the inquisitor's court and compliments his intelligence. People love to grab the spotlight, and this distraction will take the spotlight off your lack of knowledge.

at all, Hopkinson says. It's an old FBI technique: If your boss says, "We were thinking of a 5-percent raise," simply repeat, "5 percent," and be quiet. "It's a great technique where if he's nervous or thinking of a higher figure, it just makes him reveal more than he really wants to," he says. By mirroring what your boss says and then shutting up, it'll force him to fill that silence and offer you more money.

4. Anchor the Deal

Here's an alternative tactic that works every time: Throw out your figure before your boss can. "Let them know that *this* is the number you want," urges Charles Naquin, PhD, a professor of management at DePaul University and author of *The Essentials of Job Negotiations*. "Otherwise he's left in a void. You want more money, but how much is more money? So put a number out there for him to lock his mind around—as long as it's based on logic, like what your peers are getting. Be up front, be rational, and just tell him what you want."

5. Try, Try Again

If a raise just isn't happening—your company finished in the red last quarter and there's not enough room in the budget—don't let it deter you. Simply schedule another meeting by asking, "When can I talk with you again?" "The word 'no' is predicated upon conditions at a certain period of time," says Herb Cohen, author of *You Can Negotiate Anything!* "A month, 2 months, or 3 months later is different. So you persist. You come in 3 months later, tell him again what your problem is—that you'd like better compensation—and if you persevere, you'll ultimately get what you want," Cohen says.

RULE #2

You will catch a cold within a week of taking a red-eye and within 2 weeks of starting a new job.

TAKE A MENTAL HEALTH DAY

PLAN, EXECUTE, AND ENJOY THE PERFECT DAY OF HOT-WEATHER HOOKY. THIRTY-TWO PERCENT OF WORKERS PLAYED HOOKY LAST YEAR, A CAREERBUILDER SURVEY FOUND. ONE RESPONDENT'S EXCUSE WAS, "I ACCIDENTALLY HIT A NUN WITH MY MOTORCYCLE." DON'T BE THAT GUY.

1. Consult Your Calendar

Despite his comb-over, your boss isn't an idiot. To his discerning eye, a missed Monday or Friday equals a 3-day weekend. Tuesday through Thursday is your hooky safe zone.

2. Craft Your Excuse

Choose an affliction you've experienced, so you can describe symptoms. Diarrhea or food poisoning is great. "Everybody knows what it is, and no one wants to ask about it," says Kerry Speckman, author of *The Hooky Book*.

3. Stay Under the Radar

Steer clear of social media. Even if your boss isn't your Facebook friend, coworkers who are may clue him in. Don't update your status. Don't tweet about your day off. And switch off your Google account's G-chat.

4. Return to Work Safely

At the office, you may be tempted to elaborate on your story to cover your tracks—but don't. "Maintain that little bit of doubt," says Speckman. Watch your nonverbals, too. A haircut or sunburn can be damning.

How to Bounce Back from a Screwup

With eye contact and an even tone, say "I totally screwed up. I'm sorry." Then stop talking. You've owned the problem, and your brevity displays respect and sincerity. Rambling makes it about you (bad) and leads to excuses (worse).

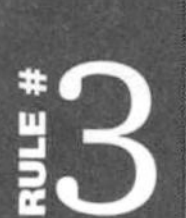

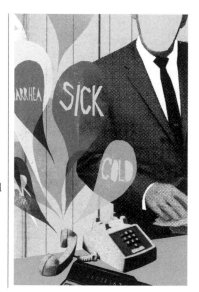

RULE #3 **Smile more. People like to be around those who smile, because it suggests not only that the person being smiled at is well regarded, but also that they'll feel better.**

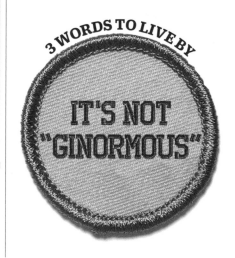

Outsmart Your Office Frenemy

DEFEND YOUR CAREER WITH TIPS FROM FATHALI MOGHADDAM, PHD, A PROFESSOR OF CONFLICT RESOLUTION AT GEORGETOWN UNIVERSITY.

Know Thy Frenemy

To gauge your colleague's trust, share some harmless but private way you've bent the rules, like how you occasionally take a personal day to golf. If the info leaks to your other coworkers, it's on.

Wield Your Words

If you're forced to work together, deploy phrases like "We make a good team," which encourages him to cooperate. Also try something like "I'm on board with that idea. It could be even better if . . ." You'll seem more focused on solutions than on fighting.

Buddy Up to the Boss

Regularly communicating with your superior gives you more leverage. Don't whine about your nemesis. Volunteer for new projects as your boss dreams them up. You'll look proactive (and promotable) and ice the frenemy out.

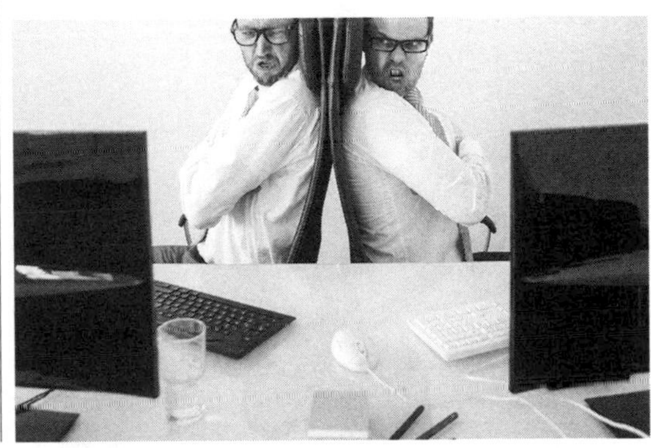

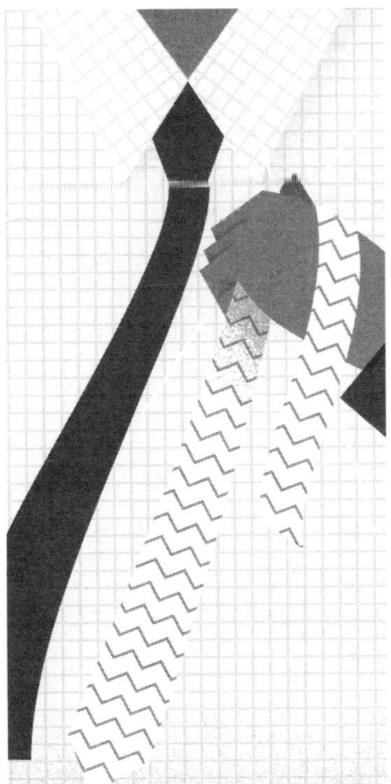

Write a Kick-Ass Recommendation

Make that reference matter, says Andrew Simmons, PhD, director of Brown University's Career Development Center.

Gather Data

Ask your colleague for a copy of the position description and job listing. Many writers repeat qualifications, flubbing the chance to extol the candidate's character traits—something a résumé can't convey.

Avoid the Spotlight

Dedicate only a sentence or two to your own introduction. Cite the number of years and capacity in which you and your colleague worked together. Anything more takes the focus off the candidate.

Tell a Good Story

If you remember your friend's game-changing idea, it'll also stand out to an employer. Write the anecdote highlighting your colleague's positive traits and how he or she benefited the company.

Whittle It Down

Keep it to one page, max. Recruiters read a lot of these. For LinkedIn recommendations, aim for a one-paragraph summary. Any longer taxes attention spans.

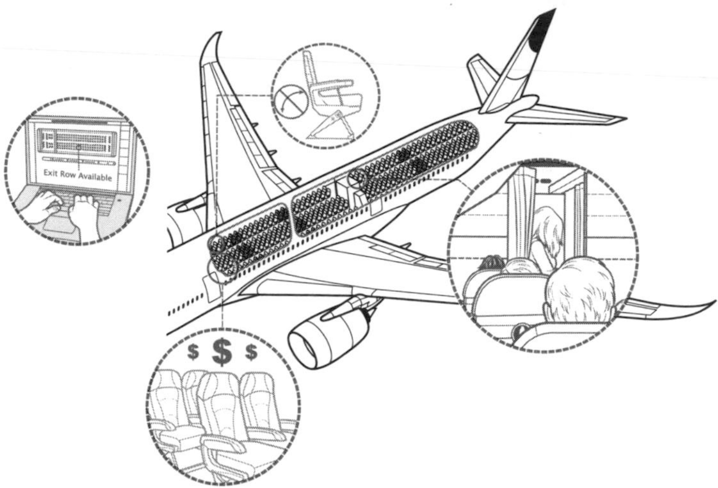

Land the Best Seat on a Plane

UNCOMMON KNOWLEDGE FOR MAKING THE BEST OF AIR TRAVEL.

Double-Check

Even if you picked your seat when you bought your ticket, check that you still have the seat a week before departure. Airlines sometimes swap planes to adjust for passenger load, resetting seat assignments.

Upgrade at the Last Minute

Go online 24 hours before your flight to check on exit-row seats. They may have opened up after the airline moved passengers who didn't fit the seating criteria (good hearing, English speaking, and so forth). If there are two back-to-back exit rows, pick the second—first-row seats often don't recline.

Forget the Front Row

Don't be fooled into picking from a section called "preferred seats" or "express seats." That's just the airline charging you extra for those front rows. Lame. Pick seats directly behind these rows; they're just as good.

Avoid Noise

If you're on a big jet and the front is booked, pick the middle of any section to steer clear of excess noise. Don't sit near the galleys, where flight attendants chat and prepare food. And avoid bulkheads (partitions between seating sections); they may have built-in baby cradles.

Have the Boss Hear You Out

Send your big ideas to your fearless leader between 6:30 a.m. and 7:30 a.m., so they jump to the top of the in-box, says Dan Zarrella, author of *The Social Media Marketing Book*. Hitting "send" late at night may annoy a recipient whose work e-mail and cell phone are linked.

How to Beat Jet Lag

- Drink plenty of water before, during, and after your flight.
- Set your watch to the local time of your destination as you board the plane and try to sleep on that local schedule.
- Don't drink caffeine after 10 a.m. the day of your flight.
- Don't drink alcohol before or during the flight.
- Don't eat during the flight. It will make it harder for you to sleep.
- Don't go to bed earlier than 10 p.m. at your destination.

RULE # 4

Never continue talking to a coworker after he enters a bathroom stall and sits down.

Make Sure Your Luggage Arrives When You Do

Over 100,000 passengers on US airlines report mishandled baggage every month, according to the US Department of Transportation. Protect your stuff.

❶ Prep the Bag

Slip your travel itinerary and contact info into an outside pocket. If the destination info is lost, baggage handlers will check there first for ID.

❷ Pack to Prevent TSA Tampering

If TSA agents spot something suspicious, they'll open your bag, which could delay it from making your flight. So help them out. Loop your cell phone charger's cord and secure it with a rubber band; that way it won't look suspicious on an x-ray. And pack fancy footwear on top for easy access. Shoes with metal supports often trip up security.

❸ Secure Your Gear

Remove any loose straps and line up zippers and locks under the luggage handle. This reduces the chance of the bag snagging on the conveyor belt. If you want to lock your suitcase, do it with a TSA-approved lock (travelsentry.org), so inspectors can gain access with their tools.

❹ Budget Your Time

Yes, you can sprint to your gate in 7 minutes. Your suitcase, however, cannot. Allow at least 90 minutes for luggage processing—and tack on 30 more for peak travel times, says Susan Foster, author of *Smart Packing for Today's Traveler.*

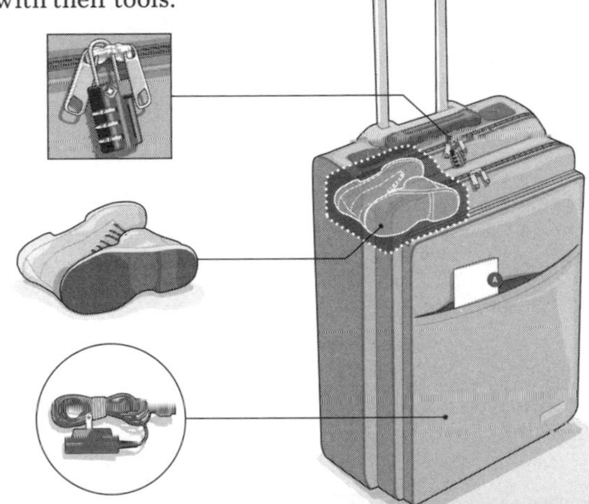

Protect Your Dress Shoes

To keep a shine and prevent scratches while traveling, wrap each shoe in tissue paper, says Alexander Mattinson, lead butler at the St. Regis Deer Valley in Park City, Utah. Your clothes won't pick up shoe polish, and your shoes won't bang around in a shoe bag. Use white tissue paper; dyes may rub off on your clothes.

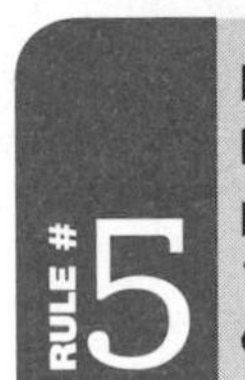

Every 5 mph you drive over 50 is like paying an additional 25 cents per gallon of gas. That means for a 15-gallon tank, doing 80 costs an extra $22.50.

SCORE A HOTEL ROOM UPGRADE

CHAIN HOTELS WANT YOU BACK TO THEIR LOCATIONS, SO IT'S THE FRONT DESK'S JOB TO MAKE YOU AS HAPPY AS POSSIBLE. THAT MEANS UPGRADING—IF YOU ASK NICELY.

Learn the Lingo

Before you arrive, look up the names of the hotel's high-end suites. If you ask for the honeymoon suite at a hotel that doesn't have one, you could strike out. But mention a specific room by name, and odds are better that the front desk will come through.

Be Specific

Instead of simply asking for a "better" room, say what you want, like a pool view. This simplifies the clerk's search. If you fail, try again later in the day. By 5 p.m., the hotel should know whether there are any great rooms to spare.

Make Friends

Your chances of an upgrade increase if it's a birthday or weekend away with your gal. Mention that you want to do everything you can to make the visit special.

Point Out Mistakes

In the Yelp era, hotels want to seem willing to accommodate if they screwed up. If your AC is stuck, they'd rather move you to a nicer room than trouble you with spot-treating the problem.

Negotiate Options

If there really are no other rooms, ask for a one-night perk, such as free Wi-Fi, breakfast, or gym access.

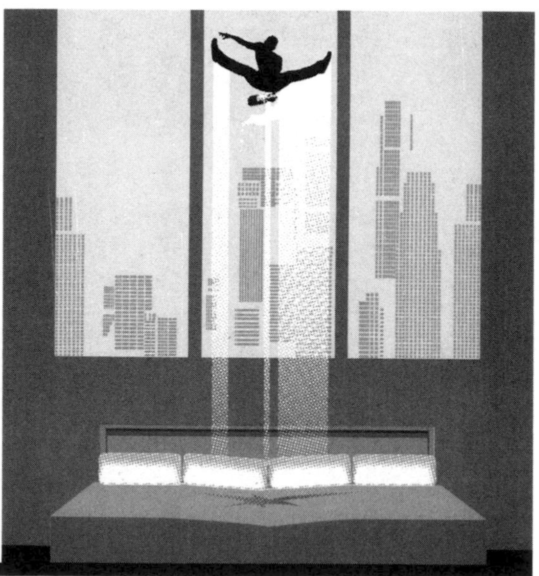

Know When to Shut Up

In these situations, it's best to zip your lip, says Teller, the silent partner in magic/comedy duo Penn & Teller.

You've Wrapped Up an Argument

Move on! Don't yield to the temptation to overapologize or ask for an apology. That always turns into "I was wrong, but I'd never have done that if you hadn't . . ." Just keep quiet and return to normalcy.

You're Tempted to Fight via E-Mail

Don't. You'll find yourself chained to the computer, trying in vain to come up with an argument an attorney would write. Incidentally, never argue with attorneys by e-mail. Arguing is their profession.

Tempers Flare in a Meeting You Lead

Take a tea break. First, you lead by example, staying polite and hospitable. Second, it suggests that you have better things to do. Third, tea—especially mint tea—has a way of bringing everybody back to sanity!

Spin a Pen in Your Fingers

Be the main distraction at your next staff meeting with this dizzyingly slick around-the-thumb maneuver.

1. Find Your Balance

A perfect pen flip is all about balance. Pen tips tend to weigh more, so place the cap on the back of the pen to even out the weight distribution.

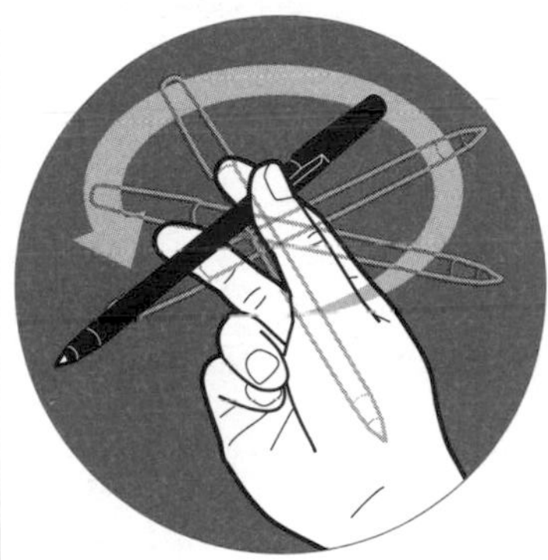

2. Form a Launch Pad

Make a peace sign with the index and middle fingers of your dominant hand, with slightly less than an inch from fingertip to fingertip. Fold down your ring finger and pinkie to keep them out of the way. Let your thumb rest naturally.

3. Center It

With palm facing up, place the pen's center of balance on the tip of your middle finger and let the rest of the pen fall onto the tip of your index finger. Place your thumb on the opposite side of the pen and grip lightly. Your thumb should be between your middle and index fingers.

4. Snap Forward

Your goal is to spin the pen counterclockwise around your thumb and then catch it where it started. To launch the move, mimic snapping your fingers—just flick your middle finger past your thumb while keeping your index finger and thumb still. The motion should sling the pen all the way around your thumb—well, after about 85 attempts.

5. Bring It Back

The catch is all about timing. After one revolution, the pen will land between your thumb and index finger. Clamp down with your index finger to stop the pen. Repeat steps 1 through 5 until your meeting is over. You'll probably need about 30 minutes of practice to nail this, so preserve your coworkers' sanity: Practice at home.

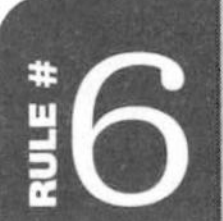

Good judgment comes from experience, and experience comes from bad judgment.

Land a Job by Voicemail

"No one has time to listen to a message that rambles on longer than 30 seconds," says Dominic Bokich, author of *Sex and Your Job Search*. After introducing yourself, say you have three recommendations on your LinkedIn profile and that you've noted your Web site on the résumé you sent last week. Short. Smart.

Streamline Your Smartphone

Most phones are optimized for thumb use, says Jennifer Jolly, host of *USA Today*'s digital video show *Tech Now*. So place your four most used apps at the bottom, where your thumbs have quick access. For more ease, name folders after active verbs ("read" for news apps, "play" for games) to connect the task with the label.

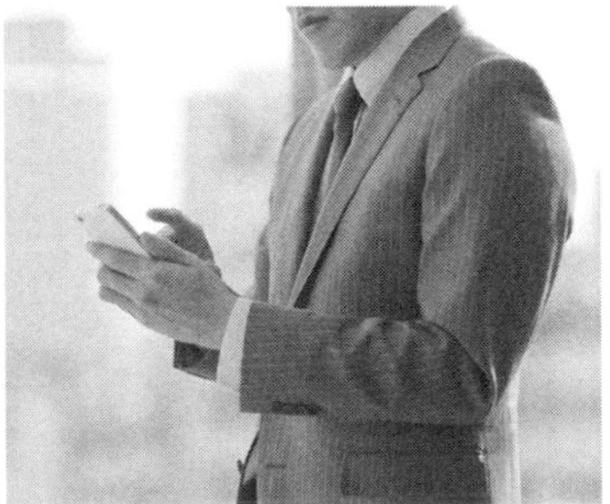

Drink with the Boss—and Keep Your Job

For Charlie Whitfield, brand ambassador for The Macallan, drinking on the job is the job. He conducts tastings on behalf of the whiskey company and has some advice for mixing work and play successfully.

1. Order Smart

The boss will probably pay, so let him order first. As a stalling tactic, ask for a drinks menu and scan it until he decides. Then order a similarly priced drink.

2. Make Fluid Conversation

Ask about his order: "I haven't had their IPA, but I love that brewery." This sort of chatting about brews and breweries can lead to other nonwork topics, such as travel and food.

3. Open the Shop Talk

Wait for the boss to bring up work, and then ease into your big idea. If he asks a tough question, sip your drink to buy time. Collaboration, not interrogation, best fits the laid-back mood.

4 Survive the Rounds

Feel the urge to overshare? Stop or dramatically slow down your intake. Remember: Your goal is to have the boss relaxed, not to have yourself relaxed around the boss.

5. Ante Up

Superiors usually pay, as the unwritten rule goes, but you should at least offer to chip in. If you really want to impress or thank the boss, excuse yourself to the restroom and pay before he has a chance to grab the tab.

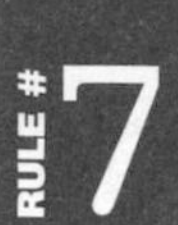

RULE # 7 Never look at a menu for longer than 90 seconds. You're picking dinner, not a business partner.

Give (and Take) Criticism at Work

There's an art to both sides. Handle each one perfectly.

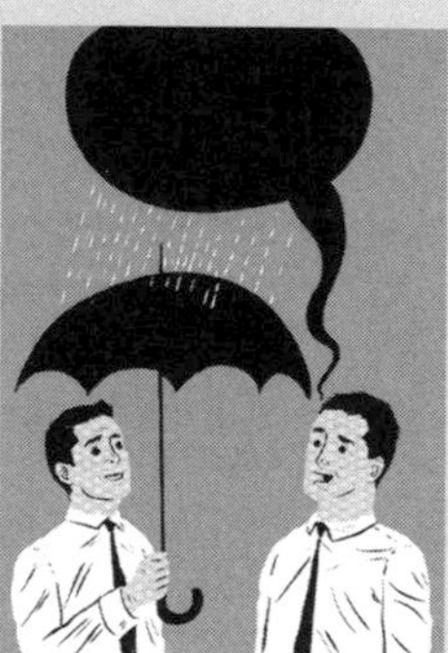

Give Criticism

Don't visit your colleague right after the misfire, says consultant Peter Bregman, author of the workplace efficiency book *18 Minutes*. He'll be stressed. Instead, set up a time to meet before the next screwup can occur. Be clear and direct, talking about the upcoming situation, not the prior mistake. Then stop talking. Silence locks in the message and allows for a response. Close with how you can best reach the goal together.

Take It

Everyone receives direct criticism, Bregman says. Accept it. Don't interrupt, be defensive, make excuses, or argue. Instead, ask questions to show you understand and want to improve. Solicit examples of ways you can work through a similar situation. Repeat advice and end by connecting your improvement to the betterment of the work. Remember: Don't take it personally. And a "thank you" doesn't hurt your reputation either.

RAISE YOUR PROFILE ON LINKEDIN

Most guys think of this social media site as a cleaned-up version of Facebook, but garnering connections is just the beginning of LinkedIn's potential. Follow these rules to build your professional persona, attract headhunters, and climb the corporate ladder.

Can the Corporate Claptrap

Unless you're CEO at a well-known company, forget about your generic title. Tell people what you actually do. You're not a "real estate agent," you find dream homes. Someone who "brings businesses together" is a stronger sell than "marketing assistant." Show that you're confident and passionate, and important people will notice.

Create an Online Portfolio

Beyond posting a photo and your most recent résumé, highlight your skills by adding your professional Twitter feed, blogs, or links to projects you've had a hand in. Seek out at least 10 recommendations. Not tight with the boss? Ask colleagues, clients, and associates for suggestions for your best work, too. A fresh perspective can help you round out your profile.

Join the Community

Making connections shouldn't be like cold-calling. Top dogs will trash unexpected LinkedIn e-mail. Instead, as a start, connect with professionals through your e-mail database. Join any groups related

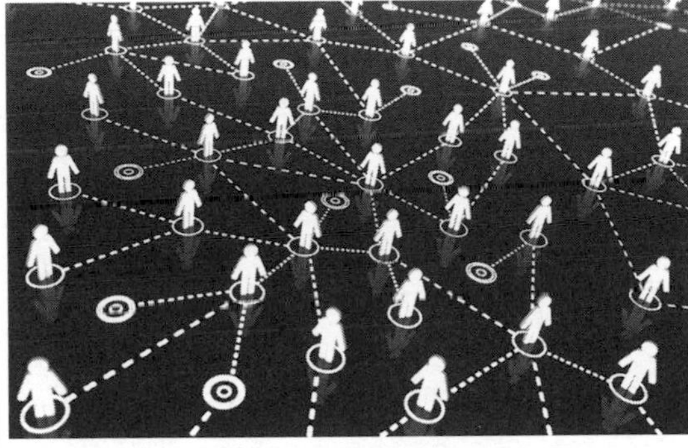

to your profession, and participate in discussions. You'll indirectly invite industry leaders to engage you, building relationships and establishing new connections.

Expand Your Career Horizons

If you're looking to make a connection, personalize the request. And keep it brief: an introduction (one sentence), a reference to a previous chat, a compliment (if it's not too over the top), and a note that you're interested in learning more about what the person does. That approach is polite and unobtrusive, and you won't sound needy.

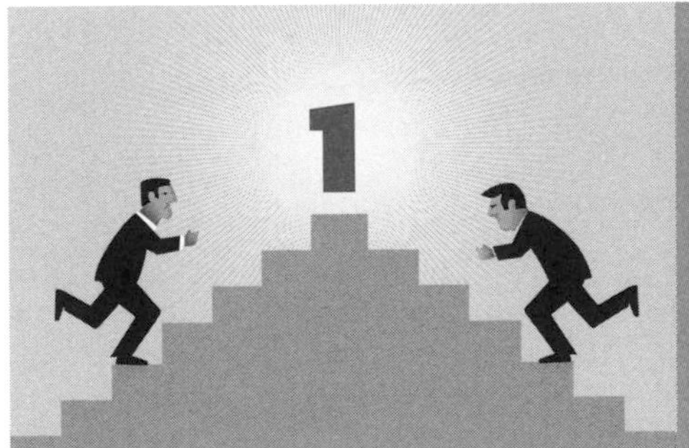

Earn the Promotion

Forget your rivals: Do your job and do it well. Where are you looking? At the scoreboard? At the other guy? Or at the assignment in front of you? In any competitive endeavor, team or otherwise, success comes down to the man in the mirror and how he completes his assignment.

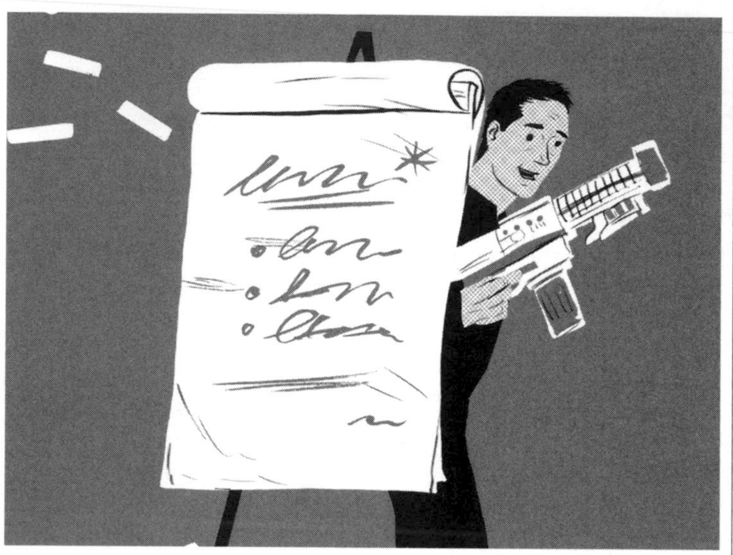

Boost Your Brainstorm

Dry-erase boards and neon-lit conference rooms are idea graveyards. Turbocharge your next brainstorm with these four tested alternatives.

Sleep on It

At Buffer, a social media startup, napping isn't just tolerated but encouraged. Mark Batey, PhD, who studies the psychology of creativity, says naps allow ideas to incubate. At rest, your brain can connect ideas in complex ways, he says. Budget for a 20-minute snooze.

Distract Yourself

Software company SendGrid gives employees time-wasters, such as video games, darts, and beer. Josh Ashton, SendGrid's director of people, says this busts routine and promotes creativity. No toys allowed? Challenge a colleague to Words with Friends.

Schedule a Deadline

Emmy winner Allison Silverman has written for *The Colbert Report* and *The Daily Show* and says she never waits for inspiration. "When I have limits, even if it's just a time limit, I can find really creative ways to tackle a problem." Set a timer and go!

Find a Novice

When Alaina G. Levine, president of Quantum Success Solutions, hits a rut, she asks someone outside her field. Think: "If I didn't have X skill or Y experience, how would this problem look?"

Try Reverse Mentoring

You're surrounded by people with darker hair (and more of it), lower cholesterol, and more energy. To adapt, identify a protégé and propose a reverse or reciprocal mentorship. This is hot at companies like Dell and Procter & Gamble. It's an informal way to encourage learning and facilitate cross-generational relationships in the office, says Lisa Quast, a Seattle-based career consultant.

Q My coworker doesn't wash his hands after using the restroom. Should I call him out?

A. Viruses can spread from a person's hands throughout an office in as little as 2 hours, so the question isn't if you should address him, but how. For a hands-off approach, just ask HR to send out an office memo, or post signs or comics about hand-washing etiquette. Comedy downgrades the situation. You can use humor, too, if you feel comfortable asking the ass-wipe to clean up his act.

Weekend Project: *Build an Indoor Oasis*

Power Plant

Ah, your office: It's probably pretty bland, boring, and . . . wait, we just fell asleep.

Thankfully, there's an easy way to liven it up and sharpen your focus, even in the dull days of winter. In a study in the *Journal of Alternative and Complementary Medicine*, people in plant-free zones rate their stress levels as nearly 11 percent higher than those exposed to plant life. Instead of tending to ever-thirsty houseplants, you can reap the same benefit with an easy-to-maintain terrarium. This resilient little glass-encased jungle waters itself through condensation. Whether you're in a window office or cubicleland, Tovah Martin, gardening expert and author of *The New Terrarium*, shows how to build some serious growth potential.

The Window Unit

In naturally lit rooms, indirect light filters through the glass, creating a warmth and humidity that mimics the environment of an equatorial cloud forest.

The Cubicle Farm

In an interior work area, fluorescent overheads create an environment similar to what you'd find in a low-light rain forest.

Materials

At a garden center, buy a pound of $^{3}/_{8}$-inch pebbles, a bag of horticultural charcoal, potting soil, and a 2-gallon glass container with a lid. For a window office, buy African violets or orchids; for a cubicle, selaginella mosses and ferns.

Sink the Foundation

Layer the materials. First add an inch of pebbles, then 1 tablespoon of the horticultural charcoal, then 2 to 3 inches of soil.

Construct the Kingdom

Remove each plant from its pot and loosen the roots with your fingers. Dig a hole deep enough to contain the plant's root system beneath the surface of the soil.

Shade Your Greens

Direct sunlight on a closed container can burn your plants. So situate your terrarium in a spot that's well lit but not in direct sun. Try a bookshelf or table that's far from the window.

Bathe in Faux Light

Mosses thrive in dimmer environments, but if the ecosystem is too dark, nothing will grow. For the best light, place your terrarium on a high shelf or an open part of your desk.

Maintain and Make Awesome

Water your plants and cap your terrarium. Every 2 weeks, take off the lid for a few hours. Then add flair with twigs, pinecones, or even tiny naked figures in Kama Sutra poses ($20, faerienest.com). Because a man at work should always be properly inspired.

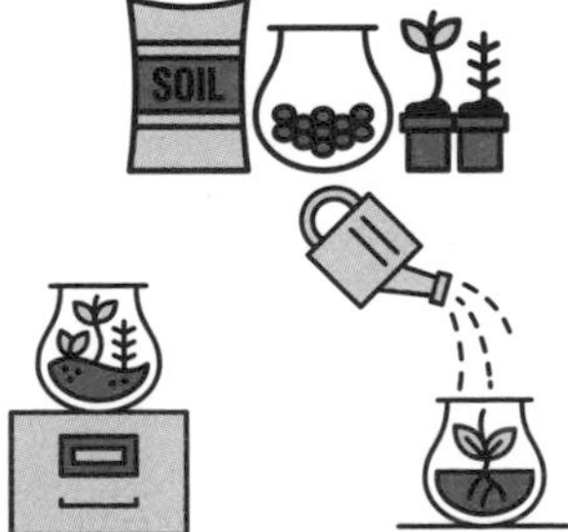

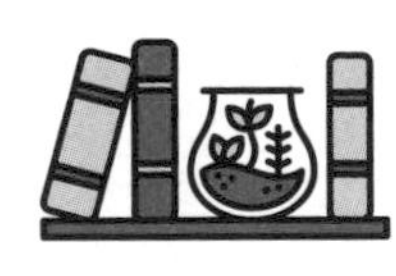

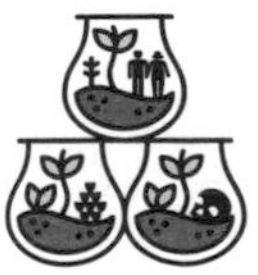

RULE # 8

Everyone sticks his foot in his mouth at work at some time or other. When you do, the best thing to do is apologize, briefly, and move on.

Calm Down or Keel Over

Chill, dude: Lose your temper and you could lose your life. An angry outburst can trigger a heart attack. In reviewing studies of behavior before a heart attack, researchers noted that people were nearly five times as likely to have an attack in the 2 hours after an angry episode. Plus, the risk of a clot-related stroke rose about three-and-a-half times. That may be because psychological stress can increase heart and blood pressure and restrict blood flow. Next time you're on the verge of a meltdown, slow your breathing—a lot. Taking six breaths a minute can reduce your blood pressure within 5 minutes.

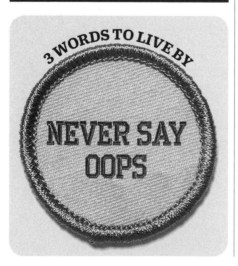

3 WORDS TO LIVE BY
NEVER SAY
OOPS

How Gnawing Worry May Shorten Your Life

Chronic work stress can raise your odds of having a stroke in the next decade, according to new research from the University of Minnesota. For every single-point increase in test scores measuring stress levels, study participants' risk of stroke jumped 19 percent. The authors speculate that chronic stress causes an inflammatory response that may impede blood flow to the brain. If you need a chill pill, try these simple ways to **BANISH STRESS IN . . .**

30 seconds Pop bubbles. We're talking about those air-filled bubbles that come in plastic sheets and are used for packing breakables. A study found that popping those plastic sheets for a while took the subjects' mind off their stressors, and they calmed down.

60 seconds Set a timer for a minute, close your eyes, and focus on breathing deeply and on observing your thoughts.

15 minutes Stretch while seated: lean forward, back, and to each side and stretch your arms above your head. Hold each pose for six slow breaths and then sit and breathe deeply with your eyes closed.

30 minutes Sweat. Just 30 minutes of exercise can reduce anxiety, and it may even help you handle future stressors.

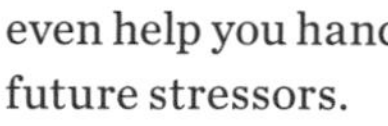

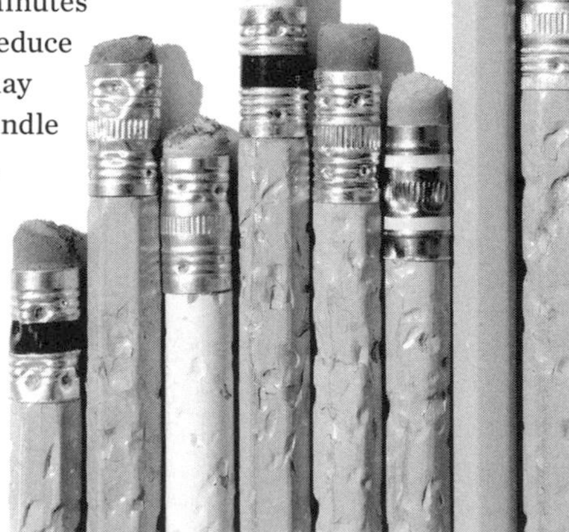

Optimize your 401(k)

How? First go to brightscope.com and see how your company's 401(k) stacks up. If it's underperforming, direct some retirement savings (after you've hit your company's match) to an IRA with a major brokerage like Fidelity or Vanguard. You'll have more options. Second, talk to your brokerage about rebalancing annually. It can reduce your risk and goose long-run returns.

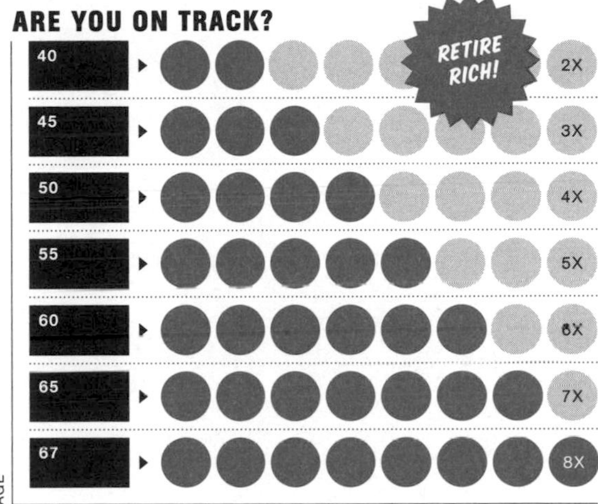

HOW TO WORK A ROOM

DON'T WING IT. HEAD INTO A WORK-RELATED EVENT WITH A STRATEGY AND YOU'LL LEAVE WITH MORE THAN A BELLY FULL OF MINI-QUICHES.

Make your must-meet list. A few days before the event, research the major players and develop talking points.

Organize yourself. Keep your own business cards in one pocket and reserve the other for cards you'll receive. This will prevent fumbling and eliminate the terrifying possibility that you might accidentally proffer a card reading "Private Masseuse—on Call."

Be on time. By being one of the first guests, you'll adopt a nearly host-like mentality, meeting and greeting rather than taking cues from others.

Infiltrate a group. This is a critical skill. Find the most animated group in the room and join in. Start by quickly making eye contact with someone from the periphery of the group, and then introduce yourself with a firm handshake. Ask an open-ended question, such as "What's your connection here?" There, you've just hooked up with the life of the party.

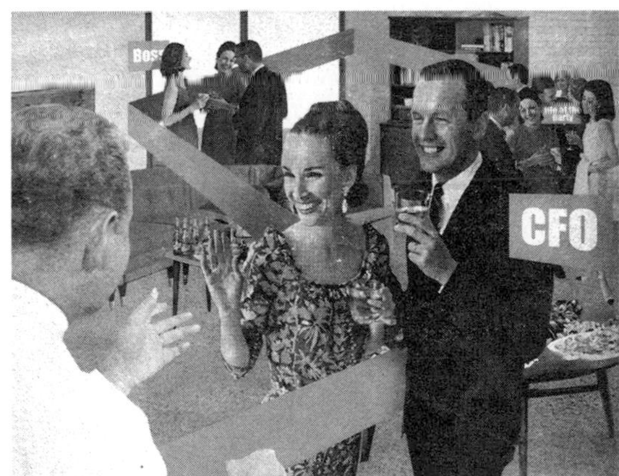

Reconnect with new connections. Before you leave, double back to a few key people. A second meeting, even on the same night, makes them more likely to remember you. Reiterate a prior talking point and say you look forward to meeting again.

Sources: Diane Darling, author of The Networking Survival Guide *and Susan RoAne, author of* How to Work a Room

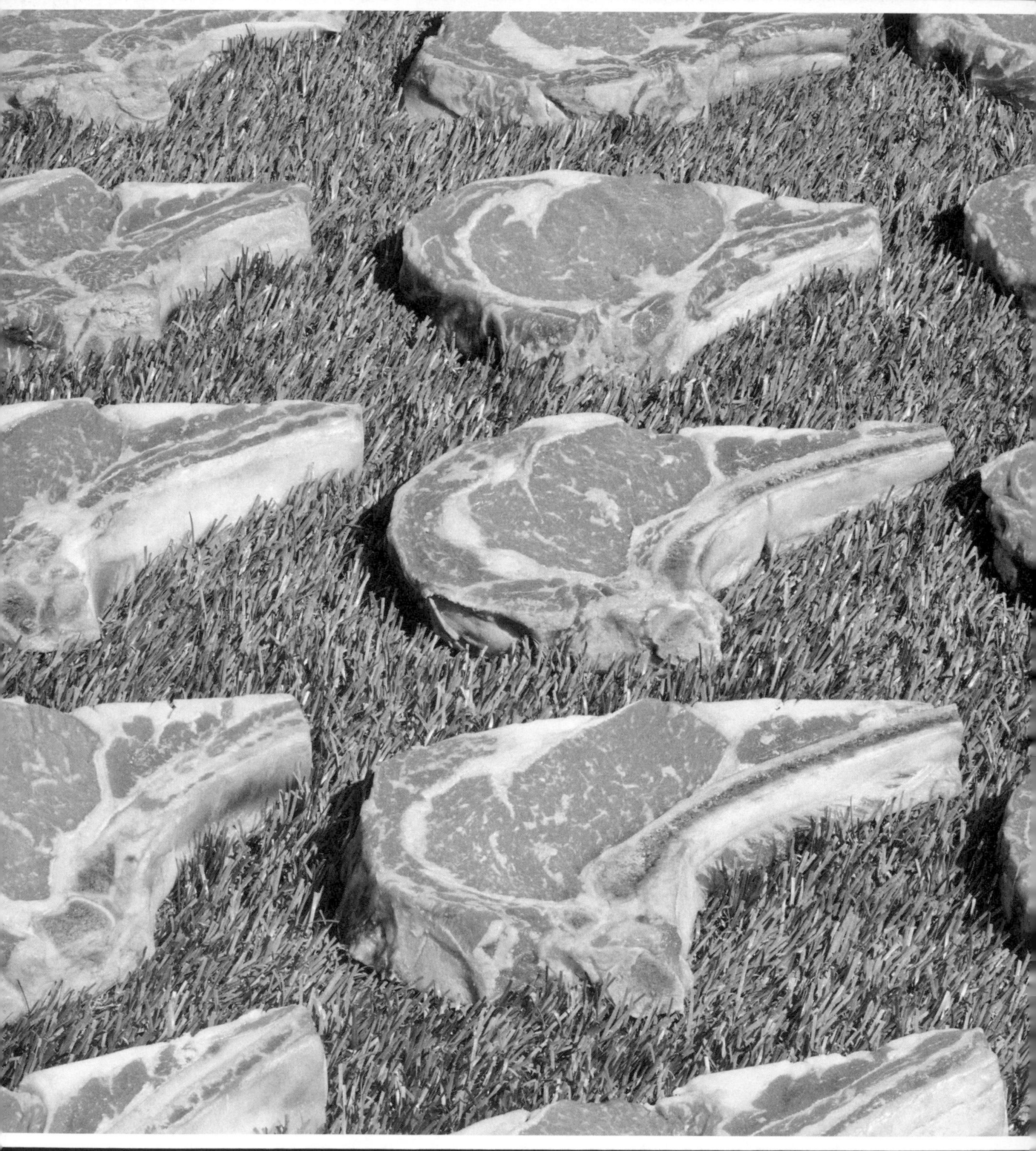

Eat like a Man

Skills, Recipes, and Other Know-How for Cooking and Enjoying Amazing Food

Man shall not live by bread alone.

He needs toast.

And for toast, he needs a toaster along with a certain level of skill to ensure he does not burn the toast. Of course, and butter.

The point is that food is no longer placed before a man, hot and bubbling, like it was done when you were 13. Today a man must hunt, gather, prepare. Or order in. The latter is bad practice because it may lead to high-calorie fried foods and the need for larger trousers.

If you would like to eat really well and stay fit and healthy, the writing is on the wall: You need to learn how to make fluffy eggs and omelets, the perfect burger, grilled sockeye salmon, pan-seared steak, and chicken soup from scratch. Developing cooking skills will not only give you a satisfied belly (and a trimmer one at that) but may also encourage further exploration of the culinary arts. You may, at some point, want to try cooking for a woman. And that's when you'd better have your shit together. Or at least know how to make toast. So let's start there—with some killer French toast.

How to Make Incredible Stuffed French Toast

Any guy can whip up a batch of scrambled eggs. But how many can delight a woman with a homemade, decadently sweet breakfast treat? Our friend Candice Kumai, chef and author of *Pretty Delicious*, walked us through this amazingly simple recipe.

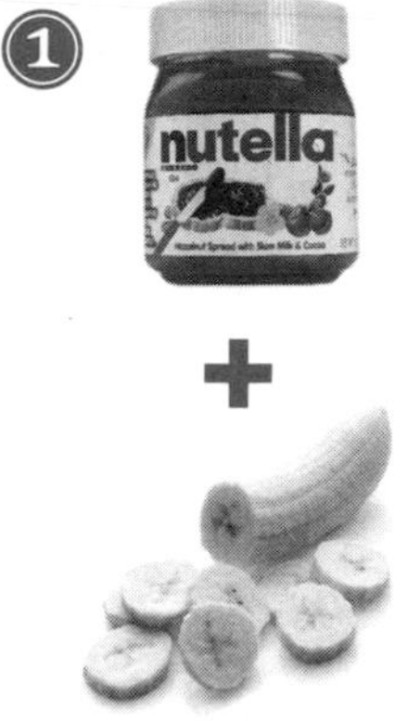

COMBO 1: NUTELLA + BANANA SLICES

Start Off Stale

Fresh bread has natural moisture that can prevent it from soaking up the egg-milk mixture. Use day-old bread for better absorption. For the best texture, try thick slices of baguette, challah, brioche, or whole wheat bread, or even a split croissant. For this recipe (two servings) you'll need four slices of bread or two split croissants.

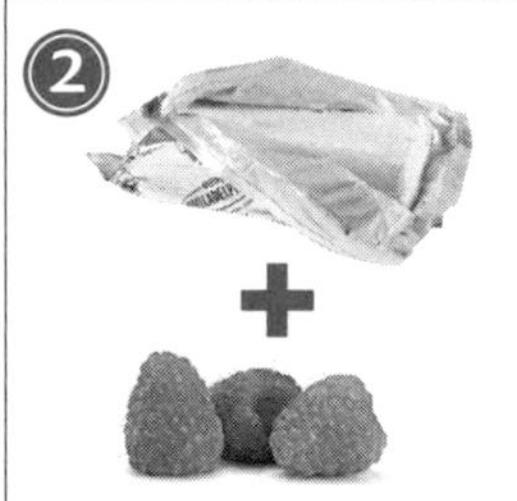

COMBO 2: CREAM CHEESE + RASPBERRIES

Stack and Soak

Top two pieces of bread with combo 1, 2, or 3. Add the remaining bread to make two sandwiches. In a medium bowl, whisk four eggs with 2 tablespoons milk, 1 teaspoon sugar or maple syrup, and ¼ teaspoon ground cinnamon. Pour into a 9″ × 13″ baking dish. Place your sandwiches in the mixture for 2 minutes, flipping them halfway through.

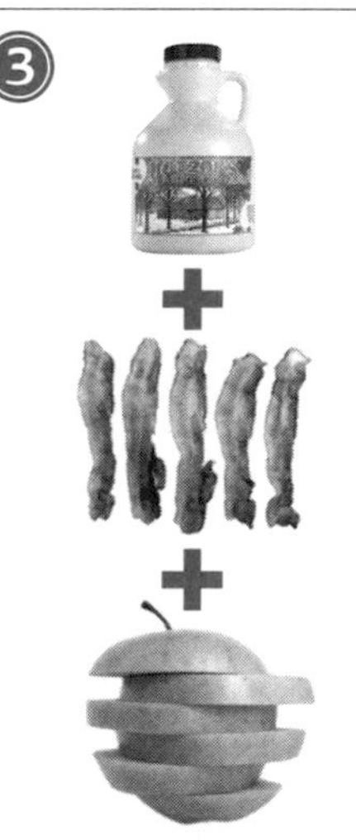

COMBO 3: MAPLE SYRUP + BACON + APPLE SLICES

Sear It

While the bread soaks, melt 1 tablespoon of butter in a medium nonstick pan over medium-high heat. Place the sandwiches in the pan and cook until golden brown, a minute or two on each side. Serve topped with powdered sugar and whatever fruit you used to stuff the French toast and maple syrup.

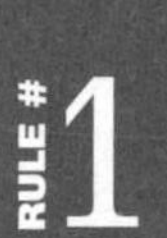

Always splurge for real maple syrup instead of the cheap pancake syrups made with corn syrup. Pure maple is loaded with healthy polyphenols. Choose grade A light or medium amber.

MacGyver a Walnut IF YOU DON'T HAVE A NUTCRACKER HANDY, HEAD TO THE GARAGE FOR A PAIR OF VISE GRIPS. THERE'S NO MORE MANLY WAY TO GET TO THE MEAT.

HONE A KNIFE IN A HURRY

According to Iron Chef Masaharu Morimoto: "If you think your knife is becoming dull, grab a well-used coffee mug, flip it upside down, and sharpen your knife by swiping each side of the blade's edge over the bottom ring of the mug several times."

Crack an Egg with One Hand

Bryan Fyler, executive sous chef at the Cosmopolitan of Las Vegas—and a man who has made many brunches—shows how to speed up (and show off!) your breakfast prep.

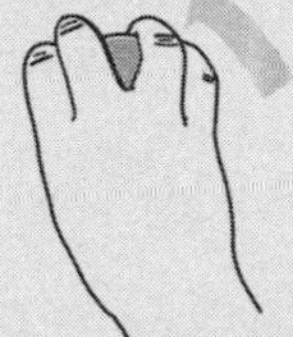

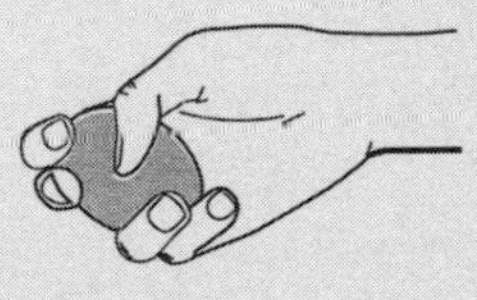

Master the Vulcan Salute

You want to pull the egg's halves apart without crushing the shell. Holding the egg in your dominant hand, spread your fingers so your index and middle digits grip the egg's left side and your ring finger and pinkie rest on the right side (or vice versa for lefties). Tuck your thumb beneath the egg for support.

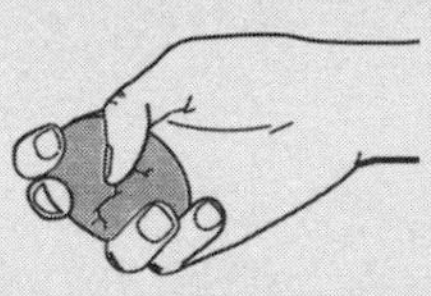

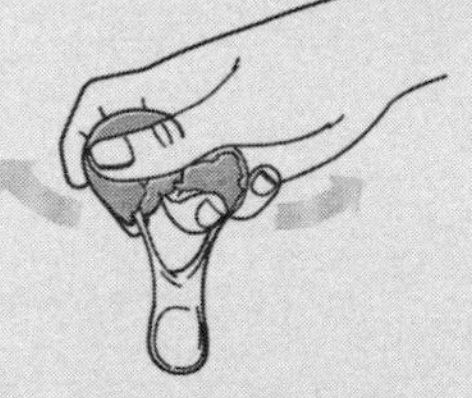

Tap That

Rap the egg on a counter near the bowl with the force of a light door knock. Done correctly, the shell should crack slightly but not split. Raise the egg above the bowl and spread your fingers outward, pulling the shell apart. If this doesn't provide enough force, use your thumb to gently pry it apart.

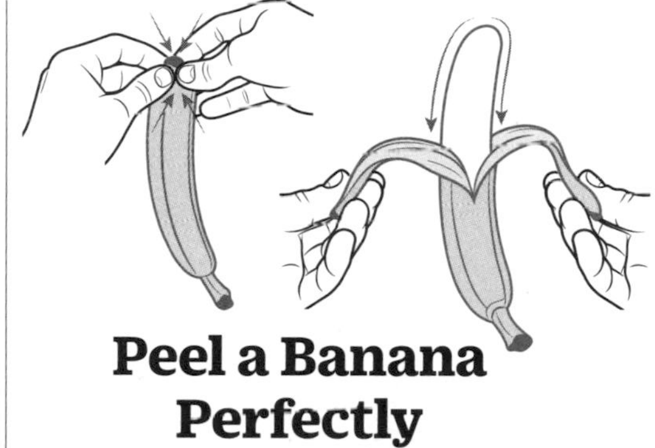

Peel a Banana Perfectly

We tested a viral video's "monkey-approved" instructions. YouTube user SomeDirection had it right: Don't start from the stem. It may not break, so the fruit could crush. Instead, use both hands to pinch the dark base and spread the halves easily apart. But we call monkeyshine on whether primates use this strategy. Our experts say they just rip it open.

MORE
PROTEIN

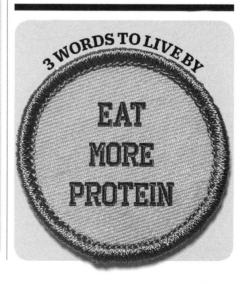

3 WORDS TO LIVE BY

Roll Your Own Sushi

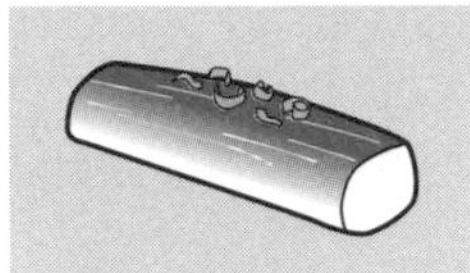

For a quick fix of Japanese without hitting the sushi bar, leave the bamboo-mat method to the skilled sushi chef and master the simple art of the hand roll.

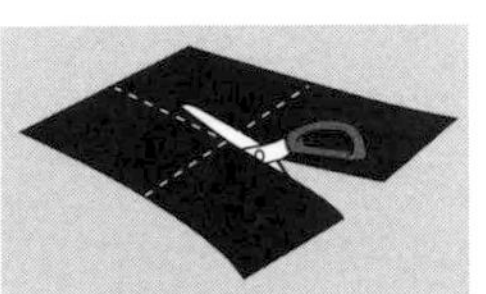

Maximize Taste

The best rolls have both texture and color. Choose from krab (fake crabmeat), enoki mushrooms, smoked salmon, cucumbers, or avocado. Select or cut your ingredients to equal size and shape so they'll fit into the hand roll.

Size the Sheets

Nori, the seaweed that holds sushi together, comes in sheets. Using scissors, cut each sheet into quarters to yield a more manageable size for the rolls.

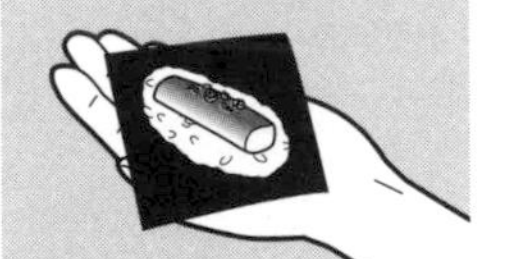

Arrange Artfully

Place the nori sheet on your palm (shiny side down) so it's in a diamond shape. With your other hand, take a thumb-size amount of sushi rice (try Annie Chun's premade varieties) and press it into the middle of the sheet, from the top of the diamond to the bottom. Line your ingredients on top.

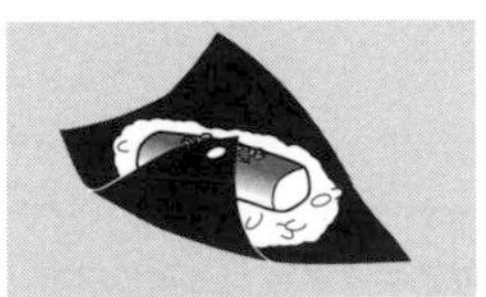

Roll It into a Cone

Slowly close the hand you're using to hold the nori to bring both outside flaps of the sheet together, sliding one beneath the other. (Put a grain of rice between the flaps to hold the roll together.) Dip the open end of the roll into soy sauce. Consume.

EAT MORE OF THIS:

Sockeye Salmon

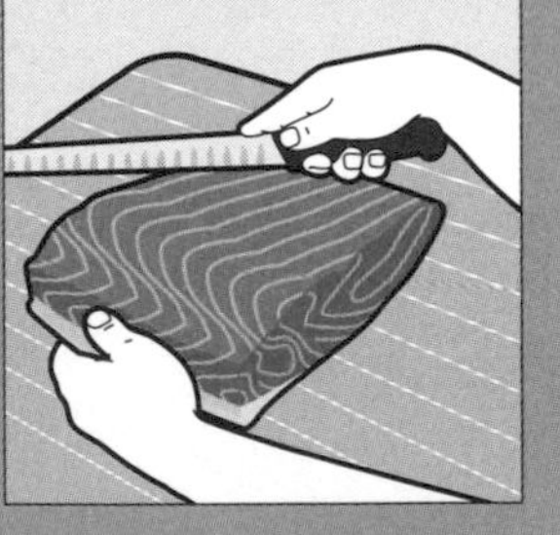

Bright orange wild-caught sockeye salmon is loaded with heart-healthy omega-3 fatty acids and offers 36 grams of protein at only 241 calories for a sizable 6-ounce serving. Plus, wild Pacific salmon has 10 times fewer "persistent organic pollutants," or POPs, than farm-raised Atlantic salmon, reports a study in *Alternative Medicine Review.*

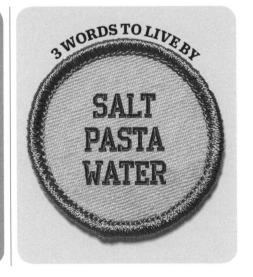

3 WORDS TO LIVE BY
SALT
PASTA
WATER

COOK IT LIKE A SUBCONTRACTOR

WHO NEEDS TO RUN TO WILLAMS-SONOMA WHEN YOU HAVE A TOOLBOX GATHERING DUST IN THE SHED? GRAB A TOOL AND BEAT YOUR FOOD INTO SUBMISSION.

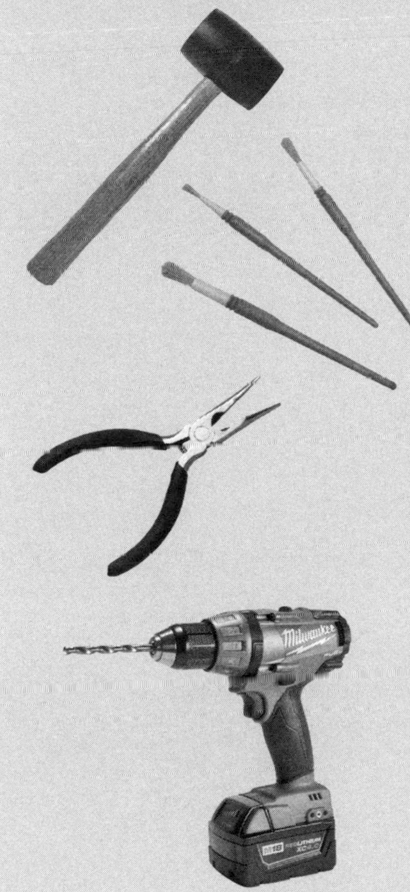

RUBBER MALLET—Use it to tenderize meats. Rinse the sawdust off first.

CHEAP HOBBY PAINTBRUSHES—To marinade roasts and clean out the coffee grinder. Use unused brushes.

5-IN-1 TOOL—Use the half-round to clean grill grates. Its angles reach places a large grill brush can't. Tap the gouger to pop a small hole on the top of a metal olive oil jug so pouring goes more easily. Use the scraper/putty spreader to remove the baked-on crud from pots or baking sheets.

NEEDLE-NOSE PLIERS—A (clean) pair can extract fish bones fast. Drag your finger along the bones to expose them and then use the pliers to pull them toward the head.

CORDLESS DRILL—Make extra-fluffy scrambled eggs by inserting a whisk attachment into the drill and beating. Unscrew the knob from the top of a pepper mill, exposing the drive shaft, and tighten the shaft into your drill to turn it into a grinder. Turn on the drill to grind a pile of pepper in seconds. (Pro tip: If not enough of the drive shaft is exposed, remove the pepper mill's head.)

PROPANE TORCH—For making crème brûlée and meringues. Just be careful out there, sport.

Makin' Better Bacon

The key to perfectly cooked bacon: Place bacon on a baking sheet and roast in a 375° F oven for 12 minutes. Bacon tends to scrunch up when cooked in a skillet, making for uneven cooking.

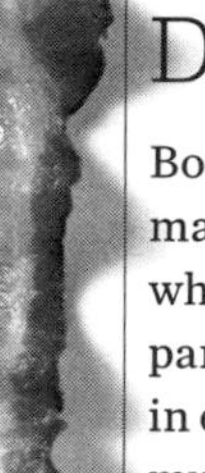

Dress Yourself

Bottled dressings are a waste of money. You can make a better vinaigrette yourself from scratch by whisking together three parts olive oil with one part balsamic vinegar, plus salt and pepper. Build in extra flavor by adding minced shallots, Dijon mustard, fresh herbs, or honey.

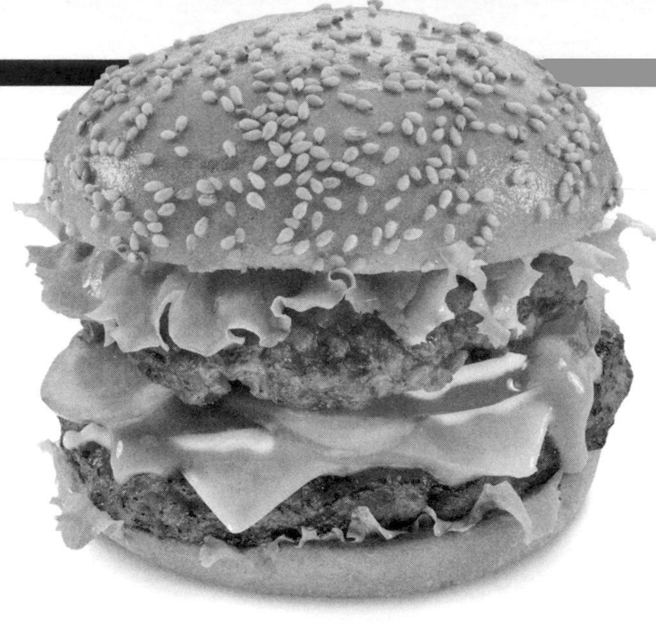

Cook the Perfect Burger

DO JUSTICE TO AN AMERICAN CLASSIC BY MAKING IT RIGHT.

Buy the Beef

For superjuicy, tender burgers, pick 80 percent lean chuck and ask for it "twice ground."

Shape the Patties

Mold, don't mix. Add nothing. If you're adding eggs or onions to your ground beef, you're making meatloaf, not burgers.

Prep the Grill

Crank the heat to high. (For a charcoal grill, skip lighter fluid. Heat coals in a chimney starter until they're lightly coated with ash.) Hold your hand just over the grill; if you can keep it there only a few seconds, it's go time.

Cook the Burgers

Salt the patties liberally and then grill them until droplets of blood appear on the raw side, about 3 minutes. Now flip. For medium rare, cook this side about 2 more minutes (or 3 more minutes for medium). Resist the urge to press on the burgers to make them sizzle. Doing that smooshes out a lot of the tasty juices.

Size it—Grab a tennis ball–size hunk of beef (about 7 ounces) and form into a loose ball.

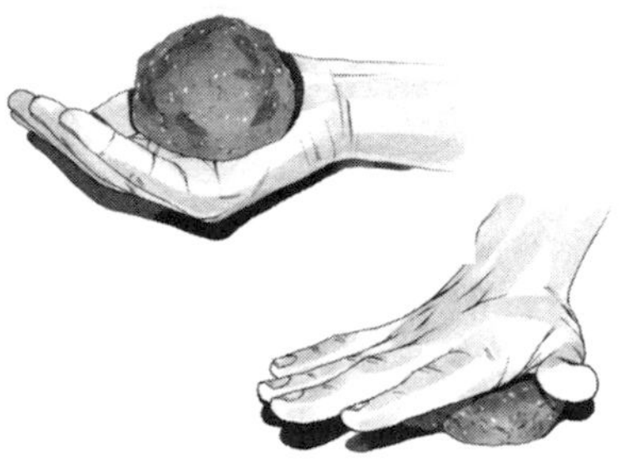

Flatten it—Place the ball of meat on a clean cutting board and press it with the palm of your hand until it's about 3/4 inch thick.

Shape it—Without completely lifting the patty off the cutting board, work your palms around the edge, lightly packing it as you rotate. Then flip the patty over and repeat. Just don't overwork the meat—too much mashing will result in a dense, chewy burger.

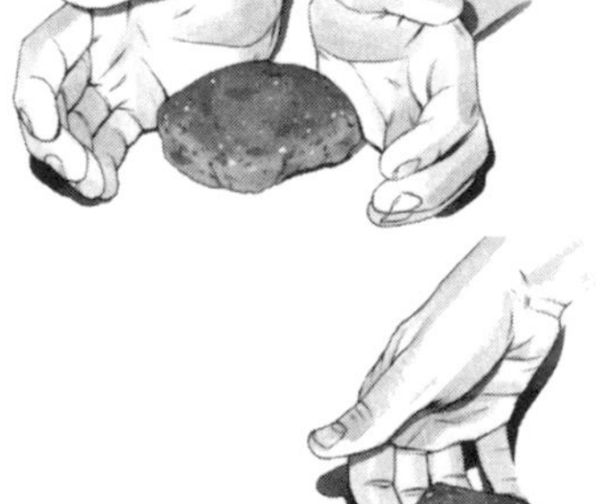

The Accessories:

1. **Bun.** For a crisp but tender bun, butter the cut sides and toast it in a pan until golden.
2. **Tomato.** The flavorful variety sold on the vine is just the right size.
3. **Cheese.** Use American, not Cheddar; the saltiness enhances the meat.
4. **Pickles.** Use to add an acidic bite to your creation.
5. **Onion.** Top the cheese with thinly sliced red onion so it wilts in the burger's heat.
6. **Lettuce.** Crisp curly-leaf lettuce on the bottom bun prevents soggy bread.

ROCK A LOBSTER

Serve up a seafood dinner that beats the shell out of that chain-joint special.

Go Live

Skip the frozen lobster. An enzyme released after a crustacean dies can degrade the meat over time, says Stuart Cromarty, PhD, an expert in lobster neuroscience at Assumption College in Massachusetts.

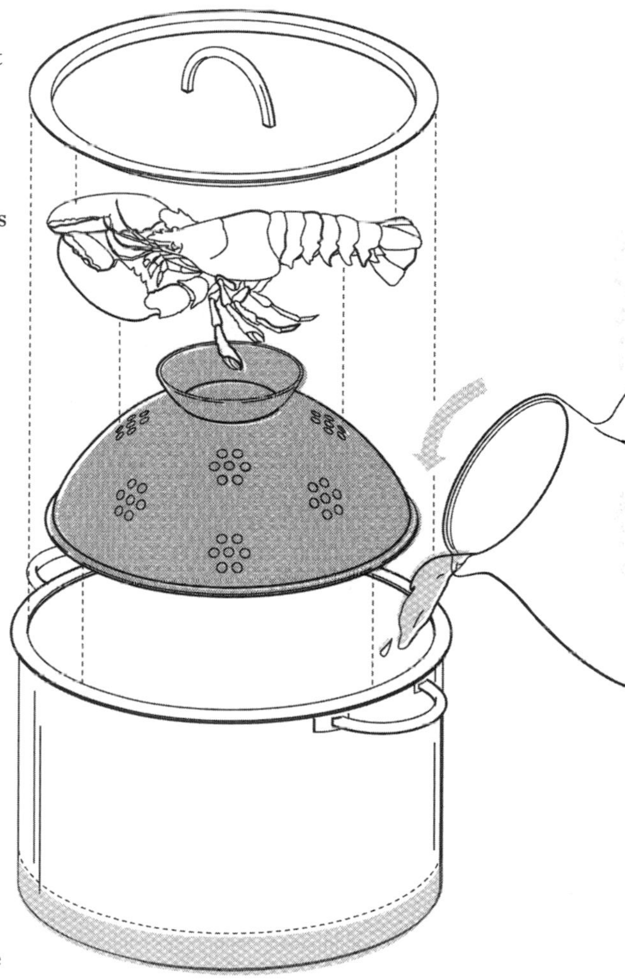

Buy Young

Look for smallish specimens weighing about $1^1/_2$ pounds, says Kerry Altiero, Maine Lobster Chef of the Year in 2012. Their meat is sweeter than that of their bigger brethren. The tank water should be clear and the lobster active when removed.

Steam It

Don't boil the lobster or you'll waterlog the meat, says Altiero. (Also, removing the meat from the shell will be messier.) Set up your stockpot and bring the water to a boil. Using tongs, grip the lobster behind its claws, pincers pointed away from you. Place it on the colander and put on the lid. Steam until the lobster is bright red, about 20 minutes.

Extract and Stand Back

Using tongs, transfer the lobster to a cutting board to sit for 5 minutes. Like other meats, lobster turns juicier when it rests, Altiero says.

Build Your Steamer

You don't need to go out and buy a specialty seafood steamer—the items you need are probably in your kitchen already. Just flip a metal colander upside down inside an 8-quart (or larger) stockpot. Add a few inches of water to the pot, making sure the water level doesn't reach the lobster.

RULE # 2 **You have about 7 days after opening a package of deli turkey to consume it safely. But always do the sniff test. Strong off-odors indicate spoilage.**

MAKE PERFECT PASTA

MOST PEOPLE SCREW IT UP, SAYS MARC VETRI, EXECUTIVE CHEF OF ALLA SPINA IN PHILADELPHIA. ALLOW THE CHEF TO SCHOOL YOU.

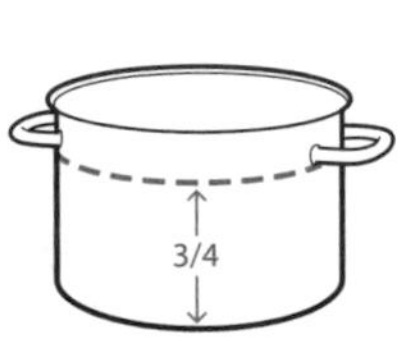

1. Go Deep

Grab an 8- to 10-quart pot for 1 pound of pasta and fill it about three-quarters full of hot water (to help it boil faster). You want enough water so the pasta doesn't stick to itself and clump.

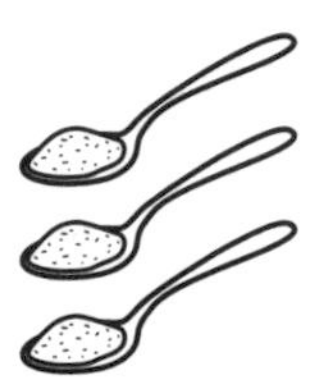

2. Add Salt

Turn the heat to high and salt the water heavily. If you're using an 8-quart pot, that's about 3 tablespoons of kosher salt. Most of the salt will stay in the water, leaving the pasta perfectly seasoned. Put the lid on the pot so the water boils faster.

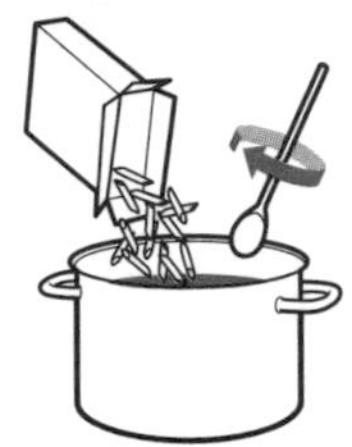

3. Drop and Stir

When the water reaches a rolling boil, add the pasta and stir immediately. This ensures that the pasta won't stick together. There's no need to add olive oil—that doesn't prevent sticking. Just stir occasionally throughout the cooking process.

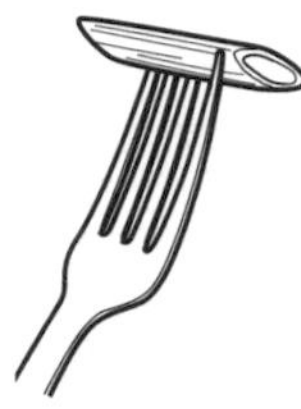

4. Test with Your Teeth

Your goal is al dente—pasta that's just tender but still has a bite. Boxed pasta usually reaches al dente about a minute before the package instructions say to cook it. The only true way to check: Pull out a piece and bite into it. If the texture feels crunchy, allow the pasta to continue to boil. Taste again after another minute or so.

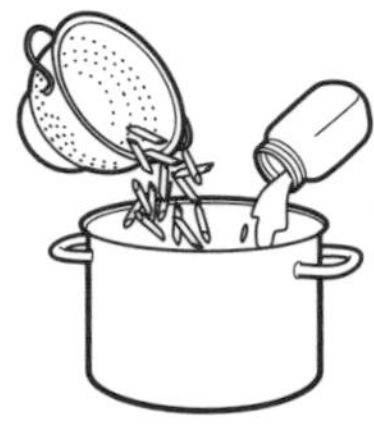

5. Finish It

Pasta should never wait in a colander—it'll go gummy. Reserve $^1/_4$ cup of pasta water and drain the pasta. Then dump the drained pasta back into the pot. Add the sauce and reserved pasta water. The starches in the pasta water help the sauce cling to the pasta, creating a creamier dish. Stir well before serving.

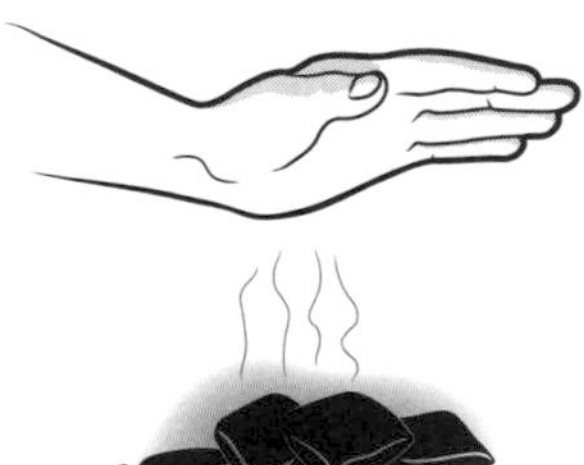

Guesstimate Grill Temp

Never press meat with a spatula to speed grilling. You'll turn it into a hockey puck. Instead put your hands to good use. Test your barbecue grill heat by placing your hand 3 inches above the grilling surface and count Mississippis until you have to pull away.

Less than 3 seconds—high heat

5 to 6—medium heat

10 to 12—low heat

The Most Nutrient-Dense Plants You Can Eat

Pick foods near the top of the list and diversify colors to boost phytochemical content.

Produce	Density Rank
Watercress	100
Chinese cabbage	91.99
Chard	89.27
Beet greens	87.08
Spinach	86.46
Romaine	63.48
Collard greens	62.49
Endive	60.44
Kale	49.07
Red peppers	41.26
Arugula	37.56
Broccoli	34.89
Brussels sprouts	32.23
Cauliflower	25.13
Cabbage	24.51
Carrots	22.60
Tomatoes	20.37
Iceberg lettuce	18.28
Strawberries	17.59
Oranges	12.91
Blackberries	11.39

RULE # 3

Eat a tablespoon of ground flaxseed daily. It's the best source of alpha-linolenic acid, a healthy fat that can help improve the workings of the cerebral cortex, the area of the brain that processes sensory info, including that of pleasure.

Gauge Your Gas

Not sure how much propane is left in your grill tank? Microwave a cup of water for about 2 minutes or until it starts to bubble. Then pour the hot water down the side of the tank. Run your hand over the wet metal; the warm part of the tank is empty, and the cool part is full.

RULE # 4

Keep meat from sticking to a grill by oiling the grates. Cut an onion in half and stick a long-handled grill fork in the round part. Dip the cut end into a bowl of vegetable oil and rub it over the grates of the grill.

How to Mince Garlic

After peeling the clove, place it on a cutting board and trim off roots. (a) Slice the clove in thin strips along its length from root to tip. (b) Turn the garlic 90 degrees and cut strips in the other direction. Sprinkle the sticks of garlic with a pinch of salt to keep them from sticking to knife. (c) Hold the garlic in place by curling your fingers under and run the knife back and forth over the sticks to mince as finely as you like.

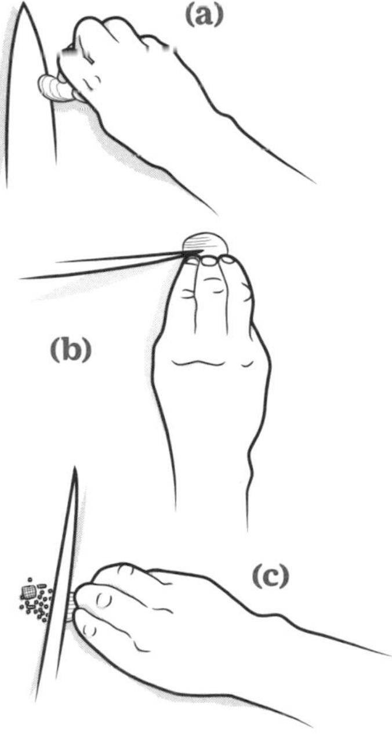

PAN-SEAR A JUICY STEAK

GRILL SNOWED IN? YOU CAN STILL ENJOY A SLAB OF BEEF FIRED TO CRUSTY-OUTSIDE, JUICY-INSIDE PERFECTION. CHEF MARC FORGIONE OF AMERICAN CUT IN ATLANTIC CITY WALKS YOU THROUGH THE STEPS.

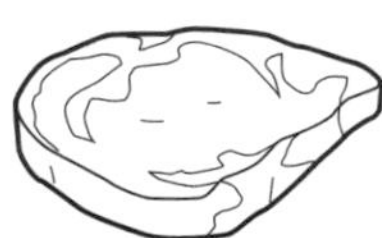

Select a Steak with Fat

Buy a 10-ounce strip or rib-eye steak; either cut will have a nice fat cap surrounding the meat to keep it from drying out and toughening up when exposed to high heat. The cap should be at least ¼ inch thick.

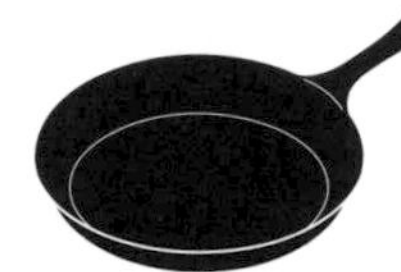

Ratchet Up the Firepower

High heat helps the meat acquire a crisp crust. The problem is that your typical sauté pan can't take high heat. So break out a cast-iron skillet or heavy-bottom metal pan. Add 2 tablespoons of canola oil and crank the burner to high.

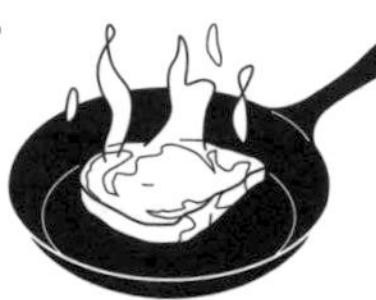

Watch and Sear

Coat the steak with sea salt, 2 tablespoons of herbed butter, and ground black pepper. When the oil smokes, add the steak and reduce the heat to medium (exhaust fan on). Sear until you see a crust form on the underside of the steak, 3 to 4 minutes.

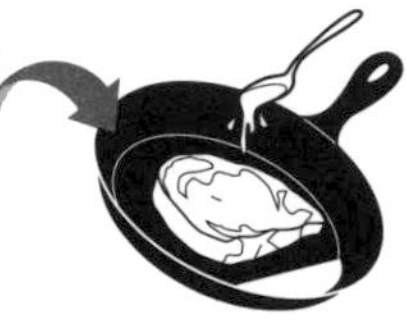

Finish with Flavor

Use tongs to flip the meat. Add a few unpeeled garlic cloves and thyme sprigs to the oil. Cook the steak 4 more minutes (for medium rare), basting it with the pan's oil. (Tip the pan until the oil pools, scoop it up, and drip it over the meat.)

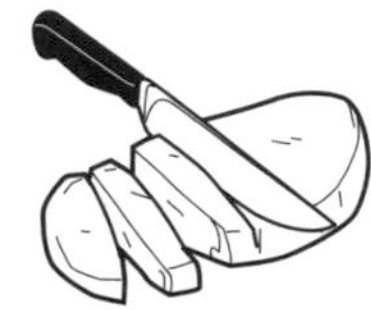

Let It Rest, Then Dig In

Remove the meat from the pan and let it sit for 10 minutes, so the juices redistribute inside the steak. Then slice it across the grain. Sprinkle on some more sea salt and serve.

Speed Your Smoothie Cleanup

Blast blender buildup with this trick from nutritionist (and avid smoothie-maker) Alan Aragon, MS: Flush out what you can using the faucet and then fill the blender halfway with hot water and a splash of dish soap. Now turn it on high for 20 seconds. Rinse thoroughly. Done.

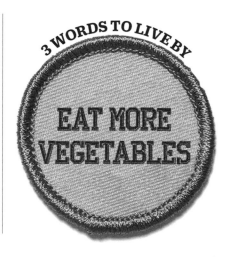

3 WORDS TO LIVE BY
EAT MORE
VEGETABLES

Grow Your Own Salsa

Cynthia James, food production specialist at the Rodale Institute Agriculture Supported Communities program, adds some spice to your garden party.

Spot Your Plot

Find a flat 4 × 8-foot soil area outside that receives at least 6 hours of direct sun daily and drains well.

Build a Raised Bed

An elevated garden is less weedy. Plus, loose soil helps plants produce more. For full plans of a raised bed like the one drawn below, head to MensHealth.com/raisedbed.

Plan the Planting

To find out when to start your garden, enter your Zip code at almanac.com/gardening/planting-dates. Plant onions at least 4 weeks before the average last-frost date. Add tomato and hot-pepper transplants on or after that date. Add cilantro seeds then too.

Circle Your Crops

Arrange the plants strategically and they'll benefit one another. Put the tomatoes and jalapeños in the center of the bed so the roots have plenty of space to spread. Plant your onions and cilantro around the edge of the garden. Their aromas will confuse insect pests.

Grow Long!

Water thoroughly after planting, and then on a regular daily schedule. Soak the plot every morning to wet the root zone. To check whether it needs a second afternoon watering, stick your finger an inch into the soil. If it's dry, drag out the hose and give 'er a soak.

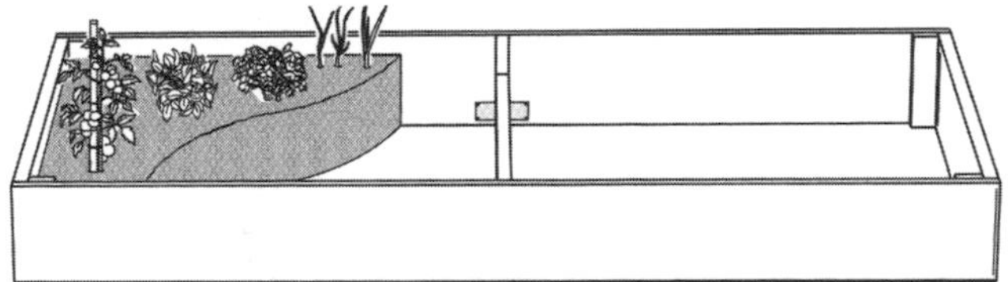

A Handy Meat Thermometer

To check doneness, poke the meat and then the fleshy area between your thumb and index finger while holding your hand in these positions, which mimic varying degrees of "doneness."

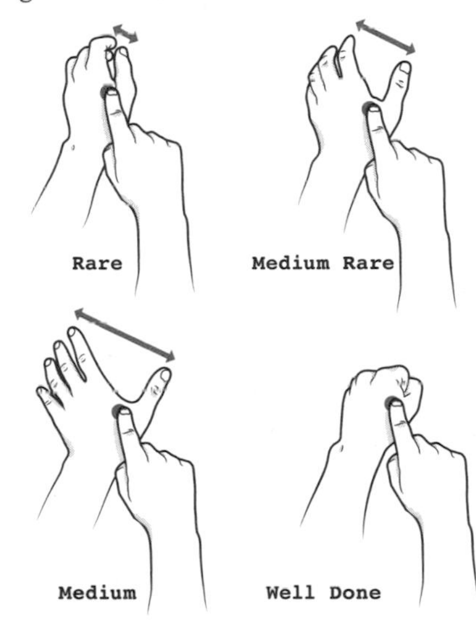

RULE # 5

Brown rice is a better choice than white because it's a fiber-rich whole grain.

Liven Up Leftovers

Think of leftovers as ingredients to build from instead of meals to eat again. Example: Chop up last night's steak and asparagus and add to a frittata. Use chili as a hot dog topper, or add roast chicken or sautéed shrimp to pizza or pasta sauce.

Make Chicken Soup from Scratch

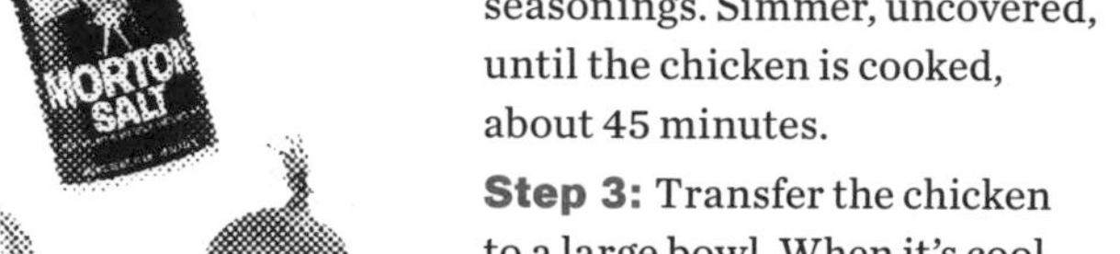

Buy the Right Bird

A 3- to 4-pound broiler (an older bird) will give your soup a strong chicken flavor and leave you with plenty of extra meat for leftovers.

Salt the Meat

For tastier soup, rub the chicken inside and out with 1 tablespoon of kosher salt and refrigerate for 15 minutes. Rinse the bird with cold water and pat dry.

Prep the Vegetables

Aromatic vegetables add a foundation of flavor. Best mix: 3 carrots, 5 celery stalks, and 1 onion (all chopped), and 3 whole, peeled garlic cloves.

Gather Your Seasonings

For a classic chicken soup, stick to subtle herbs and spices. Best mix: a few sprigs of fresh flat-leaf parsley and dill, 2 bay leaves, and $^1/_2$ teaspoon black peppercorns.

Cook Your Soup

Step 1: Place the bird in a large pot and add enough water to cover it by 3 inches. Bring to a boil and skim off any foam.

Step 2: Add the vegetables and seasonings. Simmer, uncovered, until the chicken is cooked, about 45 minutes.

Step 3: Transfer the chicken to a large bowl. When it's cool enough to handle, strip the meat from the bones.

Step 4: Return the bones to the pot and simmer for another hour. Strain the broth (discard the solids), season with salt and pepper, and add in half the shredded chicken. (Save the rest for tacos, salads, or sandwiches.) Stir in your choice of add-ins . . .

Add-ins: Cooked egg noodles, brown or wild rice, canned white beans, fresh baby spinach, chopped dill or parsley

Make It Better

For a clearer, less greasy broth, refrigerate it overnight. The next day, skim off the solidified fat and reheat.

Holy $#*! Kitchen Trick

If you have a knob of leftover ginger, submerge it in a jar of vodka and store it in the fridge. The vodka preserves the ginger for weeks without imparting any flavor. But the ginger makes the vodka taste like ginger, making it ideal for cocktails.

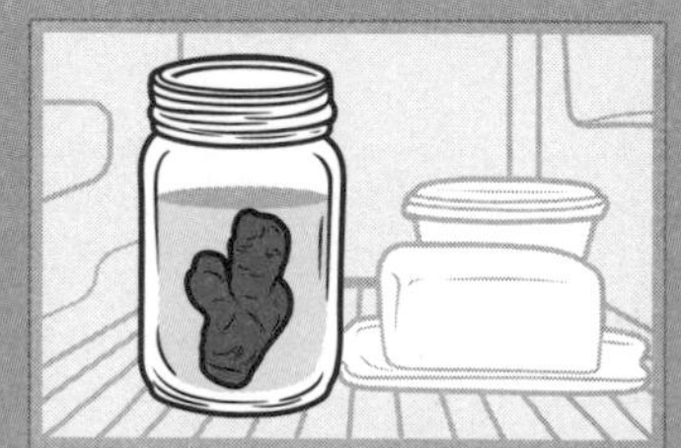

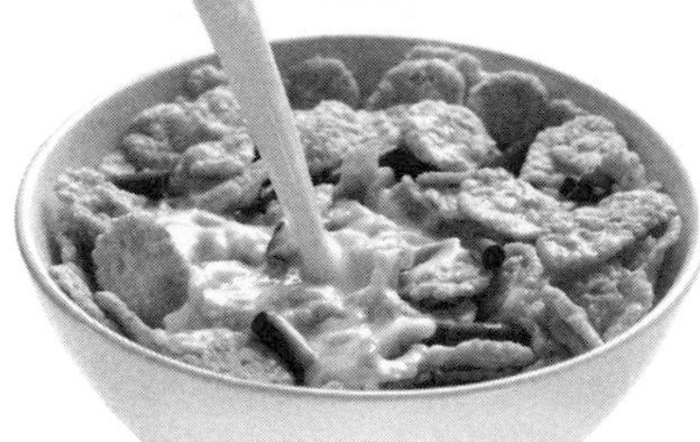

CEREAL KILLER

Want to terminate high blood pressure? Breakfast every day on high-fiber, whole grain cereal. According to a study in *Clinical Nutrition*, people who ate at least seven servings of whole grain cereal had 19 percent lower risk of developing hypertension later in life than people who ate none.

Whip Up Homemade Hummus

Use this simple technique from Michael Solomonov, executive chef of Zahav in Philadelphia, to create a tasty, silky dip that blows away the stuff in the tub.

Set the Foundation

Whole ingredients make great hummus. Save the liquid from a 15-ounce can of chickpeas—aka garbanzo beans—and rinse them. Dump them into a food processor or blender with $1^1/_2$ cups of sesame paste.

Smooth It Out

Puree with $^1/_2$ cup grapeseed oil and $^1/_2$ cup fresh-squeezed lemon juice. Slowly add the reserved liquid from the can until the hummus is creamy. Season to taste with kosher salt and cumin powder.

Top It Off

Add flavor and substance by including extras like sautéed mushrooms or sliced hard-boiled eggs. Scoop the hummus onto a plate, make a well in the center, and spoon the extras into the well. Serve with warmed pita and beer.

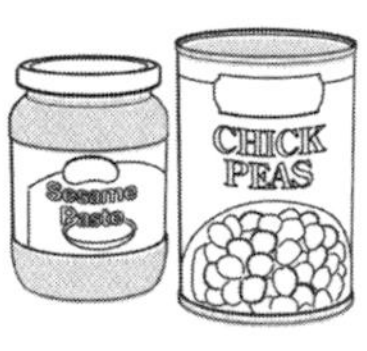

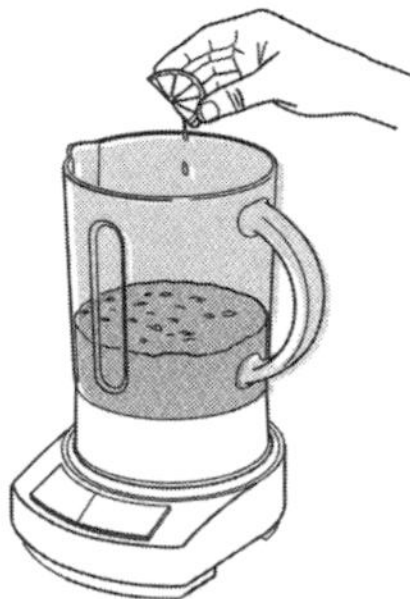

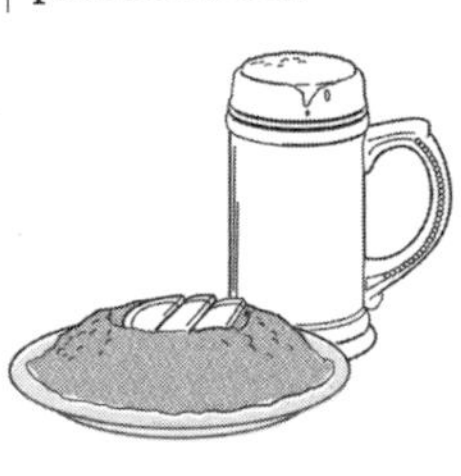

Make a Killer Tuna Sandwich

It takes more than mayo and white bread. Serve up this hearty variation with guidance from Marc Murphy, executive chef of Landmarc and Ditch Plains, both in New York City.

1 UPGRADE THE BASICS
Start with canned albacore tuna (aka white tuna)—it has the best texture and most omega-3s. Use mayonnaise made with olive oil for a richer flavor, and brighten it with a squeeze of lemon.

2 MIX IN ADD-ONS
Finely diced celery and red onion give flavor and crunch, a few capers add a salty kick, and freshly cracked pepper adds a nice bite.

3 USE DECENT BREAD
Skip the sliced sandwich bread. Choose ciabatta bread, which boasts a robust texture (or at the very least use rye bread). And always toast your bread—it creates a barrier that keeps sogginess at bay.

RULE #6

Eat the bacon. Just not too much. Fat doesn't make you fat. Too many calories does.

COOK A TURKEY IN A TRASH CAN

Trash-can turkey frees up Thanksgiving kitchen real estate, cooks quickly, and tastes incredible. Seriously.

WHAT YOU'LL NEED

Aluminum foil (two rolls of extra-wide). New steel trash can (20-gallon size). Newspaper, charcoal briquettes (three 10-pound bags), lighter fluid, matches, broom handle or sturdy stick (2 feet long), hammer, 1 turkey (about a 12-pounder), thawed, giblets packet removed, and rinsed. Large metal shovel. Heatproof gloves. Bucket of water. Fire extinguisher. Rub turkey with olive oil and 4 tablespoons chopped fresh rosemary; season all over with salt and pepper.

1. Clear a fire pit of any rocks, twigs, or other debris, and line it with foil.

2. Using a clean scrub brush and hot soapy water, thoroughly clean and rinse the inside of the can.

3. Mold a few sheets of foil so they form a bowl large enough to hold about $1\frac{1}{2}$ bags of charcoal. Place the bowl in the fire pit, off to the side. Line the bowl with several sheets of newspaper, fill it with charcoal, add lighter fluid, and light the paper. The coals are ready when they're covered with ash, after about 20 minutes.

4. While the coals are heating, hammer a 2-foot-long stick securely into dirt in the center of the fire pit. Then shove a wad of foil into the turkey's cavity and balance the bird on the stick. Gently place the can over the bird.

5. Shovel a ring of coals against the trash can's base, and the remaining coals on top of the can. Let the turkey cook until the charcoal turns to ash, about 2 hours. If the coals turn to ash and start to cool before 2 hours, shovel on a fresh layer of coals. The heat from the smoldering briquettes will light the new ones. Important: Do not lift the can to check on the turkey. Valuable heat will escape from the trash can and the turkey will require much more time to cook.

6. Using heatproof gloves, lift the hot can off the cooked bird. Stick the turkey with a meat thermometer—if it reads 165°F at the thigh, it's safe to eat. Douse the coals with water, being cautious of the resulting smoke or ash.

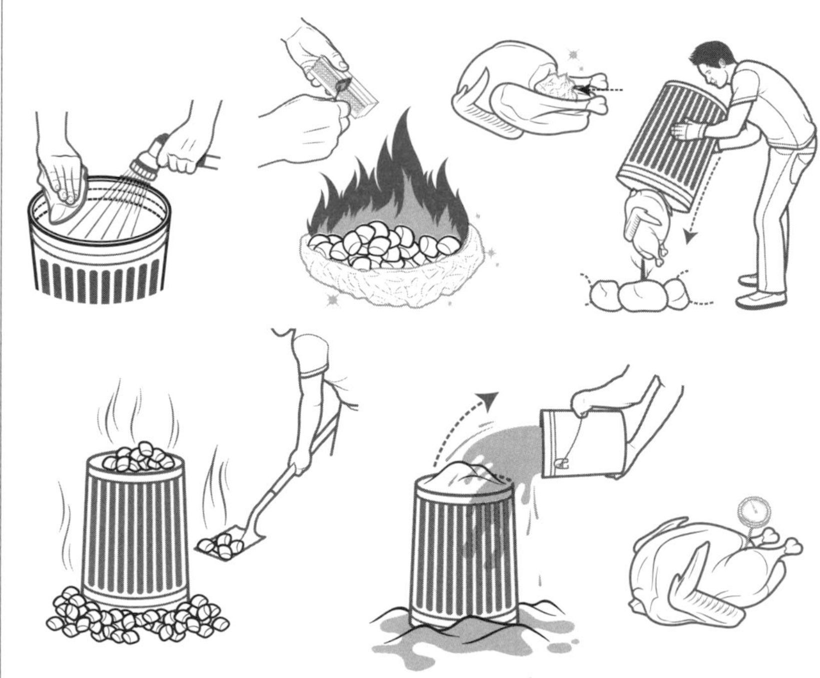

Spring-Clean Your Grill

1. Burn Off the Gunk

Crank the heat, close the grill lid, and leave it for 10 to 15 minutes. The high temperature will char food residue so it's easier to scrape off.

2. Scrub the Grates

Remove the charred residue from the grates with a semiflexible stainless-steel brush. We like the long-range Ultimate Grill Cleaning Brush ($25, Amazon.com). If the grates' undersides are greasy, remove them and wipe them down with a wet, soapy sponge. Then rinse them with a hose and towel-dry. If you have a charcoal grill, jump to step 5.

3. Attack the Burners (Part 1)

Pricier grills often have burner protectors—V-shaped pieces of metal guarding the gas jets from food drips. Remove them and use a putty knife to scrape grease off. If necessary, scrub them with soapy water, hose them off, and towel-dry them.

4. Attack the Burners (Part 2)

Clean the burners with the stainless-steel brush, using a side-to-side motion, not a lengthwise one. This helps keep debris from falling into burners' holes. Look close: Are the gas jets clogged? If so, use the tip of a wire hanger to poke through the center of each one. If the holes are rusted, it's time to replace the burners. Remove the burners for the next step.

5. Hit the Walls

Scrape the walls of the cook box with the putty knife; you want to remove carbonized grease so it doesn't affect the flavor of your food. Very filthy grills may warrant a round of dish soap and water.

6. Give It a Rubdown

Your inaugural BBQ calls for a shiny grill. If it has a stainless-steel finish, wipe the grease away with a dedicated stainless cleaner and a semisoft sponge. Warm water works fine for other finishes.

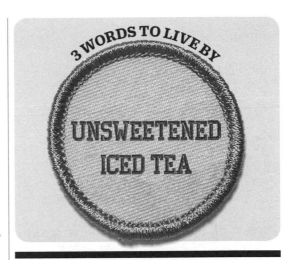

3 WORDS TO LIVE BY
UNSWEETENED
ICED TEA

Make Your Food Taste Smokier

NO NEED TO LIGHT UP THE GRILL IN WINTER. THESE INGREDIENTS ADD SMOKE WITHOUT FIRE.

Chipotle Hot Sauce

This mahogany-hued condiment adds a complex kick of heat to burritos, huevos rancheros, or roast chicken—without the need to open a can of chipotles. Tabasco makes a great version. $4, countrystore.tabasco.com

Smoked Sea Salt

For the ultimate steak, sprinkle a pinch of this seasoning on the meat before serving. Its salty/smoky combo ratchets up savory flavors better than regular table salt. Try Maldon Smoked Sea Salt on steamed vegetables, fish, and even chocolate ice cream. $8, surlatable.com

Roasted Red Peppers

These slow-cooked peppers add a sweet, lightly charred flavor to a mild-tasting sandwich (like turkey and spinach) or salad (mozzarella and basil).

MacGyver Your Bar

Hyper-decant wine

Aerating wine opens up the vino's aroma. Oenophiles do this by pouring it into a decanter, but you can aerate with horsepower instead! Pour the wine into a blender and process it on high for 30 to 60 seconds. Wait for the foam to subside, and serve.—Nathan Myhrvold, coauthor of *Modernist Cuisine*

Sip barworthy whiskey on the rocks

Make ice with water from the tap and you'll end up with cloudy cubes. For crystal-clear ice, boil the water first to eliminate the dissolved gases, and let the water cool before pouring it into trays.—Marcel Vigneron, CEO of Modern Global Tasting

Chill beer fast

Warm beer sucks. And your fridge sucks at chilling beer fast. Instead, add 1 tablespoon of salt to a large bowl of ice water and drop in your bottles. Salt lowers the freezing temperature of the water, creating a more arctic environment for your brew.—Jarrid Masse, cofounder of the Poor Porker in Lakeland, Florida

Stage a rescue operation

If the wine cork broke, fear not. Push the cork all the way into the bottle using the butt end of a butter knife. Then double-knot one end of a 12-inch length of twine and drop that end into the bottle. Tilting the bottle, use the knotted end to fish the cork toward the bottle's neck and then up and out.—Jarrid Masse

RULE #8 **Never store tomatoes, peaches, potatoes, onions, bread, garlic, or coffee in the refrigerator. Cold temps compromise the flavor and texture of these foods.**

RULE #7 **Never serve warm food on a cold plate. Heat your dishes in a 150°F oven for 10 minutes before plating a meal.**

Mix Incredible Homemade Sangria

The key? A kick of tequila, fresh fruit, and white wine. The result isn't as heavy as a pitcher of red and won't stain your lips during your backyard BBQ, says Benjamin Carrier, beverage director at Manhattan's Los Feliz restaurant.

Prep the Flavoring

Deseed three pieces of fruit, such as a peach, an orange, and a pear, and cut them into chunks. Peel a piece of ginger the size of your thumb and cut it into matchsticks. Throw everything into a large pitcher. Stir in $1\frac{1}{2}$ tablespoons of agave nectar or 2 tablespoons of sugar.

Add the Alcohol

Pour a bottle of white wine into the pitcher. (Go with a white that's light and affordable, like Vinho Verde from Portugal.) To punch up the flavors of the fruit and wine, add 2 ounces of 100 percent agave tequila to the pitcher. Try Tres Generaciones Plata ($30, finewinehouse.com) or any other tequila that's advertised as a "highland" tequila.

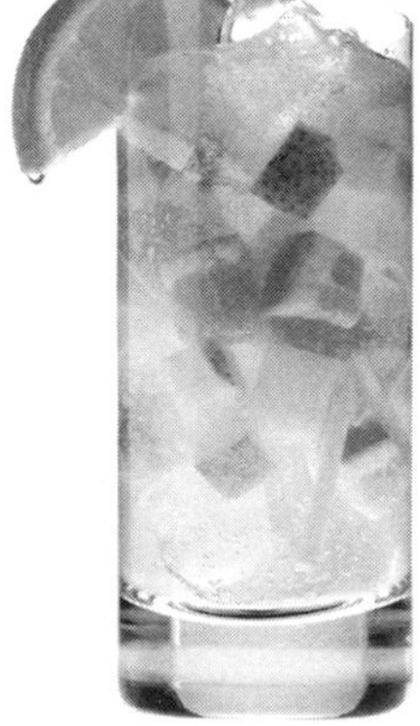

Finish the Drink

Squeeze 2 tablespoons of lime juice into the pitcher and add $\frac{1}{4}$ cup of seltzer. Stir the sangria well and refrigerate for an hour to let the flavors meld. Before serving, top it off with ice.

Make Real Texas-Style Chili

IMPROVE YOUR TAILGATE WITH A LONE STAR STATE ASSIST.

STEP 1
Make a Chili Puree

To achieve deep, robust chili flavor, Texas chili starts with dried chiles. Try two ancho, one pasilla, two guajillo, and two chipotle chiles (available in some supermarkets and from thespicehouse.com; or substitute 4 tablespoons of pure dark chili powder and three canned chipotle chiles, and continue with step 3). Making the puree is a three-part process:

Toast: Heat the stemmed chiles in a large dry skillet over medium-low heat, turning them frequently until they're fragrant and lightly charred—about 8 minutes. (A cast-iron skillet works best.)

Soak: Place the chiles in a large bowl of just-boiled water and soak them until tender, about 20 minutes.

Puree: Combine in a blender with 1 cup of brewed coffee.

STEP 2
Sear the Meat

Texas chili is made with chunks of marbled cuts like boneless beef short-rib, braised until tender. Cut 2 pounds into 1-inch chunks and brown them all over in a large, heavy pot with 2 to 3 tablespoons of vegetable oil, 4 to 5 minutes. Remove them (and juices) and set aside.

STEP 3
Assemble the Chili

Aromatic vegetables like onion and garlic round out the flavor, along with herbs, spices, and beer. In the pot you used for the meat, sauté a large chopped onion and two minced garlic cloves until softened. Return the beef and its juices to the pot and add ½ teaspoon each of ground cumin and dried thyme, and 1 teaspoon of dried oregano. Then add your chili puree and a 12-ounce bottle of beer—whatever you're drinking. Cover and simmer on low until the meat is very tender, about an hour and 15 minutes.

STEP 4
Thicken the Stew

Real Texas chili is thickened with masa harina, a type of corn flour. Find it in the international aisle of your grocery. (No go? Use finely ground cornmeal.) Ladle 2 cups chili into a bowl and stir in 3 teaspoons masa harina or cornmeal. Return the mixture to the pot. Simmer 15 minutes. Add salt and pepper.

STEP 5
Serve with Toppings

Diced red onion adds crunch, grated Cheddar adds richness, and pan-toasted corn tortillas finish the meal.

Motor Through a Sink of Dirty Dishes

TAKE DOWN A TOWER OF PLATES FASTER THAN A BUSBOY BUZZED ON DINER COFFEE.

❶ USE THE RIGHT TOOLS
Ultra Dawn detergent blasts grease and is environmentally friendly. Also buy an ergonomic bottle brush to ease your scrubbing. ($5, oxo.com)

❷ PROTECT YOUR BACK
Stand with your feet about double shoulder width apart. You'll bring your center of gravity closer to the sink, alleviating the need to bend over.

❸ BUST GUNK
For food caked onto pots and pans, add hot water and boil. Soak if necessary. Scrub with a nylon pad after the crud has loosened.

WHIP UP THE ULTIMATE SHRIMP COCKTAIL

SKIP THE BOILING AND SPIKE THE SAUCE.

Buy the Shrimp

Look for fresh, large, shell-on, deveined Gulf shrimp (head on, if possible). Cooking them unpeeled enhances their flavor. You'll need 35 shrimp of the 21/25 count size (that is, 21 to 25 per pound).

Boost Their Taste

Create a brine: In a large bowl, combine 1 cup of water, 2 ounces of kosher salt (about 1/4 cup), and 2 ounces of sugar (about 4 1/2 tablespoons). Stir until dissolved, and add about 8 ounces of ice (about 2 cups). Dump the shrimp in and refrigerate for 20 to 25 minutes.

Make Your Sauce

Blend the following in a food processor until almost smooth: 1 can (14 ounces) of diced tomatoes, 1/2 cup prepared chili sauce, 1/4 cup prepared horseradish, 1 teaspoon sugar, 1/2 teaspoon salt, and a pinch of pepper. Refrigerate.

Broil the Shrimp

Boiling leaches flavor. Instead, preheat a foil-lined baking sheet 8 inches under the broiler for 5 minutes. Rinse the shrimp, pat them dry, and toss them in a bowl with 1 tablespoon of olive oil and a pinch of Old Bay. Broil 2 minutes, flip with tongs, and broil 1 minute more. Meanwhile, wash the bowl and put it in the freezer.

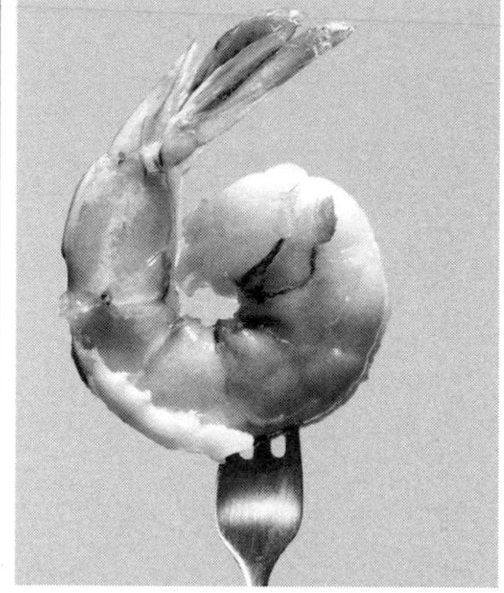

Chill 'Em Out

Put the shrimp in a bowl in the freezer. Take it out and toss every few minutes until they've cooled, about 15 minutes.

Dig Clams

Twenty small clams have only about 280 calories but pack a protein punch of almost 50 grams. Plus, clams contain high levels of vitamin B_{12}. Put scrubbed clams in a pot with white wine, garlic cloves, parsley, and black pepper. Cover and steam until they open. Hit them with lemon juice.

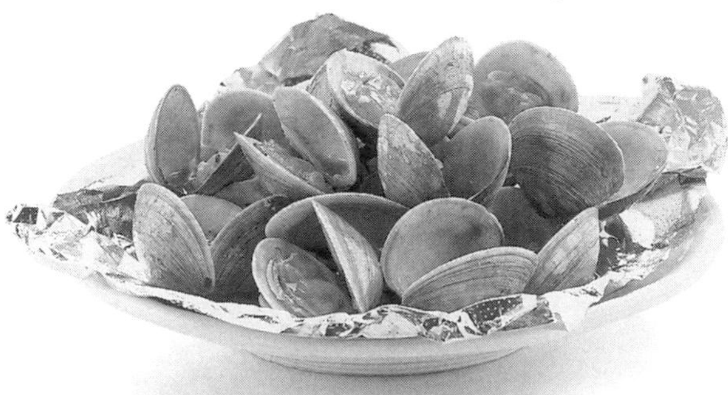

Q I'd eat more broccoli if I could get over the taste. How can I do that?

A. Mustard. Mix the yellow with the green and the result is a tastier broccoli. It'll also be more nutritious, says Elizabeth Jeffrey, PhD, a professor of nutritional sciences at the University of Illinois. "Mustard triggers the release of sulforaphane and indoles, compounds in broccoli that help your liver destroy carcinogens and other toxins." Other flavor-masking tricks: Toss the florets in olive oil and 1 teaspoon of sugar and roast for 10 minutes at 450°F—the broccoli will caramelize, becoming less bitter.

SHUCK AN OYSTER—
with a Screwdriver

IF YOU DON'T HAVE A SHUCKING KNIFE TO POP OPEN THIS DELICIOUS INSTANT APPETIZER, HEAD TO THE TOOLBOX.

❶ SET THE STAGE

Grab a clean flathead screwdriver, a cutting board, and a kitchen towel. Fill a platter with ice to chill the ready-to-eat oysters. Scrub them under cold running water with a vegetable brush.

❷ LOCK AND POP

Look for the hinge—where the shells meet at the tapered end. Tuck the oyster into the towel with the hinge end exposed and the cupped side of the oyster down. Holding the oyster with the towel, place the screwdriver tip between the shells at the hinge. Twist the screwdriver until the top shell pops from the bottom.

❸ FREE THE GOOD STUFF

Pry the halves apart with the screwdriver. Find the adductor muscle (toward the rounded end) and scrape it until it detaches. Chuck the top shell. Clean any debris with your thumb. Separate the muscle from the bottom shell by scraping the tool beneath the meat.

❹ ONE LAST THING . . .

Just remember that eating raw oysters can increase your risk of foodborne illness.

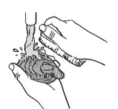

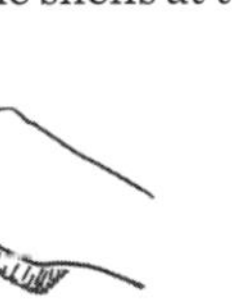

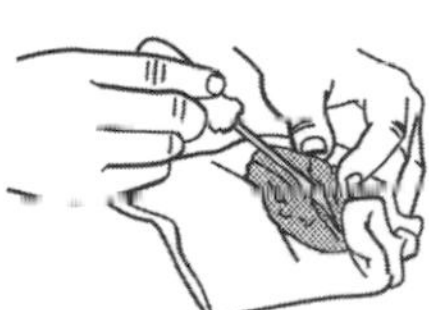

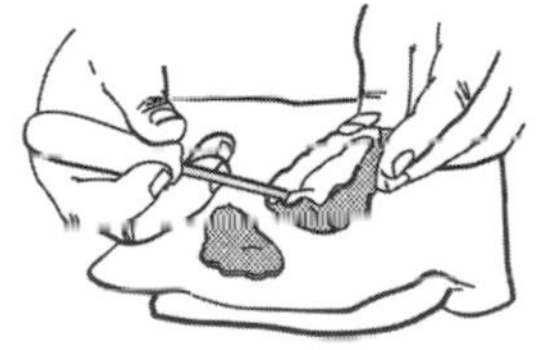

Know Your Oysters

EAST COAST		
Malpeque	**Wellfleet**	**Blue Point**
Prince Edward Island	Cape Cod	Long Island Sound
Small because they grow slowly; light, clean taste.	Rich, flavorful brine with mild mineral notes.	Firm texture; salty with mild mineral notes.
WEST COAST		
Olympia	**Pacific Kusshi**	**Kumamoto**
Olympia, Washington	British Columbia	California and Oregon
The only native West Coast variety is petite and tastes smoky.	Pacific oysters are the most common; Kusshis boast a pillowy texture.	Tiny, so it's a good beginner oyster; notes of melon and cucumber.

Go Saucy

Bottled cocktail sauce doesn't taste as good as the fresh stuff, so make your own: In a small bowl, mix together ½ cup ketchup, 2 teaspoons prepared horseradish, 2 tablespoons lemon juice, 1 teaspoon Worcestershire sauce, and a pinch of freshly ground black pepper. Serve with freshly shucked oysters or cooked, chilled shrimp as a simple appetizer.

RULE #9

Never nuke your lunch in plastic. Even if the container is BPA-free, phthalates can still leach into your food, potentially damaging sperm and altering hormones, says the National Institutes of Health. Transfer the food to glass before microwaving.

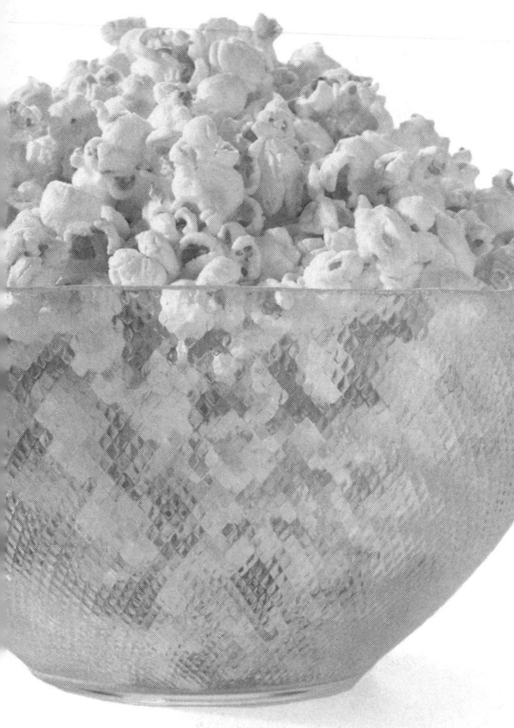

Pop a Perfect Bowl of Popcorn

USE THE STOVETOP, NOT A MICROWAVE, FOR FRESHER-TASTING, MORE THOROUGHLY POPPED KERNELS.

STEP 1:
Prep Your Pot

In a large pot, heat 2 tablespoons canola oil and a few popcorn kernels on medium high. When the kernels begin to pop, the oil is hot enough. Remove the pot from the heat and add 1/4 cup popcorn kernels and 1/2 teaspoon kosher salt. Put on the lid and count to 20, allowing the popcorn and oil to reach the same temperature; otherwise some of the kernels will burn.

STEP 2:
Steam and Shimmy

With one hand, gently move the pan back and forth over the burner; with your other hand, hold the lid like a shield over the pot, leaving it slightly ajar. The idea is to let the steam escape without letting the popcorn kernels leap out. Heat the popcorn until you notice a delay of several seconds between pops, about 3 minutes total. Transfer to a bowl.

STEP 3:
Coat the Kernels

In a small pot, melt 2 tablespoons unsalted butter and, if you want, add additional flavors (below). Once the butter is melted, pour it over the popcorn, cover the bowl with a dinner plate, and give it a few shakes to coat evenly. Serve immediately. Makes 5 to 6 cups of popcorn.

Superior Seasonings

Sweet Bombay
2 teaspoons hot madras curry powder + 2 teaspoons sugar + 3/4 cup toasted, flaked, unsweetened coconut

Salt Rim Margarita
1 tablespoon tequila + 2 teaspoons chopped pickled jalapeños + 1 minced garlic clove + zest and juice from one lime

Caesar Crouton Flavor
1/4 cup grated Parmesan + 1 teaspoon fresh thyme leaves + 1 minced garlic clove + 1/2 teaspoon freshly ground pepper

Take Two Blueberries and Call Us in the Morning

A couple handfuls of fresh blueberries can help you snack your way to better heart health. A Harvard study found that people who consumed the most anthocyanins—found in high amounts in blueberries and strawberries—had 12 percent lower risk of developing hypertension than those who consumed the least.

Roll the Perfect Burrito

The Goal: Arrange ingredients to turn your tortilla into a perfect specimen. Follow these tips from Nate Appleman, culinary manager at Chipotle.

1. Go Big

A 12-inch tortilla lets you stuff your burrito with ingredients yet still provides enough room to wrap it tightly. (Or try a whole wheat wrap for more fiber and a nutty flavor.)

2. Heat Your Tortilla

Don't warm tortillas in the microwave—they'll turn soggy. Instead, heat them in a dry skillet or nonstick pan on medium high until puffed and pliable, 30 to 45 seconds a side.

3. Set a Foundation

Line the tortilla with rice first, to soak up the other ingredients' juices. Leaving 3 inches around the perimeter, layer your rice, beans, and protein in a line.

4. Apply the Finishing Touches

Add sour cream, salsa, or guacamole in a line beside (not atop) the lines of ingredients. Otherwise you risk blobs, which make for inconsistent mouthfuls. Add loose ingredients (lettuce, cilantro, sliced jalapeños, shredded cheese) last so they can adhere to the sour cream and guac.

5. Secure the Burrito

With the line of layered ingredients oriented top to bottom, fold the tortilla's left side just over the ingredients. Then fold the bottom up about an inch. Finally, finish rolling the burrito tightly from left to right. The top remains open. Now chow down on your creation, stain-free.

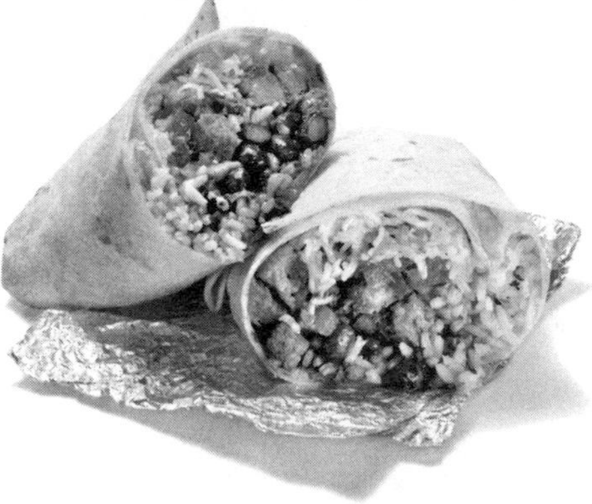

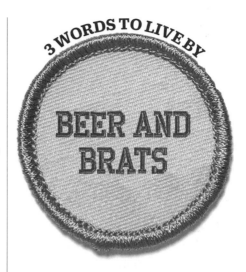

3 WORDS TO LIVE BY
BEER AND BRATS

How to Resuscitate a Dying Broccoli

Nothing's worse than a limp stalk of broccoli. Check that, there are some things worse. But you can perform CPR on almost any wilted vegetable. Simply drop your elderly produce in to a bowl of ice water before cooking. The cold water will penetrate the plant's cells to restore crispness.

Holy $#*! Health Trick

Sprinkle some vinegar on that sandwich bread. Scientists in Sweden found that when people consumed 2 tablespoons of vinegar with a high-carb meal, their blood sugar was 23 percent lower than when they skipped the vinegar chaser.

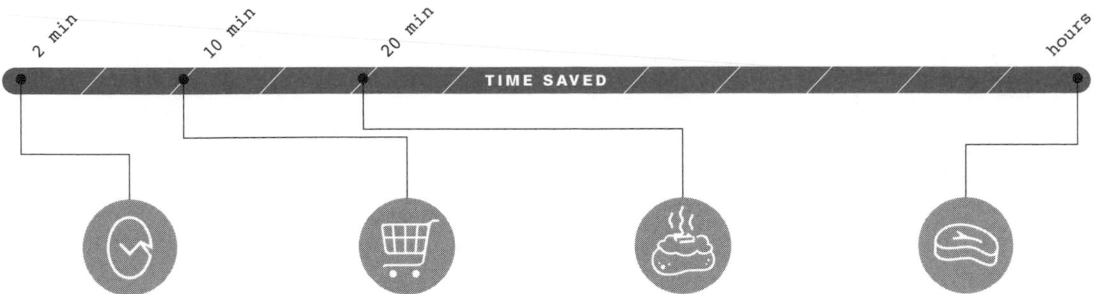

How to Be a Faster Foodie

Cook Quick-Peel Eggs! The fresher your eggs, the harder they'll be to peel. Make hard-boiled eggs easy by adding a bit of baking soda to the water before you turn on the heat. The baking soda penetrates the eggs, preventing the albumin in the whites from sticking to the shells.

Shop the Salad Bar Stir-frying happens quickly, but the prep work can be a slog. For any recipe that requires lots of sliced vegetables, raid your supermarket's salad bar. Not only are the ingredients precut, but you can also buy the exact amount you need.

Speed Up Spuds! For faster baked potatoes or sweet potatoes, start them in the microwave on high for 1 minute. Then transfer them to a preheated oven. You'll cut the time in half while maintaining the fluffy texture that only baking can provide.

Thaw Food Faster! Don't place that frozen T-bone on the counter to thaw—that's how bacteria multiply. Instead, seal meat in a zip-top bag and drop it into a bowl of cold water in the sink, according to the USDA Food Safety and Inspection Service. Change the water every half hour until the meat thaws, 2 to 3 hours for a 3- to 4-pound package.

5 Belly-Filling Foods

Each of the following contains hunger-fighting doses of protein, along with fiber or fat, to help keep you full long after you've eaten.

ALMONDS · OATMEAL · SALMON · QUINOA · BLACK BEANS

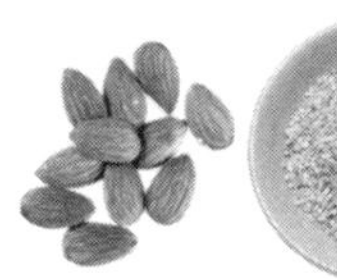
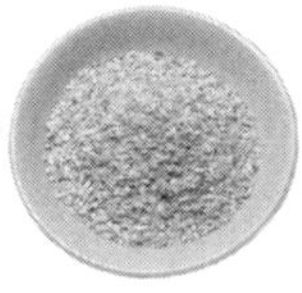
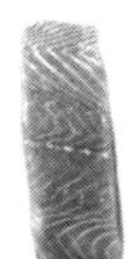
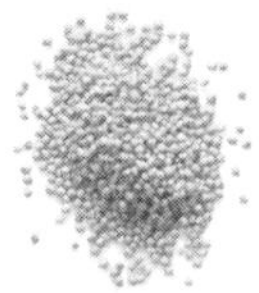
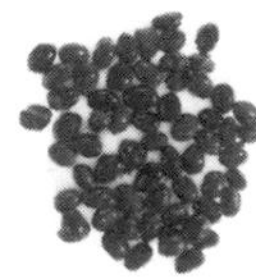

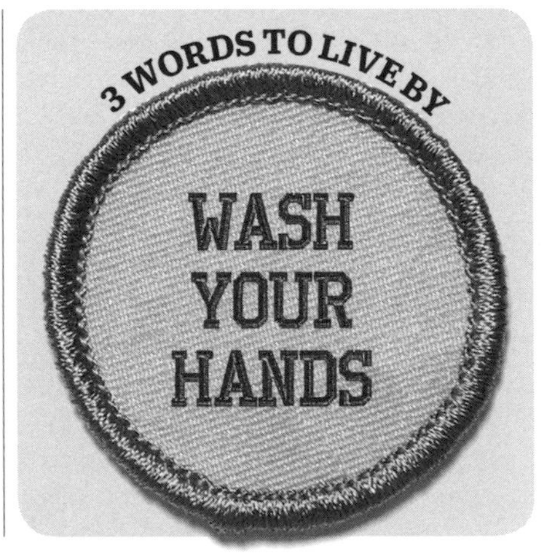

Best Ballpark Foods

Crackerjack Options to the Ubiquitous Dog

CITI FIELD, QUEENS

Pulled Pork Sandwich

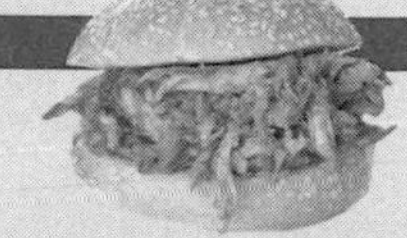

MILLER PARK, MILWAUKEE

Cheese Curds (fried chunks of cheese)

U.S. CELLULAR FIELD, CHICAGO

Mexican-Style Elote Corn (corn tossed with butter, lime, chili powder, mayo, and cheese)

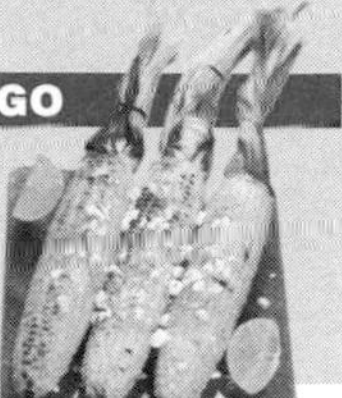

AT&T PARK, SAN FRANCISCO

Dungeness Crab Sandwich

TARGET FIELD, MINNEAPOLIS

Turkey Leg

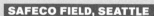

SAFECO FIELD, SEATTLE

The Ichiroll (sushi roll of spicy tuna with daikon radish sprouts and black sesame seeds)

MINUTE MAID PARK, HOUSTON

Fajitas

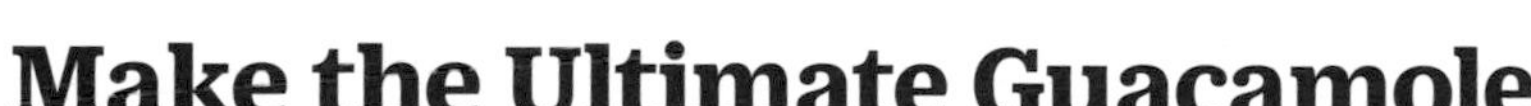

Make the Ultimate Guacamole

GREAT GUAC DOESN'T REQUIRE TOMATO OR MAYO—THAT'S JUST HOW RESTAURANTS SAVE MONEY BY USING LESS AVOCADO.

The Avocado

Buy the pear-shaped, rough-skinned Hass variety. (Its texture is best.) If the fattest part yields slightly when you squeeze lightly, it's good. If it's soft, has brittle skin, or the small button up top is gone, it's brown inside.

The Guac

Peel and dice three avocados. In a bowl, combine them with a small handful of chopped fresh cilantro, ½ cup chopped white onion, one minced jalapeño or serrano chile, a squeeze of lime juice, and salt to taste. Mix vigorously.

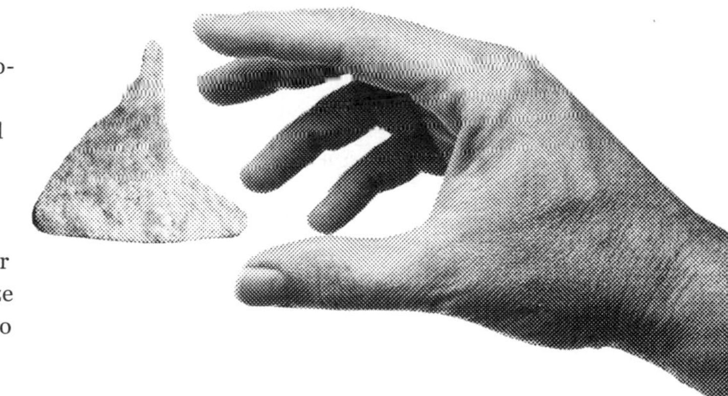

Scoop the chopped onion into a strainer and run it under cold water for 30 seconds. This removes sulfurous compounds that can overpower the guacamole's taste.

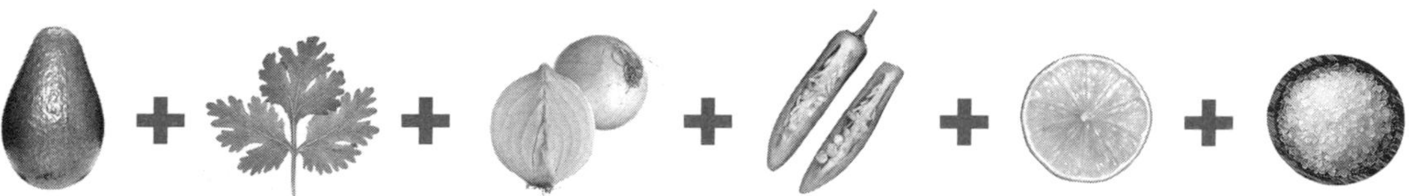

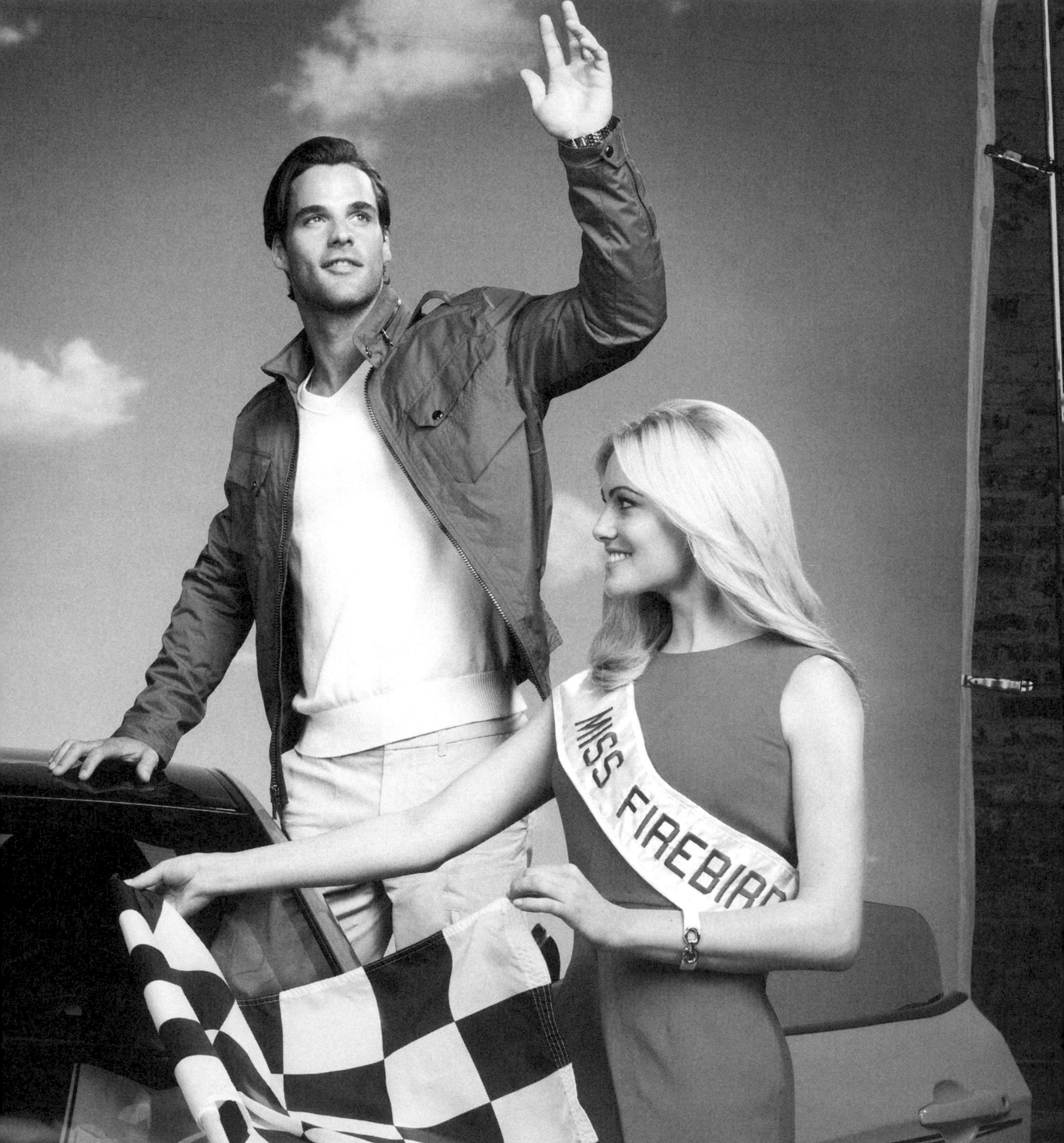
MISS FIREBIRD

How to Win at Everything

You Need Skill, Knowledge, a Few Tricks, and a Little Luck to Triumph. Find Three of Four Here.

Many very smart people have said about winning that the real reward is found in the struggle and effort you make as you strive toward greatness. That's all true. We have great admiration for the man who has left it all on the field at the end of the game even if he has no points on the scoreboard. But on the flip side, let's be honest: Nobody wants to be labeled the runner-up, a sister-kisser, a loser.

We like to win. So whatever you're competing for in life, no one will ever tag you with those descriptions again thanks to this chapter. From winning the wishbone to bar bets, Scrabble to golf, pickup basketball to Rock, Paper, Scissors, and everything in between, we know how to put 'em in your "W" column.

Kick Butkus in Flag Football

Leave defenses bewildered and quarterbacks dizzy with this playbook from Jerry Johnson, 2004 US Flag & Touch Football League National Hall of Fame inductee and head coach.

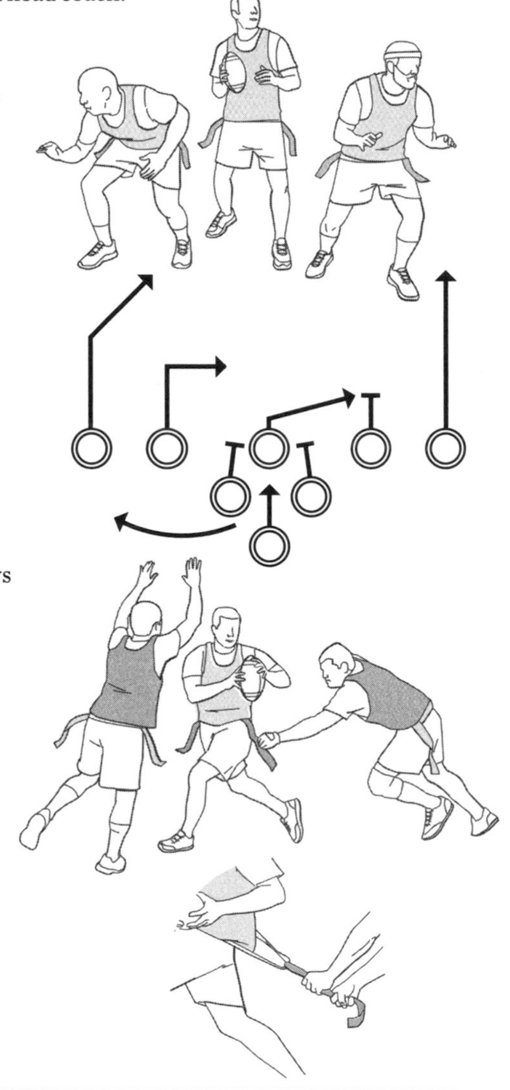

Own the End Zone

Flag football is a faster game than tackle. With more rushing, success depends less on pass plays, which can result in interceptions. Instead, protect the QB's runs with two good blocking backs, or move your slot receiver into max protection as the third blocker to attempt a deep pass.

Steal This Play

To rack up points on offense, call a "throwback" maneuver: After the snap, the quarterback steps up 3 yards and then throws to his man in motion. The quarterback then becomes a potential receiver sprinting along the sideline. It'll work as long as Big Uncle Bubba isn't your QB.

Solidify Your D

Most flag football teams expect the pass, so they overcover the potential receivers. You can break up more plays by always blitzing at least two rushers on each play to contain the QB, designating the fastest defender as a power rusher to swat down hurried passes or make the sack.

Bonus:

SNAG THE FLAG

Don't blindly swipe at the flag. Square your shoulders and reach toward the runner's waist while keeping him directly in front of you. This will slow him, giving you extra time to get help from your teammates or grab the flag belt, yanking it off in one swift motion.

RULE # 1 **Encouraging yourself with non-first-person pronouns ("You can kick his ass") is more effective than using first person ("I can kick his ass"), according to the *Journal of Personality and Social Psychology.***

Win the Wishbone

1 Retrieve the wishbone. Place the bird on its back and locate the V-shaped valley between the breasts. Gently pull the wishbone from beneath the middle muscle flap. Rinse the grease off the bone and give it some time to dry.

2 Choke up. Grasp the wishbone between your thumb and forefinger as close as possible to the base of the V.

3 Let your opponent do the work. Simply hold the wishbone—the other guy can tug. He'll probably pull out and up, which will shift the breaking point from the center to his side. Stand firm and you should watch the bone break in your favor most of the time.

How to Win an Argument

Let your foe present his entire argument without interruption. Allowing him to blow off steam will make him more receptive to your point. Then restate his view before you present your case to show that you understand him; he'll be more likely to be swayed by your calmly presented logic. Never get personal. It'll only piss him off and make him less willing to concede.

Score on the Fast Break

Finish strong with advice from New York Knicks guard Arron Afflalo.

If You Have an Open Court. Make a run for it using the fewest dribbles possible. NBA pros can make it to the hoop from half court with two or three strong dribbles. If you minimize the number of times the ball hits the floor, you'll book it to the basket faster.

If One Man Is Guarding You. Keep your man backpedaling—he can't jump as high to block your shot. Protect the ball with your free forearm as you jump and bank the ball off the top corner of the square.

If They Caught Up and Pushed You to the Baseline. The defender isn't as threatening as his backup. If they're both on the strong side, go up and under for a reverse layup. If they're watching the weak side? Hit a quick jumper.

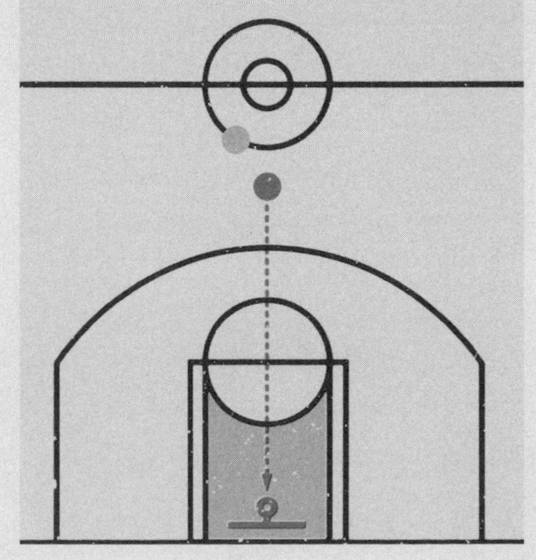

Rule the Pool Table

Pool hustlers know that "grip it and rip it" doesn't work. Start your games using these smart break strategies from Max Eberle, creator of the *Powerful Pool* DVD series and head instructor at ProPoolAcademy.com.

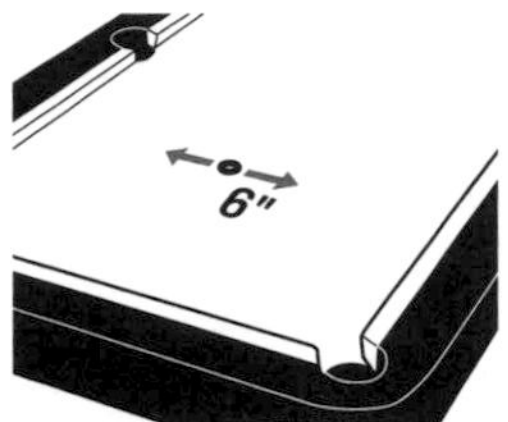

Prepare the Ammo

Your goal is to blast the cue ball into the head ball at an angle that forces all the balls to explode outward from the point of impact. To do this, place the cue ball within 6 inches to the left or right of the head spot (the bull's-eye on the table's felt), depending on which side feels most comfortable.

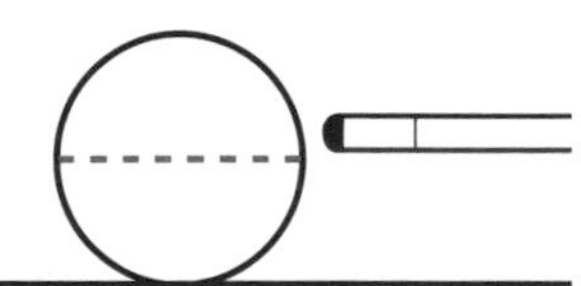

Plan the Break

Adjust your hand bridge to aim your cue $1/16$ inch above the cue ball's center; this will make it stop in the center of the table after the break. Hold the cue loosely with your back hand. A too-tight grip tenses the muscles in your arm and shoulders, increasing your risk of a wayward break.

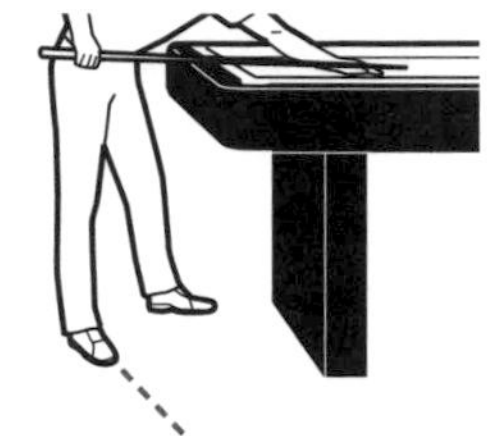

Approach the Table

For a powerful break, you need a powerful stance. Position your forward foot beneath the line of your cue to help stabilize the shot. Step back with the other foot so your feet are beyond shoulder width apart; at the same time point your toes a little less than 90 degrees from the line of your cue.

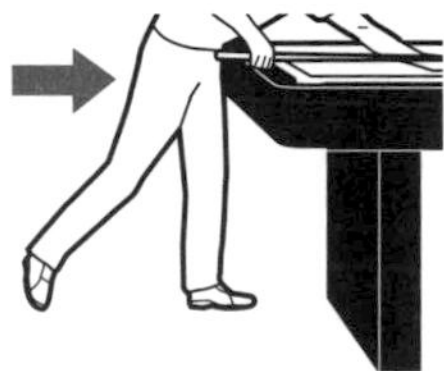

Execute the Break

To keep your stroke smooth, cradle the cue in the pads of your fingers. Rest your weight on your back foot and then forcefully transfer the weight to your front foot. Keeping your elbow tucked next to your side, hit the ball as hard as you can, following through for greatest accuracy.

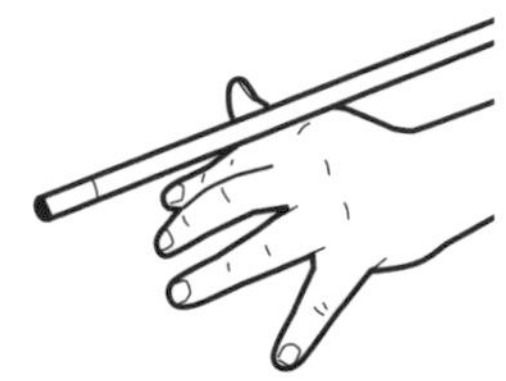

Build a Bridge

Newbs move their stabilizing hand when they shoot, causing the cue tip to swerve. Put your lead hand on the felt, keeping the heel of your palm flat and your fingers fanned and extended to form a bridge. Tuck your thumb to your index finger and tent your hand. Rest the cue in the crook that forms.

Chalk It Up

The blue stuff helps create friction between the tip and the cue ball for more accurate shots. Most people spin the tip in the chalk; this prevents the chalk from sticking, resulting in a slippery tip. Instead, stroke the cue tip with the chalk for better edge coverage (three to five times around). Always apply chalk before you break.

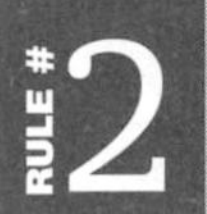

When betting on horses, it's wiser to consider the horse's trainer's winning percentage over the jockey's.

Jump a Ball

This trick can rescue you from one of the toughest spots on the billiards table, says Shanelle Loraine, a pro player with Dragon Promotions.

Change Weapons

It's best to use a jump cue, which is a shorter stick. Hold it loosely, for fluidity and control. Set a sturdy base grip with a traditional open-hand bridge.

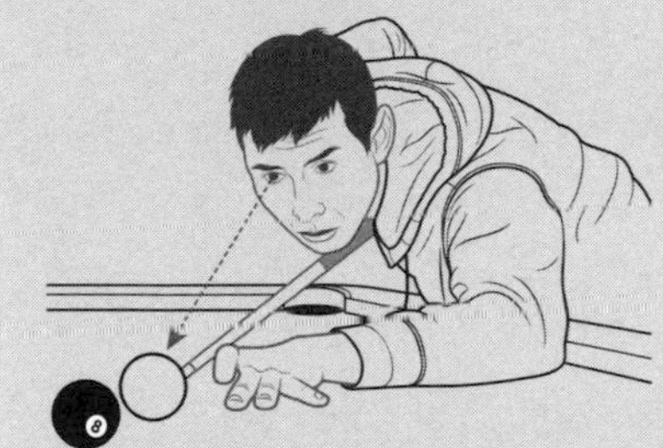

Aim Down

Your cue and line of sight should point downward, with your cue angled 30 to 45 degrees—much higher than normal. Don't target the bottom of the ball—you risk scooping (an illegal hit) or worse, tearing the cloth. Instead, imagine you're piercing through the center of the ball.

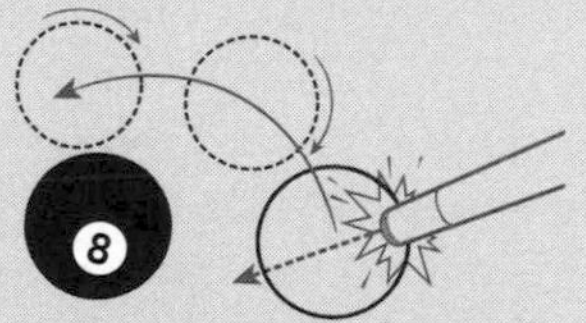

Fire Quick

Strike the ball hard with a sharp movement. The slight downward motion provided by your stance should be enough to propel the ball over the obstacle ball with a little backspin.

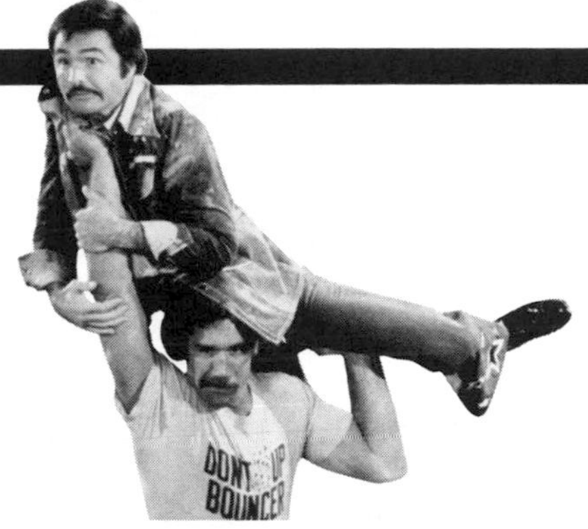

Win Any Bar Fight

The principle is "distract and conquer." There's a reason why a magician waves a wand. It allows him to move the other hand more freely undetected while the audience is focusing on the wand. You can use this bit of magic to your advantage in a bar fight. Here's how: If some punk backs you into a corner, first fake a roundhouse right. Then hit him with a fast left jab. He'll be so focused on following the big curved move that he'll miss the straight attack. While the jab isn't very powerful, he won't see it coming, and then you can follow with a hook. Presto-change-o! Now you've taken him to school . . . and he's learned a lesson he won't soon forget.

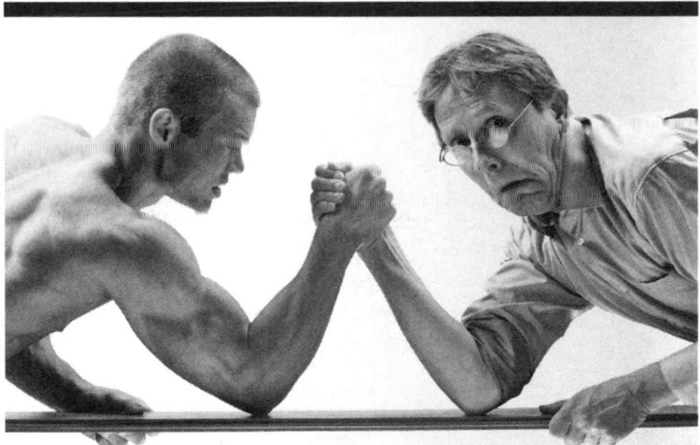

Win an Arm-Wrestling Match

THINK: HIGH, TIGHT, AND FAST.

Grip high on your foe's thumb to increase your leverage.

Stay tight by keeping the distance between your hand and body as close as possible.

Move fast at the start. The player who makes the first strong move usually wins. Few arm-wrestling matches last longer than 10 seconds.

Beat a Speeding Ticket

Start Off Right

Pull over as soon as you see the officer's lights. Turn on your interior light if it's dark out, and have your license and insurance card ready. This will put him in a good mood.

Don't Hem and Haw

Officers are lied to so often that it's refreshing when someone just fesses up. Acknowledge where you erred and promise you'll be safer. Throw in an apology as well.

Cop a Plea

Now that you've proved your sincerity, ask for a break: "I earned that citation, but would you mind issuing me a warning instead? It won't happen again." Being direct may work.

Win in Court

If you do get a ticket, consider lawyering up. A good attorney can turn a six-point "30 mph over" ticket into a four-point "unsafe lane change" ticket—and you won't have to go to court.

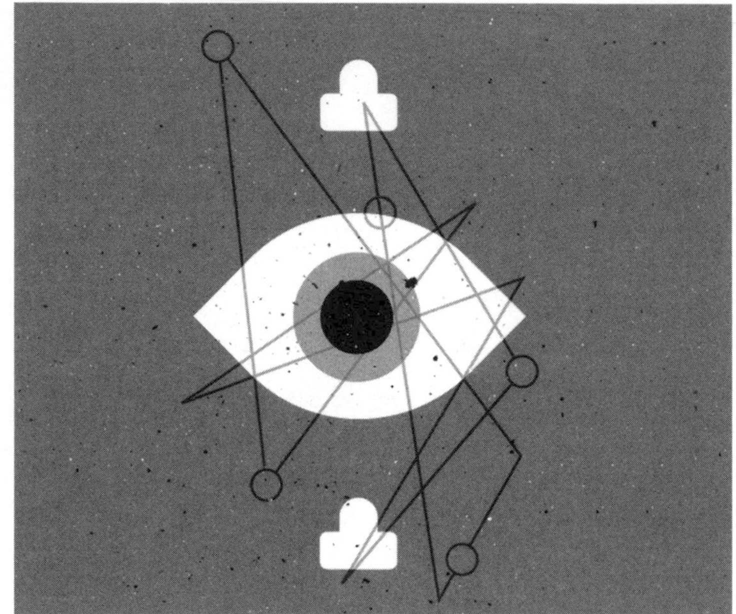

Beat Anyone at Air Hockey

Don't smash the puck and hope for the best. Slow down, study your opponent, and wait for your time to strike.

The Grip

Plant your index and ring fingers firmly in the groove between the knob and the rim of the mallet. Your middle finger should bend slightly, with the knuckle touching the knob. Your thumb and pinkie should rest outside the mallet. Move the mallet by turning your wrist, not your hand. This allows you to react faster to the puck.

The Defense

Hold the mallet about a foot from the goal, and don't sweep too far to chase the puck—you'll leave yourself open. When you block a shot, tap the puck lightly to keep it on your side. Then look at your opponent's position before firing back.

The Offense

If you find your opponent guarding the goal closely, attack him with straight shots to either corner of the goal. If he usually keeps his mallet out away from the goal, bank the puck off the side rail so the puck travels around and behind the mallet before he can bring it back to block the goal.

Win Scrabble *Every Time*

Hammer the competition with these strategies from three-time national Scrabble champion Joe Edley.

Run the Board

Yes, early in the game (or later on, if you're losing), you want a "bingo" that uses all seven tiles, racks up 50 bonus points, and crushes your opponents' hopes. But if you're ahead by more than 70 points, go into defensive mode: Block, or use double- or triple-word-score tiles wherever possible.

Balance the Rack

Think "entrails." Its letters (in order, SRNTL for consonants and EAL for vowels) are the most versatile bingo builders in the game. Those high-point tiles (Q, X, Z, J)? Rookies may bogart them, but you know better. Get rid of them quickly (see "Go Small"), because they're tough to use in long, game-changing words.

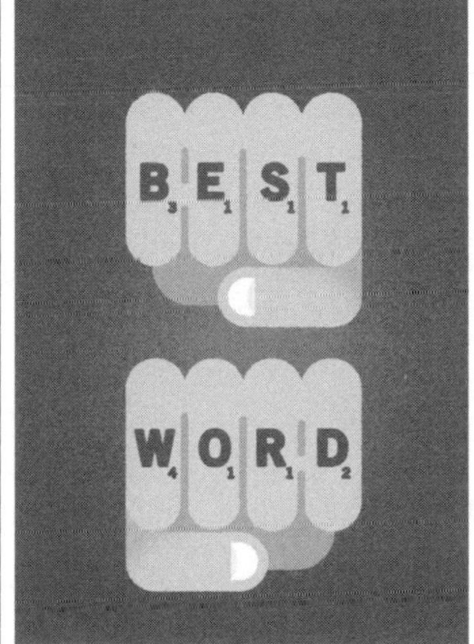

Use Word Extenders

To build those bingos, you'll need to manage your tiles. Try to keep your balance of vowels and consonants relatively equal. Cultivate prefixes (pre-, over-) and suffixes (-ing,-able,-ive). Then deploy them on the board to create common words such as overcome, staying, capable, or preface.

Go Small

Most players associate long words with big points, but unless it's a bingo, stretching letters across the board gives your opponent access to scoring points from the bonus squares. Short words (ZA, QI, AX, JO, XI) boost your score, use up tough-to-play letters, and help you keep the game under your control.

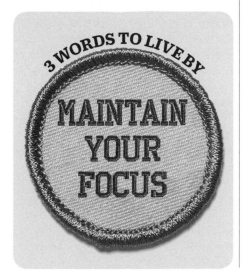

Rock, Paper, Scissors, WIN!

Boost your odds of winning with tips from the scientists at China's Zhejiang University who completed a large-scale study of player behavior in the timeless playground game. The researchers found some typical patterns of player behavior emerge in the second and third rounds of the game:

- If a player wins, he will usually play the same item. (Win with Scissors, he'll play Scissors again.)
- If a player loses, he will typically switch to the next item in the sequence of the name of the game. For example, if he loses with Rock, he'll usually pick Paper. If he loses with Paper, he'll pick Scissors. Loses with Scissors, he'll pick Rock.

You can gain the advantage by understanding this and quickly predict your opponent's next choice.

Shred the Air Guitar

Tips courtesy of William Ocean, 2009 US Air Guitar Championship winner:

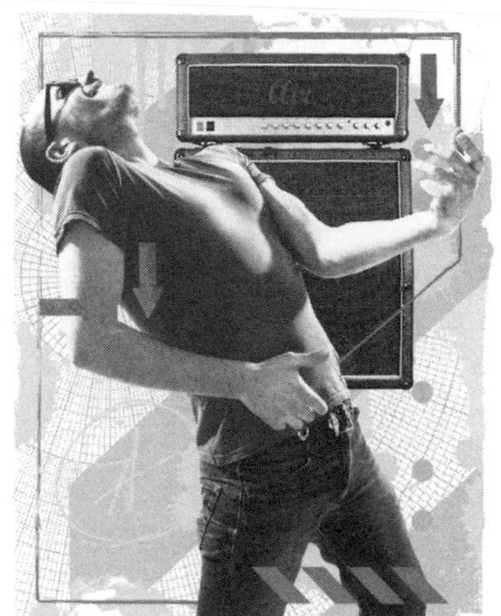

1. Envision Your Ax

If you can't picture your guitar, nobody else can. Put the strap over your head and don't forget to tune. You'll set parameters for the guitar's size.

2. Hold It Right

Rest your dominant hand across your waistline, about 4 inches from your body. Your other hand should hover at least 2 feet up the neck.

3. Time Your Fingers

Strumming is boring. Instead, time your finger movements to major key changes in the music—and nod or thrust forward as you do so people can see that you're synced with it.

4. Pace Yourself

Walk and purse your lips—but space out the arm swings and jumps, or you'll look spasmodic.

WILLIAM OCEAN'S TOP THREE FACE-MELTING AIR-GUITAR TRACKS

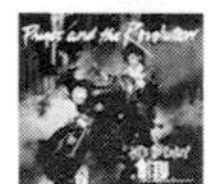

"Let's Go Crazy," Prince & the Revolution

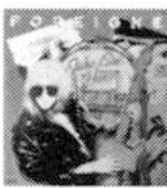

"Juke Box Hero," Foreigner

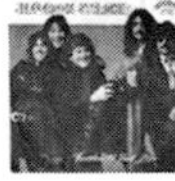

"Jane," Jefferson Starship

Win a Bar Bet

Put a couple of pints on someone else's tab with The Dime-Drop Deception.

Bet This

You can drop a dime, suspended above a beer bottle with only a toothpick, into the bottle. And you'll accomplish this feat without touching the bottle, toothpick, or dime.

Do This

Fold a toothpick in half, making a V, and then rest it on the mouth of the bottle so the toothpick is parallel to the table. Then carefully place a dime on top of the folded toothpick so it rests slightly off center over the mouth of the beer bottle.

Now slowly drip a few drops of water onto the fold in the toothpick. The water will gradually cause the wood to expand, making the toothpick spread outward and allowing the dime to drop into the bottle.

Remember: You lose valuable points if your beer bottle isn't empty.

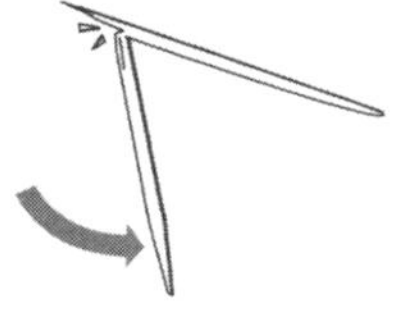

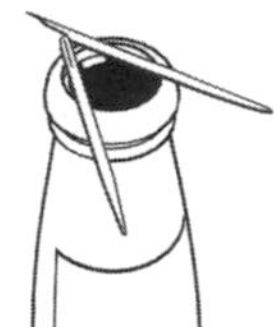

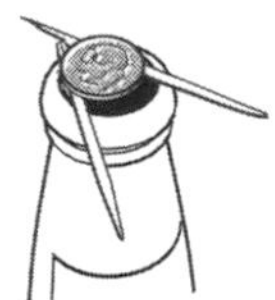

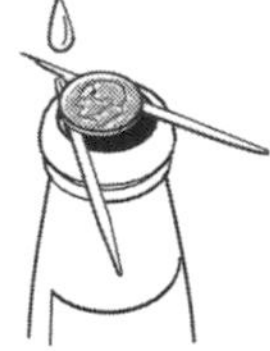

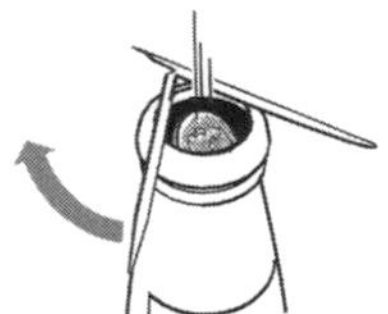

How to Punt a Football High and Deep

Former Dallas Cowboys All-Pro kicker Shayne Graham helps you put the foot in football.

Take Your Position

Deep, accurate punts require controlled form. Grip the ball with your dominant hand as if you were giving a handshake, nestling it between your thumb and fingers. Extend your arm forward as far as you can and hold the ball horizontally, with the nose pointing slightly to your left (or to your right if you're left-handed). Keep the laces up.

Make Contact

Starting with your kicking foot, take two steps forward to build momentum and then swing your foot out to meet your hand. Make contact with the ball as late as you can so you're almost kicking it straight out of your fingers. If you drop the ball too early, you're more likely to have a wayward punt. A smooth kick will fly farther than if you simply blast the ball.

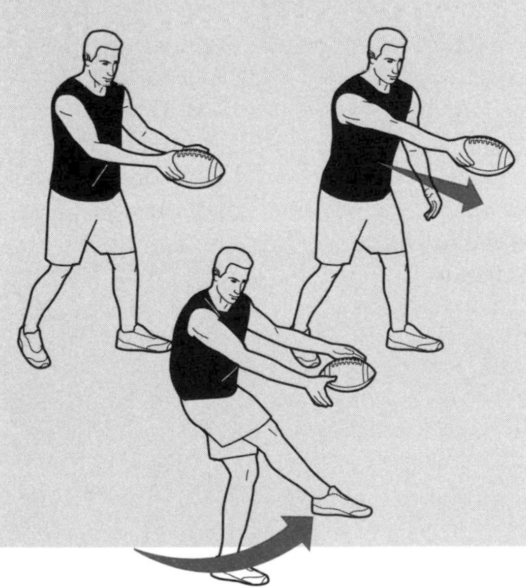

Win at the Casinos

Look at the house edge and the speed of the game, says Frank Scoblete, author of *Beat the Craps out of the Casinos*. "How many games you play per hour and how many decisions you have to make can determine how fast the casino's edge adds up." Blackjack might give the dealer only a 0.5 percent statistical advantage, but you'll play as many as 100 hands per hour. Roulette is slow-paced, but the dealer has a whopping 5.26 percent advantage. Scoblete's advice: Join a packed blackjack table so the dealer can't churn through cards as fast, or belly up to a craps table, which offers some of the best odds in the casino. Forget about the patchwork quilt of betting options and lay down $6 "place" bets on both the 6 and 8. Whenever someone rolls either of those two numbers, you'll win $7 for every $6 you wager. Odds dictate what will happen 10 times out of 36 rolls. "You're getting a lot of action without being involved in all the decisions," says Scoblete. "That's a lot of entertainment for your money."

RULE # 3 **Even bad card players get good hands from time to time.**

Run Farther
THAN YOU DID YESTERDAY

Instead of taking on an extra quarter mile at the end of your regular route, begin your run a few blocks ahead of your usual starting point. By the time you reach your regular turnaround, your mind has all but forgotten that you've actually gone farther than normal.

Pull Off an April Fools' Prank

Punk like a pro with these practical-joke tips, courtesy of Streeter Seidell and Amir Blumenfeld, collegehumor. com staffers and hosts of *Pranked* on MTV.

RULE 1:
Keep It Simple

The more complicated you make the prank (multiple people, intricate plans), the tougher it will be to pull off. Think: Stick a stuffed dead bird in your buddy's favorite cereal box, rig a camera, and watch him have breakfast. Surprising. Easy. Hilarious.

RULE 2:
Have Your AV Setup Down

It's the YouTube age: Pranks must be shared. Crisp video quality can add drama. Stabilize the camera with a discreet mount; the flexible GorillaPod Video tripod ($30, joby.com) can fit into good hiding spots.

RULE 3:
Be Mean

Don't hurt anyone, but great pranks often involve some kind of temporary emotional stress. It's why a whoopee cushion pales in comparison to responding to your pal's snarky e-mail about a colleague with, "Hey—did you mean to cc him on this?"

Fresh out of prank ideas? Try these.

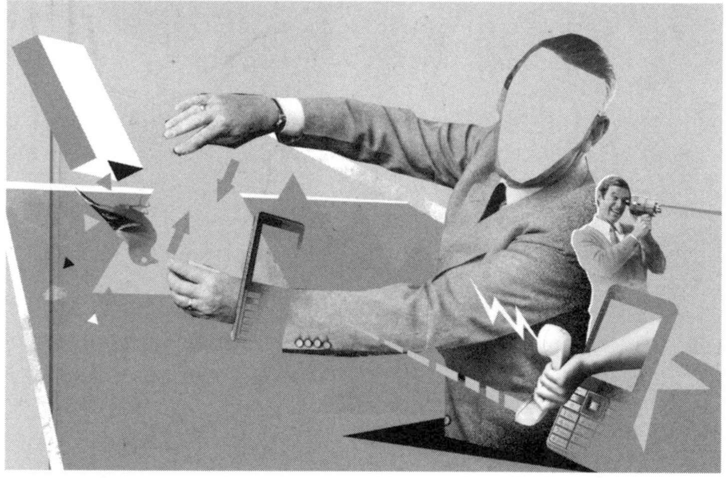

AT WORK:
Idle Hands

In a public place, challenge a coworker to a coordination test: Tell him to close his eyes and move his hand vertically up and down between both of your hands, which you're holding about a foot apart—but he must do it without hitting your hands. As soon as he starts, quietly step away and leave the room.

HANGING WITH BUDDIES:
Cell Phone Swap

Ask your friend if you can see his phone for a sec. (Say yours is dead and you want to check some scores.) While entrusted with his phone, change his ex-girlfriend's number to your own. Throughout the day bombard him with "Call me now!" texts. When he calls back, start laughing at him.

AT WORK:
Mouse Gremlin

Place a Post-it Note under a colleague's mouse so it blocks the laser. (Trim the edges so it's not visible.) He'll spend a good 15 minutes struggling with the mouse, cable, and computer before finally turning it over.

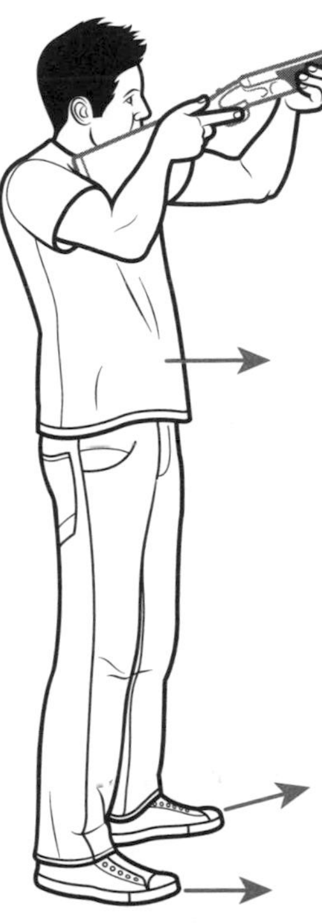

FAKE YOUR WAY THROUGH

Sporting Clays

Know the game: You yell, "pull!" and the guy operating the target release hits a button launching a clay "bird" target (or two) for you to blow to smithereens.

Ready . . .

Have the course guide release a practice target so you can see its path. (Don't shoot at this one.) Square your hips in the direction you'll be shooting—typically the high point of the target's arc.

Plant the butt of the gun into the pocket of your shoulder firmly enough that it can't slip—this will soften the recoil.

Aim . . .

Point your barrel about halfway between your estimated firing spot and the launcher. Keep both eyes open for maximum accuracy. After calling "pull!" spot the target in your peripheral vision and start trying to "cover it" with the muzzle. Don't play catch-up—if anything, stay a bit ahead of the target.

Fire!

When the target reaches your firing point and your muzzle's over it, pull the trigger—but don't stop your movement. Maintain your follow-through for greater accuracy.

RULE # 4

Stay with the gun. In skeet shooting, one of the most common mistakes shooters make is taking the gun off their shoulder too quickly. That breaks the gun's momentum and wastes the tail end of the shot. Try staying with the target after you pull the trigger before lowering the stock.

10 RULES OF SAFE GUN HANDLING

1. **Always keep the muzzle pointed in a safe direction.**
2. **Firearms should be unloaded when not actually in use.**
3. **Don't rely on your gun's "safety".**
4. **Be sure of your target and what's beyond it.**
5. **Use correct ammunition.**
6. **If your gun fails to fire when the trigger is pulled, handle with care!**
7. **Always wear eye and ear protection when shooting (unlike the clown above).**
8. **Be sure the barrel is clear of obstructions before shooting.**
9. **Don't alter or modify your gun, and have guns serviced regularly.**
10. **Learn the mechanical and handling characteristics of the firearm you are using.**

Dominate the Pub Dartboard

Lesson one: Don't throw anything if you can't focus on your bull's-eye. Also ...

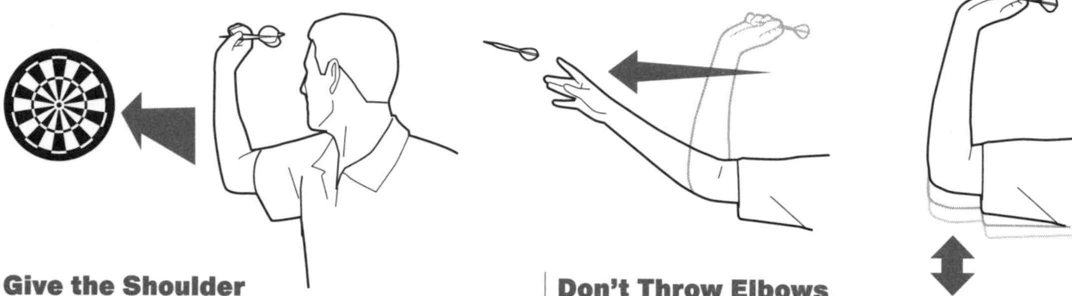

Give the Shoulder

Newbs usually face the dartboard, a stance that allows for errant throws. Instead, stand with the shoulder of your throwing arm facing the board. This locks your arm, ensuring darts fly true.

Plant Your Feet

If you lunge (or worse, jump) in an attempt to add oomph to your throw, you'll send your dart off course. Your throwing power should come from your biceps, elbow, and wrist. Keep your body rigid to create a good foundation.

Don't Throw Elbows

Your elbow should naturally move slightly upward or downward to adjust to the height of your target on the board.

Ease Your Grip

The tighter you clamp down on the dart, the harder it is to transition into a quick, smooth release.

Stay Focused

Aim for an exact point on the board—not a section. The more focused your eyes are, the less space you subconsciously allow your arm to move and cause a miss.

Conquer Carnival Games

Want to win the giant bunny for your date? Your best odds of winning are with balloon darts (57 percent), skee-ball (46 percent) and water gun races (36 percent); ring toss on the soda bottle is nearly impossible at (2 percent).

Balloon darts: Aim at the shiniest balloons; they're reflecting light because they're the most inflated, or ready to pop. Throw hard, arcing your dart so it's more likely to hit the top of the balloon, where the latex is stretched tightest.

Skee-ball: Don't waste shots on hard-to-nail 100-pointers. Shoot for the 40-point center. If you miss, you'll still score.

Water gun races: Watch a race to pick the most accurate gun. Then pay for two games up front. Calibrate your aim that first game. Then maintain that firing position for the next one.

Basketball shooting: The rim is squeezed slightly, so you'll miss with anything but a swish. Since the hoop is also closer than typical free-throw distance, a higher-than-usual trajectory will increase odds that it will fall through.

Nail the Chip Shots

Shave strokes around the green with an assist from Mark Wilson, one of the best short-game players on the PGA Tour.

Club Down

For a less risky shot, "bump and roll" the ball between the edge of the green and the hole. Don't be afraid to use a pitching wedge or 9-iron (or lower) to start the shot.

Set Up Your Shot

Using a narrow stance, align the ball with your back foot's big toe. Place more weight on your front foot. The shaft should lean so your hands are ahead of the clubface. Keep a short backswing, wrists locked.

Hit the Practice Green

Pick a few pins on a practice green. Take nine balls and hit toward a pin, never aiming at the same pin twice in a row. Add up the distances the shots sit from their pins. More than 90 feet? Try again.

Survive a Rough Patch

If your ball is buried, break out a higher-lofted sand wedge or lob wedge to make sure the ball lifts in the air. Use the same mechanics as normal and let the club do the work.

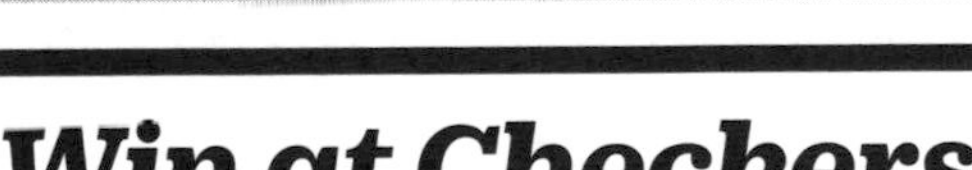

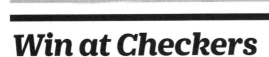

Win at Checkers

- Get a king ASAP, even if it means sacrificing a few pieces to open a path.
- Push through the center to disrupt your opponent's forces.
- Call up your back row quickly. Don't wait to develop those pieces.

Source: U.S. checkers champ Ryan Pronk

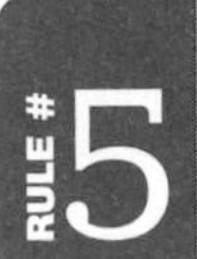

You can never practice too many long putts.

Be a Foosball Wizard

Raw power doesn't bring victory—speed, control, and shot setup do. Let Ryan Moore, world-ranked table soccer champion, help you dominate.

A. Learn Ball Control

Position your index finger and thumb in the indents of the handle. A closed-fist grip limits your range of motion and slows you down.

B. Serve—to Yourself

When you serve, place your index finger on the right side of the ball in the serving hole and gently flick it as you release. This adds spin. The ball will exit at an angle—straight toward your players.

C. Perfect the Stop

If you stand firm, the ball will bounce back to your opponent. Instead, turn the handle toward the ball so your little dude's foot traps it underneath.

D. Develop Surefire Attacks

Pass shot: Opponents expect direct shots, so pass between players on the same rod before shooting.

Side sweep: Center kicks are easily blocked. Move the ball to the edge of the table and have the player brush the side of the ball for an angled shot.

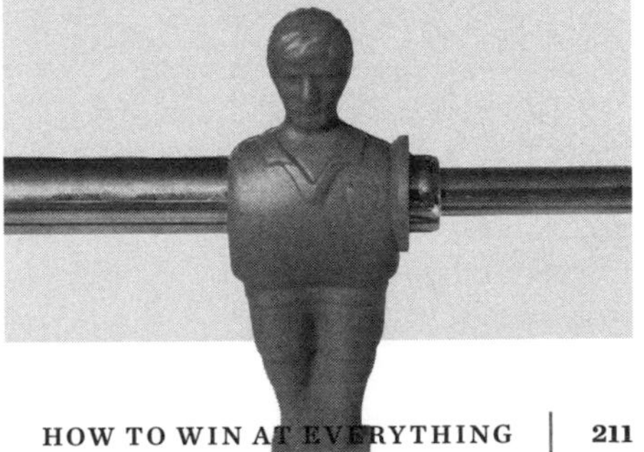

Tackle Mini Golf like *Nicklaus*

We asked two pros (yep, they exist) how they attack the three hardest shots in the game.

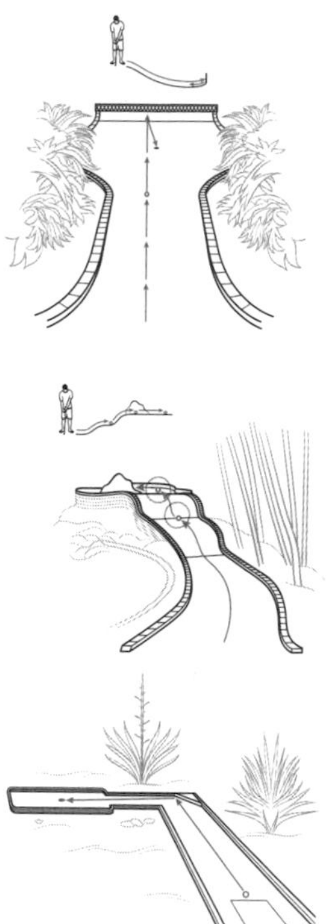

The Downhill

A straight-line hole-in-one is nearly impossible here—the ball picks up too much speed. Aim for the back wall slightly to one side of the hole. The ball will rebound and roll back toward it. With the right touch, you may stop close or even sink one.

The Double Uphill

Powering up both hills in one shot is too risky. Aim your first putt to one side of the "fairway" so that it banks and slows to a stop on the first tier. Repeat to position the ball safely on the second tier. If an obstacle sits on the top tier, aim for the rail behind it. That way if the bank goes awry, the obstacle will keep the ball from sliding back to the tee.

The Diabolical "L"

Most people bank the ball off the middle of the diagonal in the corner. This causes the ball to ricochet between the rails. Instead, hit the ball off the far end of the diagonal; it will kick once off the rail and coast toward the hole.

Bonus

Find quality mini golf courses at prominigolf. com/uscourses.html, or try the iLocate Mini Golf app ($2) on your iPhone.

Source: Matt McCaslin and Tim Tally, of the U.S. ProMiniGolf Association

Beat Your Last 5-K Time

Lose weight. For every pound of fat you lose, you can shave 2 to 5 seconds off every mile, says Jeff Galloway, running guru and author who trained with Steve Prefontaine and Bill Rodgers.

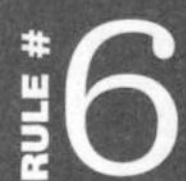
RULE #
6

If you want to win an eating contest, keep the food moist and don't chew, just swallow.

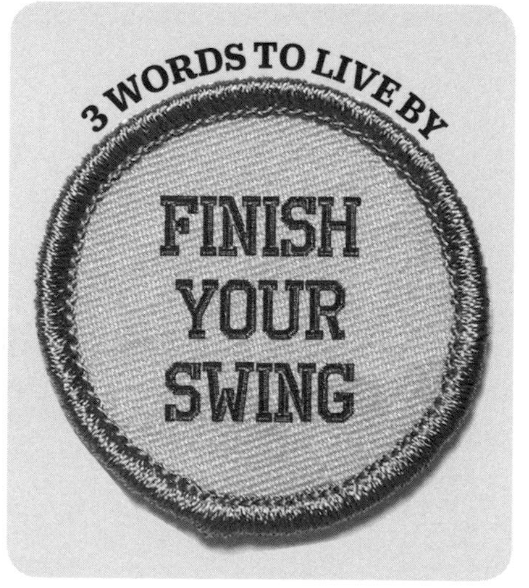
3 WORDS TO LIVE BY
FINISH YOUR SWING

How to Slam a Table Tennis Serve

Start with Perfect Grip

Hold the paddle as if you're shaking hands—with your fingers wrapped around the handle. Place your slightly bent thumb along the side of the handle that faces your opponent. Lay your index finger across the base of your side of the paddle. This grip provides you with greater control. Now add a dose of unpredictability with a little spin:

Topspin

Hold the paddle at a 45-degree angle so the top edge is tilted toward your opponent. Start the stroke below the ball and swing up and forward.

Backspin

Hold the paddle at 45 degrees so the top edge is tilted away from your opponent. Start the stroke above the ball and brush it down and forward.

Sidespin

With the paddle and your index finger parallel to the table, swing sideways to brush the ball.

For All Spins

The closer the ball is to the tip of the paddle, the more spin it will have.

Drill Your Tennis Serve

It's key to elevating your game, says pro player Michael Russell.

Harness the Racket's Power

Use a "continental" grip: Hold the racket like an ax, with the face in line with your forearm. Move the heel of your hand to the base of the grip, with your pinkie on the bottom of the handle.

Align Your Body

Stand with your feet shoulder width apart, your dominant foot parallel to the baseline, and your other foot angled 45 degrees toward the line. Place slightly more weight on your dominant foot.

Don't Overtoss

To create forward momentum, toss the ball to an apex 6 to 8 inches in front of you, and 1 to 2 feet higher than where your racket would strike it. Don't throw higher and try to hit it on the way down.

Smash It

Bring the racket behind you in one big arc and strike the ball with the racket angled slightly downward, toward your opponent. Don't bend your elbow or jump, and don't take your eye off the ball. Follow through with your swing.

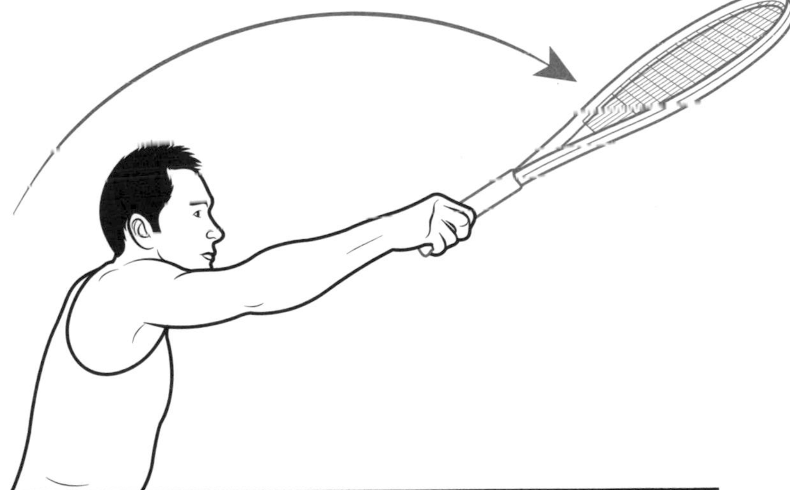

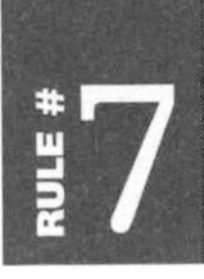

Let out a grunt whenever you hit a tennis ball. A study in the *Journal of Strength and Conditioning Research* found that the ball travels 4 percent faster through the air when you do.

Ace Your Fantasy Football Draft

ESPN's gridiron guru Matthew Berry, author of *Fantasy Life*, shows you how to draft smart and school your league.

Scout Preseason Games

They're not riveting, but watch anyway—especially the third game, when starters play the longest. Note which receiver draws the most QB looks and which runner carries the must-make plays. Those clues could be better than the stats inside a draft guide.

Stick with Proven Players

Veterans with solid track records tend to outperform young, unproven players with hype. Many veteran second-tier TEs will score you points.

Pick Your Defense Last

Select one earlier and you're wasting a pick. The points a defense scores can vary wildly each game, so you're better off nabbing a new D from your league's waivers every couple of games based on weekly matchups. Ignore the "No. 1" defense. In recent years, that squad has failed to finish on top.

Make Things Interesting

Personalize your league by instituting goofy rules and punishments. Drafting with old friends? Every team has to be named after a high school girlfriend. Beer buddies? The league loser buys the winner a case of suds of their choosing. Remember: In fantasy, camaraderie counts just as much as football.

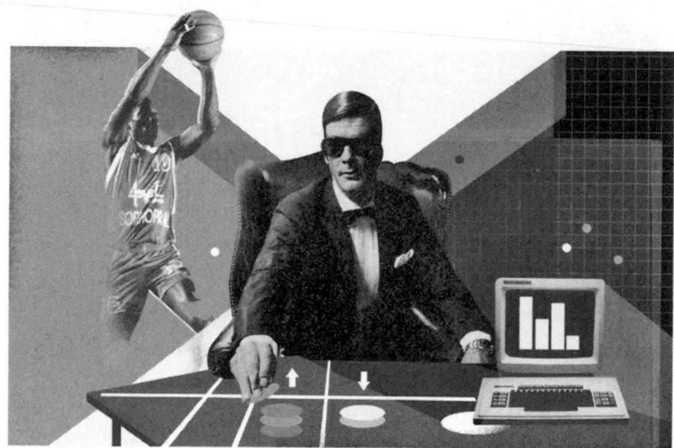

Pick NCAA Bracket Busters

Most March Madness fans assess the seeds, select an upset or two, and throw down their picks. Here's a more informed way to increase your odds:

Look to Last Year

Bracket builders tend to focus on the current tournament and forget the teams' past performance. Look for last year's sleeper teams that played hard and lost in tough games but retained the same coach and many players. Bonus points for teams now stocked with seniors.

Scan the Score Lists

Head to ncaa.org to check out scores for the current season. Blowout games can help you pick winners, but pay more attention to close games from underrated teams. Those are your upset-bound picks.

Analyze the Stats

Come tournament time, check out usatoday.com for its in-depth look at detailed stats behind the points. Notice a team that's ranked 60th in three-pointer defense playing a team in the top three for sinking the trey? Lock down the bracket.

Check the Odds

Even if you're not a betting man, see what Vegas has to say about the spread. Vegas plays it safe, and if it's saying the opposite of what most sportscasters are predicting, consider siding with the house.

Win at the
GO-KART TRACK

Make like Kyle Busch and leave your competitors chasing your tiny tire tracks.

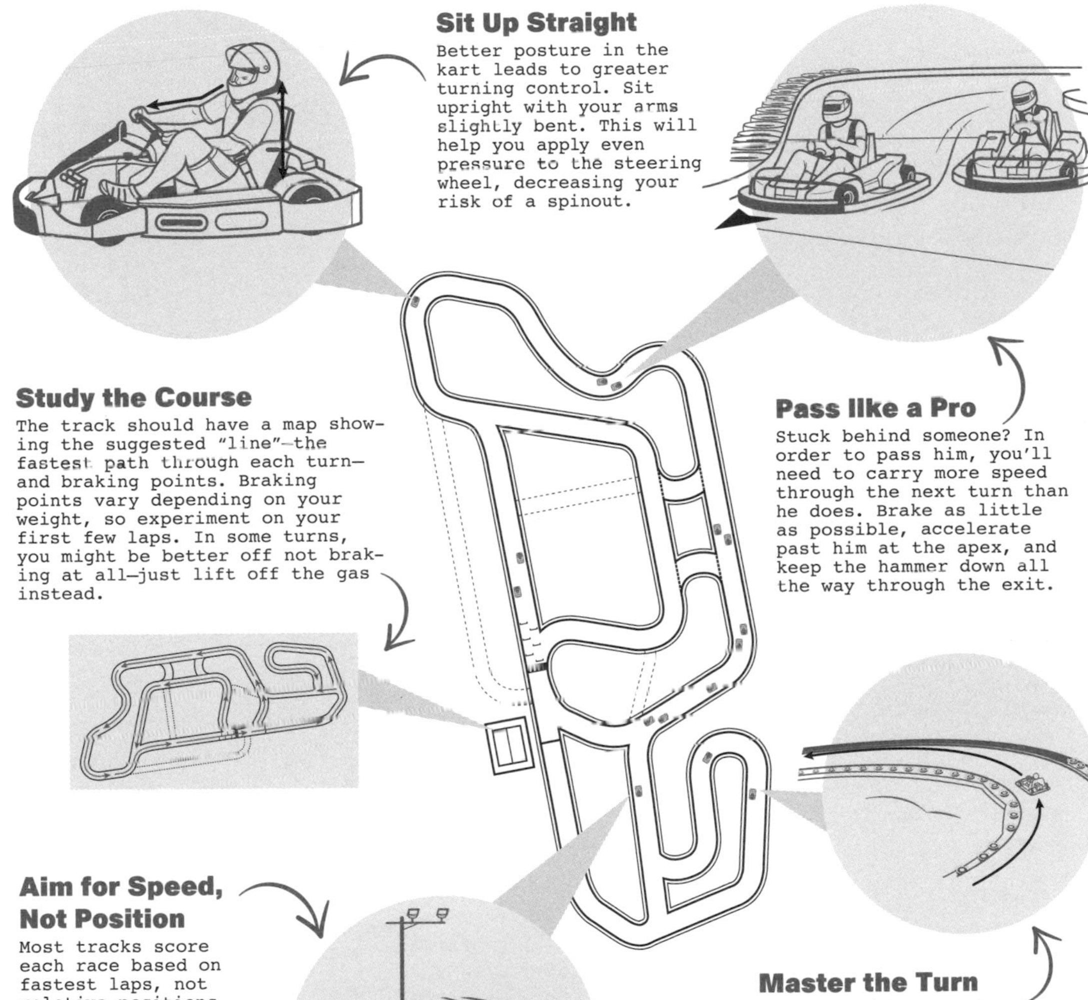

Sit Up Straight

Better posture in the kart leads to greater turning control. Sit upright with your arms slightly bent. This will help you apply even pressure to the steering wheel, decreasing your risk of a spinout.

Study the Course

The track should have a map showing the suggested "line"—the fastest path through each turn—and braking points. Braking points vary depending on your weight, so experiment on your first few laps. In some turns, you might be better off not braking at all—just lift off the gas instead.

Pass like a Pro

Stuck behind someone? In order to pass him, you'll need to carry more speed through the next turn than he does. Brake as little as possible, accelerate past him at the apex, and keep the hammer down all the way through the exit.

Aim for Speed, Not Position

Most tracks score each race based on fastest laps, not relative positions. If that's the case, hang back so you have a clear track to produce the best time, or stick behind the fastest guy so you can follow his line and stay motivated to pass him.

Master the Turn

Brake or lift your foot off the gas before the turn. Stay on the inside of your lane, accelerate as you exit, and allow the kart to drift to the outside. You'll cut seconds off your time.

Catch Fire at Arcade Hoops

Tim Legler is a former NBA player and current NBA studio analyst at ESPN. He's also got serious arcade-hoops game. Here Legler breaks down his can't-miss strategy.

1. Go In Close

Stand with your thighs pressed against the front of the machine. You'll stabilize your stance and position yourself closer to the hoop, so making baskets will be easier.

2. Double Up

Grab a ball in each hand and shoot them one at a time. By using both hands, you increase your odds of scoring.

3. Be a Softy

Use a slight wrist flick to send the ball toward the hoop. The lighter your touch, the lower your odds of chucking a brick.

4. Don't Bank It

The best way to score is by swishing the ball or giving just enough oomph to nudge it over the front of the rim. Flimsy backboards will sometimes misdirect banked shots.

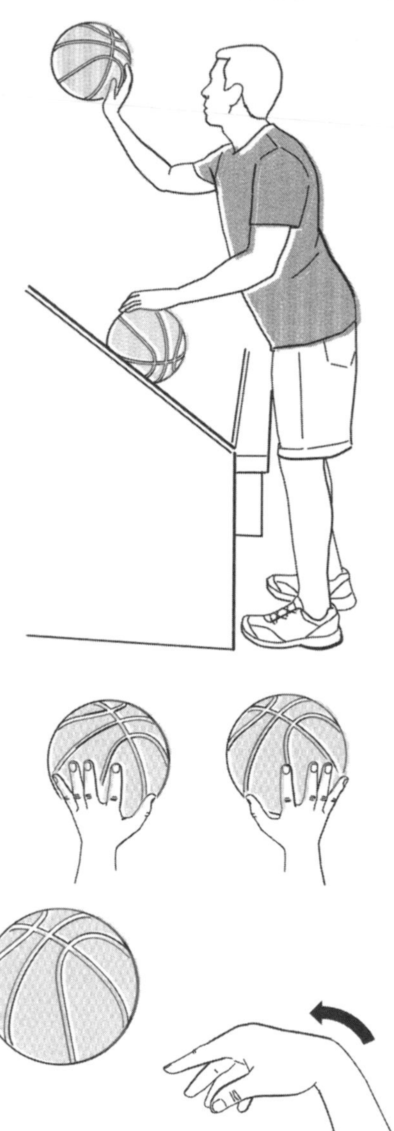

Perfect the Running Hook

1. Catch the ball on a pass and fake to the baseline.
2. Spin back and dribble toward the middle of the paint.
3. As you cross the paint, jump up, and while your inside arm helps clear space, make sure you keep it in (so as not to foul), and shoot with your outside arm.

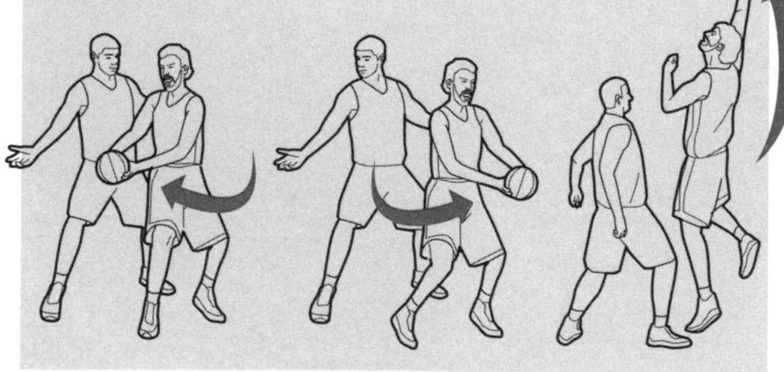

"The man who complains about the way the ball bounces is likely the one who dropped it."—Lou Holtz

Crash the Front Row at a Concert

Leave the binoculars at home. Use your brains (and beer!) to work your way to the best view of the band with this concert navigation guide from Matt Jordan, a music photographer and blogger for youaintnopicasso.com.

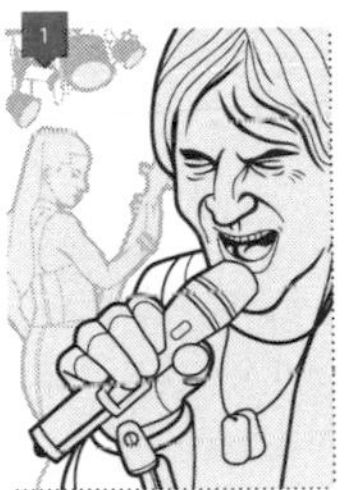

1: Arrive for the Opening Act

The best time to score a choice spot for a headliner is when the opening act is about to wrap. Folks will want to grab a beer (or pass their last one) during the break between acts. So buy your beer when the band announces its last song; that way you'll be back when the crowd starts leaving.

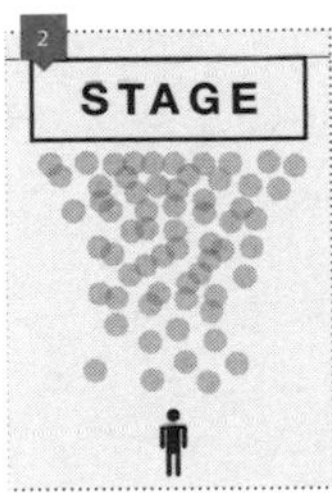

2: Work the Edges

If you arrive later and try to blitz up the middle, you'll hit a blockade. Crowds tend to be weakest toward the sides of the stage and by the walls (especially at indoor concerts), so you'll make faster progress by working the perimeter. Once you're 10 rows or so from the front, start heading diagonally toward the stage.

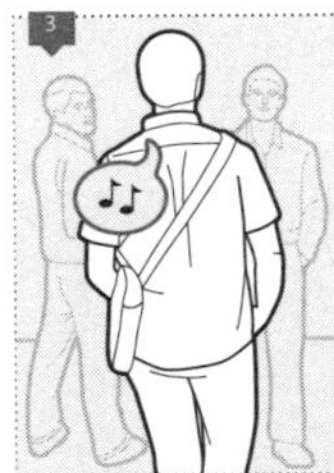

3: Make Friends

Close quarters can make navigating a crowd fraught with flare-ups. The best way to slide through trouble spots? Be sociable with the folks around you. Strike up a conversation about the last time you saw the band, or talk about your experience with the venue or this part of town. Share your excitement.

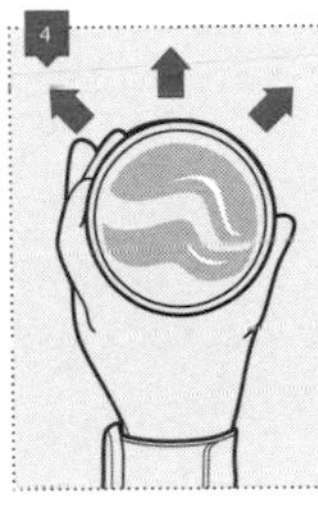

4: Be Moses

Don't underestimate the fear of beer. You can use that beverage you bought to part the crowd. (People will see the cup and move out of the way for fear of being spilled on.) Keep your body sideways, with the shoulder of your beer hand pointed toward the stage. And don't be touchy. That's weird, dude.

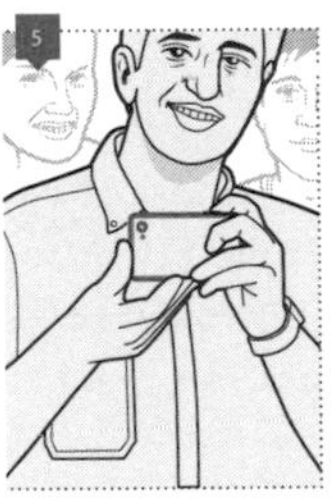

5: Go Easy on the Photography

If you tick off your fellow fans, you could find yourself dead in the water. One of the dumbest moves concert-goers make: reaching up over their head to take snapshots. If you really want a photo of the band, just keep your camera at chest height so you don't hit anyone in the head.

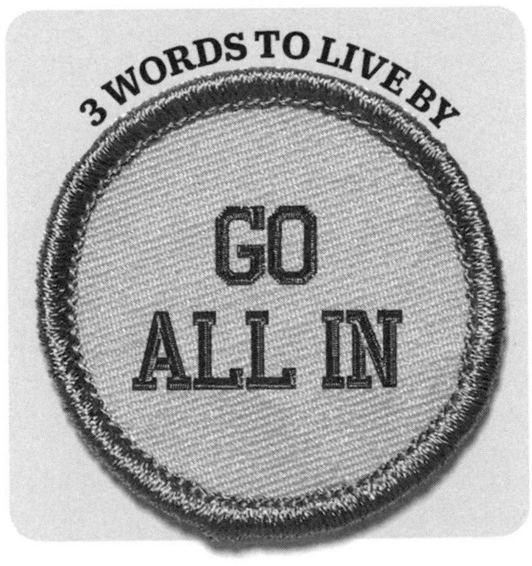

Wow the Crowd at *Karaoke Night*

Sing your way to a standing O with crooning tips from Josh Scholl, 2011 Karaoke World Championship USA winner.

Tune Your Pipes

So you're no Michael Bublé. Don't let that stop you. The crowd should be able to hear you above the track. Sing with gusto, but don't roar into the mike. If your voice is bad, admit it and laugh it off. The crowd will too.

Time It Right

Before you pick a song, survey the scene. See how the crowd responds to a few acts and then put your request in when the room hits its sweet spot: People are rowdy but still watching the stage (i.e., not wasted).

Pick a Hit

Select a high-energy track you can at least sing the chorus to—or better yet, that the crowd can sing the chorus to. Some ideas: "Jump Around," by House of Pain; "Wannabe," by the Spice Girls (sing it for the ladies, of course); or "Ignition (Remix)," by R. Kelly.

Fire Up Your Audience

Most guys just stand around until the lyrics hit. Use that time to connect with the crowd. Bring the banter: "Where are all my Journey fans?" Start a clap. Dedicate the song to your mom. (Yes, even if it's "Baby Got Back.") Funny is good. Don't apologize—it's insecure. Remember, it's never about the song; it's about the performance.

Close Out with Confidence

Bows are boring. To end a song, drum the air to the last few beats, placing heavy emphasis on the last one. If it's a dramatic ending, drop to your knees and throw your fist in the air. When you leave the stage, go sit next to the woman you took notice of onstage. Or end with a joke like, "Shots on this guy!" and point to your buddy who was too chicken to sing.

Bonus:

CROWD-PLEASING ROCK MOVES

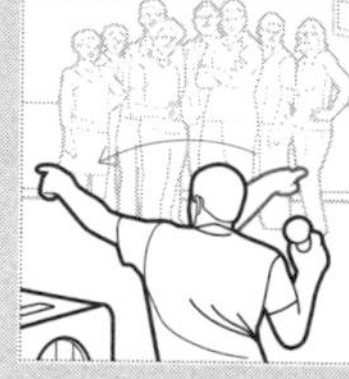

The Finger

Simply pointing to the crowd can fire people up. During grand moments in the song, like a key change or the first chorus, take a knee, extend your arm, and point your index finger, sweeping from one side of the bar to the other; then pop back up on both feet.

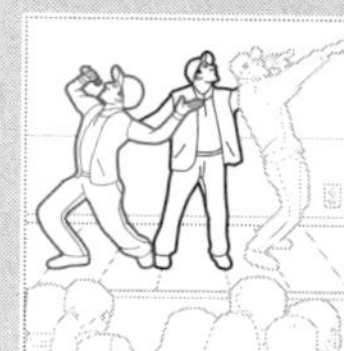

The Catwalk

Move from one end of the stage to the other, strutting a few steps and then stopping. Sing while executing fist pumps, snapping your fingers, or hoisting your rock horns to the beat. Punctuate with rock kicks at your discretion.

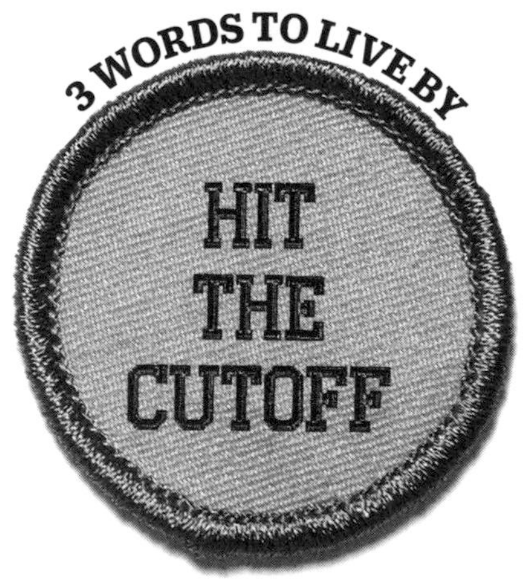
3 WORDS TO LIVE BY
HIT
THE
CUTOFF

Bowl More Strikes

Clear the lane with these tips from Chris Barnes, former Professional Bowlers Association World Champion.

Choose Your Rock

Your fingers should fit snugly into the holes but not so snugly that you can't extract them easily. To find a ball that fits comfortably, insert your thumb and stretch your fingers over the top of the ball. Your knuckles should line up with the middle of the holes. Pick the heaviest ball you can swing while still keeping your shoulders square.

See the Strike

If you're right-handed, place your right hand beneath the ball at the 6 o'clock position and use your left hand at 8 o'clock for support. (Left-handed? Use 6 and 4 o'clock.) Start four steps back from the foul line, plus an added half step for the slide at the end. Use the lane's targeting arrows as a guide. For the most effective angle, straddle the first dot to the right or left of center and aim between the second and third arrow from the gutter—that's the lane's sweet spot for starting a chain reaction of tumbling lumber.

Load the Shot

With your elbow flush against your body, make a right angle with your forearm and biceps. Move toward the foul line at a brisk walking pace, your knees slightly bent, leading with your dominant hand and foot. As you move forward, shift your weight to your other foot and let your other hand fall away so the ball swings freely. Aim with your shoulder, letting your arm relax and swing back to shoulder height.

Unleash the Fury

As the ball reaches the top of your backswing, slide into your final step. Swing the ball forward, and as it passes your ankle, turn the ball so your thumb points at 10 o'clock, giving the right amount of spin. For more spin, rotate your hand from 12 to 10 o'clock when it crosses your ankle.

Score Better on a Timed Test

Place a green apple on your desk and dab some vanilla extract on the inside of your wrists. Studies at the Smell and Taste Treatment and Research Foundation in Chicago have found that men were more relaxed and performed better under time pressure after sniffing those scents.

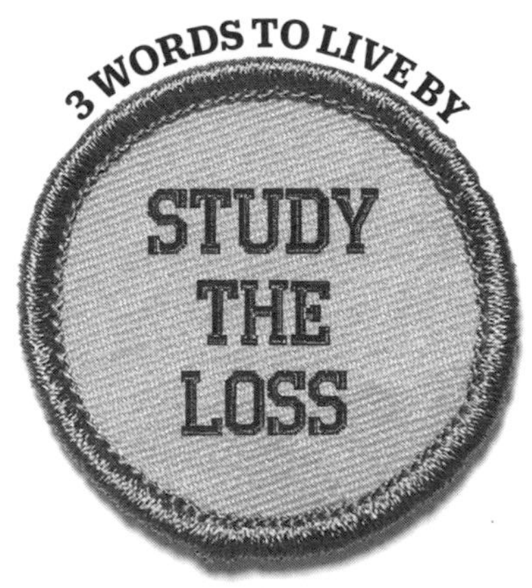
3 WORDS TO LIVE BY
STUDY
THE
LOSS

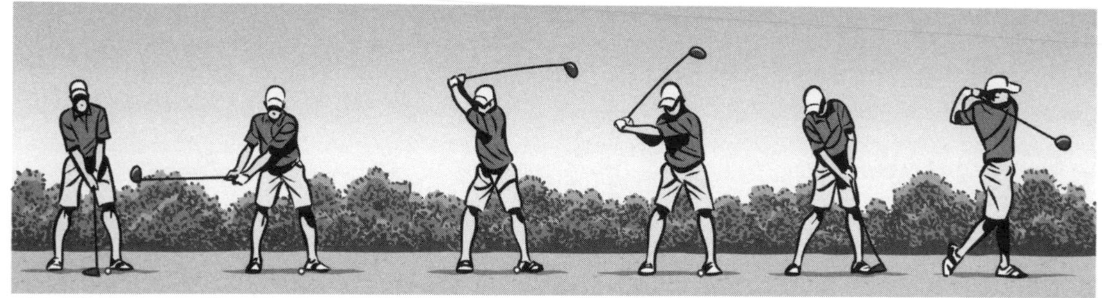

Kill the Bogey Monster

Improve your drive and you'll dramatically improve your game. The key is to keep things simple. Clear your mind and swing easy with driving tips from Mike Bender, the director of the Mike Bender Golf Academy at Magnolia Plantation Golf Club in Lake Mary, Florida.

Address

Feet are just wider than your shoulders, left arm aligns with shaft, ball lines up with left armpit.

Takeaway

Keep the clubhead low as you first take it back. Do not "pick up" the club quickly.

Turn

At the top, you should feel a slight tilt to the right as you load up before the downswing.

Transition

Arms accelerate and weight starts to transfer. Feel your feet pushing into the ground.

Impact

Now rip it—don't "flip" your hands. They stay ahead of the clubhead until after impact.

Finish

Try to stick your landing, weight on your left side, right toe pointed, no wobble. Nice shot!

Behave like a Golf Regular

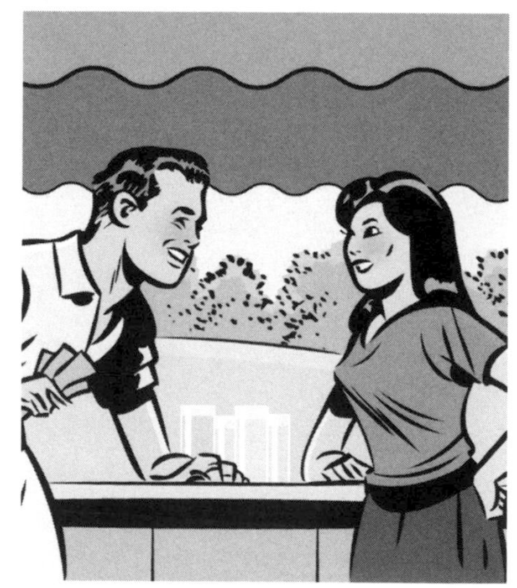

Even if you don't play golf often, you can appear to know what you're doing.

Know the rules. You must tee your ball behind the markers. On the green, slide the marker behind your ball without touching it.

Keep play moving. In a serious competition, the player farthest from the hole hits first, but in a regular round, if you're ready, hit.

Watch your step. Don't walk where another guy's putt will be going.

Tip the cart girl. Whoever approaches the drink cart first offers to buy for everyone—it evens out in the end. Mild flirting is permitted if your tip is generous.

Sink More 10-Foot Putts

Start draining shots you should be making with this advice from Zach Johnson, PGA pro and 2007 Masters champion.

1. Practice Smarter

For every ball you blast off the driving-range tee, set one on the practice green later. Nearly half of your strokes come from your putter, so if you neglect to warm up your short game, you'll have a poorer sense of the speed of a course's greens—and speed is a key to mastering clutch putts.

2. Develop Precision Control

Before your game, drop a few ball markers on a practice green at different distances from the hole, and place a club 2 feet behind the hole. Hit three balls toward the hole from the closest marker, but try not to hit the club. Move to the next marker only when none of the balls hit the club.

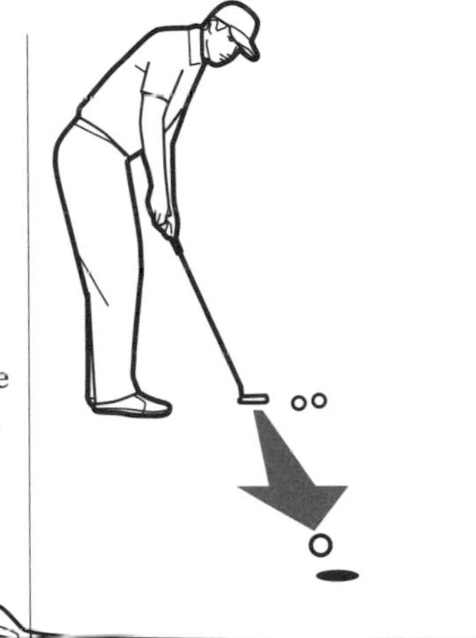

3. Adjust Your Eyes

No matter how straight the shot is, aiming directly for the cup is more likely to cause you to lose focus. Instead, visualize a "track" you see the ball taking to the hole, according to your read and breaks. For greatest accuracy, line up your feet 90 degrees to the starting point of that track.

4. Ditch Your Doubt

At each hole, take the same amount of time to survey the green, and the same number of practice strokes. Then take a moment to clear your head. You're developing habits that can carry a stressed brain through high-pressure situations. Don't think of the outcome (I need to make this!). Just putt.

Simplest Way to Improve Your Drive in Golf

Loosen your grip. Clubhead speed, which is what generates power, is unrelated to your strength, so a death grip isn't necessary. In fact, it can undermine your drive. Many pros will tell you, "Hold the club as if it were a tube of toothpaste." You don't want a gob of Crest on your new golf shoes, do you?

3 TIPS FOR CUTTING STROKES

1. **Sidehill downhill putt:** Place your feet in the direction of your line, not toward the hole, and follow through. Put more weight on your leading foot.
2. **Short chip from a tight line:** Don't choke the club and scoop the ball. Use soft hands and hit the ball with a square face. This keeps the ball low—the safest bet.
3. **Drive into the wind:** Don't hit the ball hard; that'll create spin, allowing the wind to catch it. Instead, tee the ball lower than usual and back in your stance. You'll produce a low, straight shot.

Win at Pickup Basketball

According to former Oregon State University basketball coach Craig Robinson, author of *A Game of Character* (and Michelle Obama's brother) . . .

Play Low-Scoring Games

Robinson prefers playing to seven baskets. "Each point is more meaningful," he says. "When you play to 32, it's easy for the game to be a blowout, and then you're not working."

Make It, Take It

If it's a half-court game, the scoring team should start with the ball. It'll force you to play good defense (something guys often go lax on), which practically doubles your workout.

Play All Positions

Cut hard and run to spots you normally wouldn't: Big guys should go outside, and small guys to the key. Even if you're not as effective there, it makes you less predictable to defend.

Run to the Foul Line

Don't hang back when the other team is on a fast break. Your goal: On every play, run at least to the other end's foul line. You'll build conditioning so you can run the court.

Score a Spot on a *Game Show*

Earn a chance to win it all with these behind-the-set secrets from Mike Richards, executive producer of *The Price Is Right* and *Let's Make a Deal.*

Stand Out in the Crowd

Snagging a spot isn't as simple as just showing up—it's an interview process. First, reserve your tickets online up to 60 days ahead. On taping day, line up outside the studio at least a few hours before. That's when you're likely to score a 30-second interview with the producer.

Look the Part

Watch old episodes to see how those contestants dressed. Now give it your own personal touch.

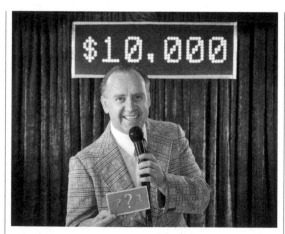

Refer to the show with reverence or be unique (black clothes, big magnet, tiny toy chicks for *Let's Make a Deal*). And no overt sex jokes, okay?

Go Nuts—but Not Too Nuts

During the interview, pump up your energy by a third. You want to show passion, not craziness. Speak loudly and clearly, be gracious, and drop in a line about how excited you are to win prizes.

Stay Pumped

Made the cut? Great! But as you file into the studio, don't fall out of character—the producers are watching you here too. Hamming it up during the interview and then wiping the smile off your face demonstrates that you're just putting on a show of your own.

RULE THE *Shuffleboard Table*

Rule the shuffleboard table with these strategies from pro player Dave Shewbridge, president of the Table Shuffleboard Association.

Take a Strong Stance

The weight will travel in the direction you're facing. Stand with your dominant hand and foot in front and your lead hip turned inward toward the board. Rest your other hand on the outer rail of the table's frame for balance. Use your arm and wrist to push (not toss) the weight.

Devise a Game Plan

Try to score two points. One point isn't risky enough, and three makes you easy prey.

Work an Open Board

Use spin to slow the weight to a stop. Make the thumbs-up sign with your shooting hand, keeping your fingers loose. Place your thumb in the center of the weight, allowing your bottom two knuckles to rest on the board. Then push the weight forward.

Respond to a Score

Blast away! Grip the weight with your thumb over its center and your index finger supporting it from the side. In one swift motion, extend your arm and open your hand to fire the shot toward the sitting weight.

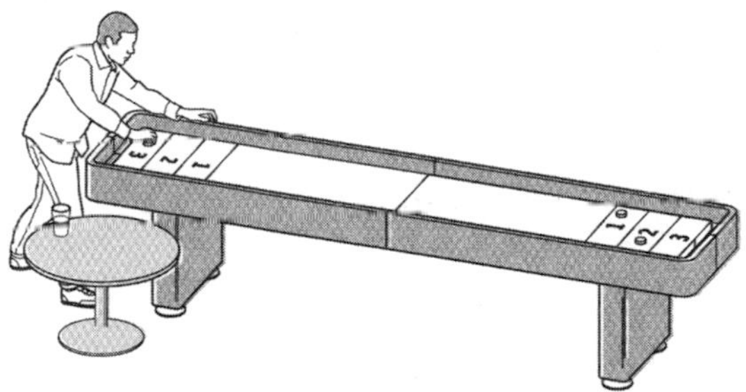

Execute a Perfect 10 Flip Dive

MAKE A SPLASH AT YOUR NEXT POOL PARTY WITH A FORWARD 1½ TUCK DIVE.

Approach the Board

Most divers either take off running or start with their toes gripping the edge of the board. Don't do either. Instead, walk down the board until you're a foot from the end. Jump and land an inch from the edge. That's where the board has the most spring, which will help with takeoff.

Jump with Leverage

Don't double-bounce—you could lose control. To gain momentum and maintain balance, start by squatting until your knees are bent 45 degrees. Then, in one smooth, quick motion, jump and swing your arms up over your shoulders. Aim to jump about 3 feet outward and upward.

Spin with Precision

About halfway before the peak of your jump, tuck your legs into a somersault position, reaching for your shins. You'll rotate naturally in the tucked position. Keep your head and neck aligned straight, looking over your knees to see the water; don't tuck your chin or you risk overspinning.

Don't Make Waves

For a smooth entry, straighten your legs and extend your arms above your head to finish in a flawless dive. Come up for air and wink at that bikini-clad spectator.

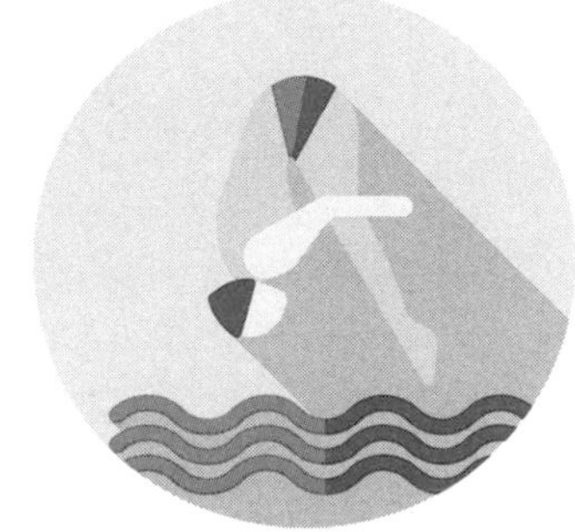

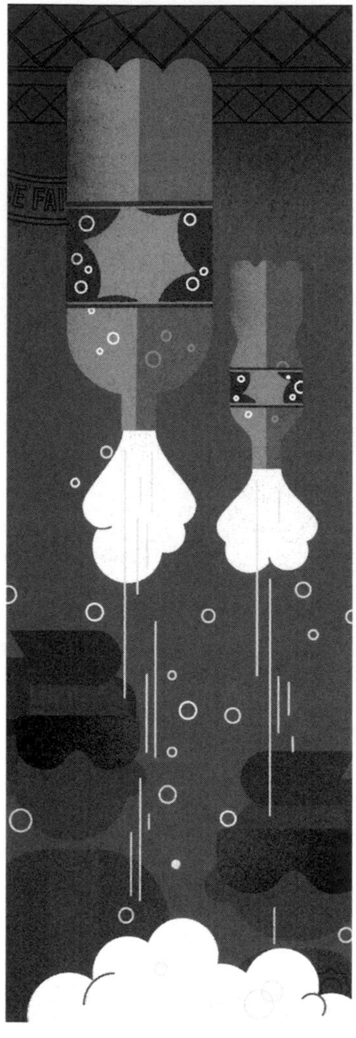

Help Your Kid Win the SCIENCE FAIR

Bill Nye the Science Guy tells you how to assist your son or daughter in wowing the judges and landing the blue ribbon.

Guide Inspiration

Fourth-graders don't have to experiment with yellow-cake uranium. Ask your kid to look around the kitchen with a questioning eye: Why is soda bubbly? Why do some bottles have caps and others corks? Comparing items shows the type of critical thinking that judges value, so try to go beyond simple observation.

Step Back

Once your child has settled on a subject, it's time for you to back off. Judges can tell when an adult has interfered too much; besides, the child will learn more by taking the reins. Request a simple assignment instead. Say you'll be the "assistant" to set the tone. Ask questions instead of providing explicit instructions.

Follow the Method

Judges will look to see if the student stayed with the scientific method. (Hypothesis, experimentation, refine the idea, experimentation, final statement . . . remember?) If your child becomes upset because the experiment isn't playing out perfectly, just say it's part of the process. After all, that's how science works.

Present with Style

Solid science beats a loud, flashy display every time. Keep the presentation to a trifold, going easy on the neon and glitter. And resist the urge to edit: You can point out glaring errors in the report, but don't sweat the occasional stray comma or sloppy letter. This is one time when too much perfection can thwart success.

Bonus:

THREE A+ SCIENCE FAIR IDEAS

1. Test different dishwashing soaps on greasy plates to see which ones clean best. Are manufacturers' claims correct?
2. Put tea leaves in a cup with water, and stir. The leaves aren't thrown to the outside as you'd imagine, but move to the middle. How come? Compare with other things like peppercorns or sunflower seeds.
3. Test how texting affects critical thinking. Ask your child to solve problems while texting and not texting and note the elapsed times. Then have him or her replicate the experiment with other people. Why are the results the way they are?

Pick Stocks That Soar

The secret to choosing a wealth-building investment is to read the market and do a bit of essential homework, according to Damien Hoffman, the editor-in-chief of *Wall St. Cheat Sheet.*

Target Up-and-Coming Products

Some growth is product-driven. Pick companies that have promising merchandise and big launches in the pipeline. Anticipated releases from Apple, for instance, add to its balance sheet, bottom line, and income statement, making it a hot stock. Read blogs that track businesses you're interested in and watch firms' investor-relations centers for products in development.

Anticipate Scandal

The easiest way to avoid busted business schemes is to make sure A-level management is running the show. Check the Web for the CEO's track record—not just at his or her current company but also with previous firms. Make sure the company hasn't had

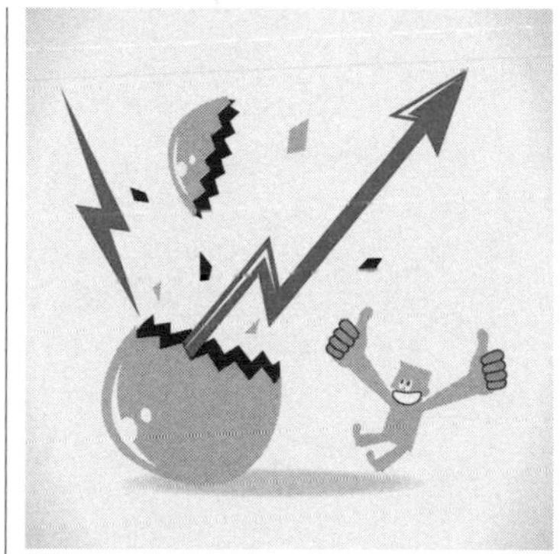

inquiries from the Securities and Exchange Commission in the past 10 years. Any such scrutiny should raise a red flag; for the safest bet, select a company with zero inquiries on file.

Denounce Debt

Look for companies that are relatively unburdened by large debt loads, which could hamper their operations. In a slow economy, they'll more easily thrive than operations that have to cut big interest checks for the bankers. The good news? That information is public. Visit sites like Yahoo Finance to check a company's stock quote page and see how much (or little) debt it's holding. Less debt? Better bet.

Be Tough on Overall Performance

The simplest way to verify that a company is technically sound is by looking at its stock chart. Jagged shark teeth, flat lines, or long descenders? Not good. You want a stable, boring, ascending line from past to present. It doesn't have to be a drastic "hockey stick" formation—some of the best companies are steady and slow growing. Look at the past year's stock performance for an idea of the current trend.

Conquer a Mountain

Climb the toughest of mountain bike trails with these tips from Todd Wells, Olympic mountain biker:

- Set your tire pressure to 30 psi, which gives your tires flexibility to grip the trail.
- For a stronger climb, pedal at the same rate the whole time, saving a few low gears just in case. Don't stand; you'll lose rear tire traction.
- Power over obstacles. As you approach rocks or logs, center your weight over the rear tire. Lean slightly over the handlebar so your front end doesn't lift. Raise the bar just enough to initiate a climb over the obstacle. Avoid bunny hops.
- Control your descent by feathering the front brake with small pumps. Keep your feet level so your weight stays transferable.

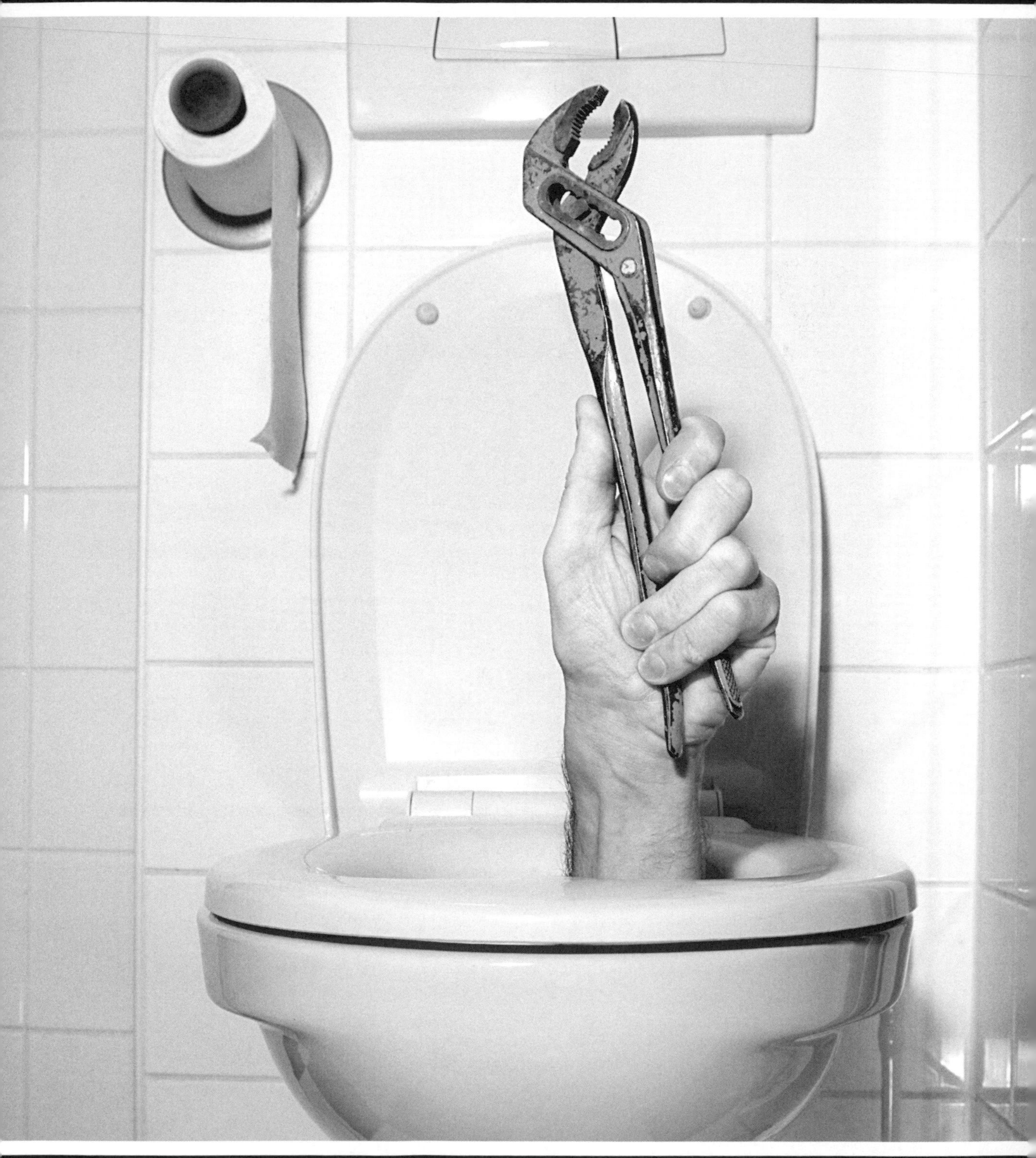

Your Cave

Su Casa is More Than a Roof Over Your Head. It's a 365-Day-a-Year Work in Progress. So Here are Some Upgrades and Fun Ways to Make Your Home Reflect Your Style.

Many moons ago, when our homes were made of sticks and bark and interest rates were really, really low, a man didn't have to worry much about domestic upkeep. If the roof leaked, he threw on another hide. If the herd moved to greener pastures, he simply left home A standing and built home B with new sticks and bark. RE/MAX had yet to be invented.

Today, homesteading is far more complicated, even if you rent a one-bedroom apartment. So much can go wrong in your quest for comfort and style. And now with HGTV, Houzz, and Zillow, you can't escape images of handier-than-thou handymen and palaces that shame your humble abode in size, open concept, and a great outdoor living space. Uncommon Knowledge is what you need. And a heavy-duty reciprocating saw.

Break into Your Own Home

Slam! Click. Ohhh, crap.

When you're locked out of the house, eternal shame isn't the only reason to bypass the locksmith. The Federal Trade Commission warns that some locksmiths lack professional training, and many states don't require formal licensing. And even with the creds, an inexperienced operator may choose brute force over finesse and insist on drilling your lock out. So first, try this: Make a key with help from master lock picker Eric Michaud. You could be back inside in 5 seconds.

1. Lucky you! You've already stashed two bobby pins in a secret place near the door. (If not, ask the neighbor lady for some.) Convert these into two lock-picking tools—a torque tool and a pick. To make the torque, scrape the rounded edges off the first pin and bend it into a smoother U shape. Bend the tips 90 degrees [A].

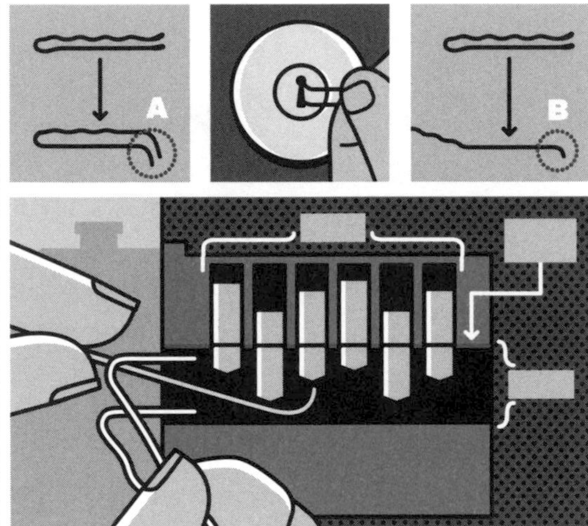

2. Turn the torque tool parallel to the ground (round end pointed away from the latch) and insert the prongs into the lock. Keep pressure on the torque in the direction you want it to turn. (Locks on the left side of a door open clockwise; locks on the right go counterclockwise.) Leave the torque in this position. There's another tool to make.

3. Time to create your pick: Open the second pin, scrape the rounded edge off the tip of the straighter side, and bend the same tip up just slightly so it resembles a very shallow curved fishhook [B]. Insert the hook end into the keyhole; then pull the pick up toward the top of the chamber. If anyone passes, just say "It's cool! I live here!" If a cop stops, drop your pick and raise your hands.

4. Keep light pressure on the torque with one hand; use the other to push the pick deeper into the keyhole. Inside, five to six small locking pins line the roof of the tunnel. Each needs to be shifted upward to catch a higher rung, mimicking what happens as a key slides in. Use the hook's edge to lift the pin with the most resistance first.

5. As each locking pin moves up, the lock will loosen, turning slightly in the direction it should open, and another pin will become resistant. Bounce up the last one, and you'll feel the torque tool turn toward the direction you've been keeping pressure in, springing open the lock. Restash the tools before entering, just in case.

Locate a Stud without a Stud Finder

Turn on an electric shaver and run its base across the wall. The pitch will dip when you pass over a stud.

Build a Sturdy Workbench

Here's a project for all your projects. This one will cost you about $125 in materials and you'll have nothing left over, says Dan Faires, host of HGTV.com's *Danmade*.

WHAT YOU'LL NEED

Circular saw; 1 sheet of finished plywood (3/4" × 4' × 8'); two 2 × 4 studs (each 10' long); four 2 × 4 studs (each 8' long); 1 box of 2½" screws (1 lb); 4 clamps; wood glue; level

1. Carve 'Em Up

Cut the plywood down its length into 24-inch by 8-foot and 18-inch by 8-foot pieces. Save the leftover 6-inch piece. Cut one of the 10-foot 2 × 4s into three 32-inch pieces and one 21-inch piece. Cut the other into one 32-inch piece, two 21-inch pieces, and three 15-inch pieces. Sort them all into like-size piles.

2. How to Take It to the Top

Set the 21-inch cross braces between two of the 8-foot 2 × 4s (one on each end and one in the center). Screw the pieces together, creating a rectangle the same size as the 24-inch by 8-foot plywood. Glue the top of the frame, put the plywood on top, and secure with screws.

3. Add Storage

To make a shelf, repeat the frame-making step for the tabletop using the other two 8-foot 2 × 4s and the 15-inch cross braces. Apply glue to the top surface of the frame, and then place the 18-inch by 18-inch plywood piece on top and screw it to the frame. Set the shelf aside.

4. Give It Legs

Flip the tabletop over so the plywood side faces down. Position a 32-inch leg in a corner so that the wider side of the 2 × 4 faces the long side of the frame. Hold the leg tightly against the corner and secure it to the frame with one screw. Repeat with the other three 32-inch legs.

5. Install the Shelf

Turn the table over and slide the shelf between the legs. Using pieces of scrap wood, prop up the shelf to your desired height. Clamp the corners of each leg and make sure the shelf is level. Secure each leg to the tabletop frame with two more screws. Remove the clamps.

6. Finish It!

Glue, clamp, and screw the 6-inch by 8-foot plywood piece to the back of the tabletop at your desired height. Now you're ready to work. Customize in any of these ways: Run a router over the edges, putty the screw holes, sand, lacquer, prime and paint, install locking casters, or add a vise.

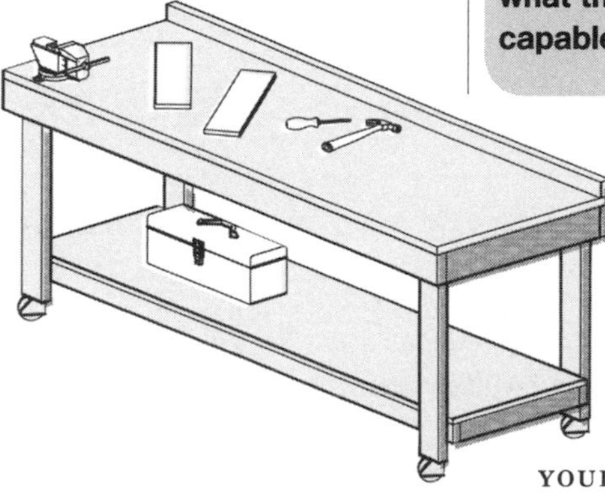

Fix a Leaky Showerhead

Wrap the fixture's nut in electrical tape for protection, then unscrew it with a wrench. Pop out the gasket with a screwdriver, clean out any buildup in the pipe, and drop in a new gasket. Wrap the threads in Teflon tape and reinstall the showerhead.

RULE #1

Circular saws are like big dogs: If you treat them right, you needn't really fear them, but you should never forget what they are capable of.

Tune a Muffled Mower

"Before you do anything, remove the spark plug so the mower doesn't accidentally fire up while you're working on it," says Tom Shotzbarger, the president of the Lawn Care Association of Pennsylvania. Follow his tune-up drill to make your mower start faster and run smoother.

1) Empty the fuel tank.

Gasoline degrades as it ages, so drain any fuel left over from the past season. Replace the oil, too—microscopic contaminants can build up in the oil, reducing its viscosity and grinding against the engine's parts.

2) Lose the grime.

Use a degreaser on the engine housing to remove grime, which can contaminate the filters, fuel, and oil. Extreme Simple Green Motorsports Cleaner & Degreaser (simplegreen.com) is an eco-friendly option.

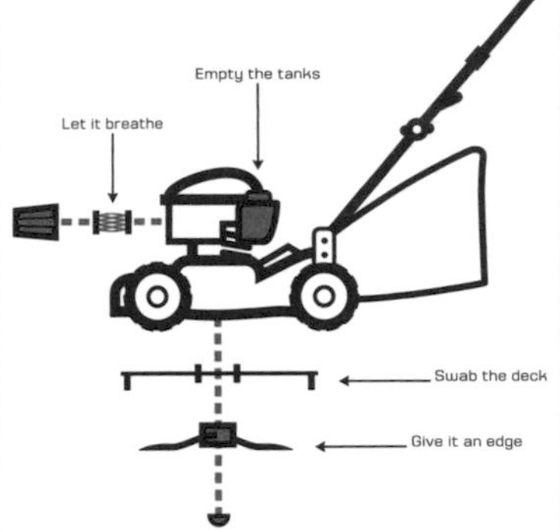

Empty the tanks
Let it breathe
Swab the deck
Give it an edge

3) Let it breathe.

Install a new air filter. "The engine needs clean airflow to burn fuel most efficiently," says Shotzbarger. Change the spark plug, too. It can rust or wear down, also causing the engine to run inefficiently.

4) Clear the deck.

Pry any caked-on grass from the underside of the deck using a putty knife. "If there's too much stuck on there, it will interfere with the cutting," says Shotzbarger.

5) Give it an edge.

If the blade is bent or dinged, buy a replacement for $15 to $20 at a hardware store. If it's just dull, take it to a lawn and garden center to have it sharpened. You'll pay about half the price of a new one.

RULE # 2

Cut mowing time in half. A 36-inch walk-behind mower does the job in half the time of an 18-incher. If you have 2 acres, get a rider with a deck that is 42 to 48 inches wide.

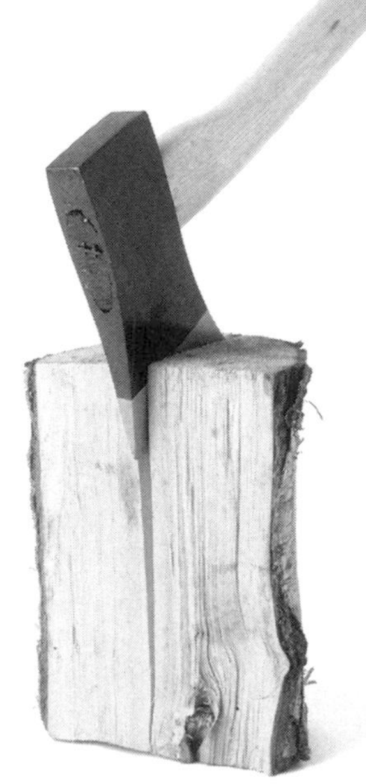

Split a Log in One Blow

"This isn't about brute force; the correct blade angle adds all the power you need. Step an ax handle's length away and swing the ax so the blade head comes down in line with the grain. Just prior to impact, let your wrists collapse like you're hammering a big nail. You'll hit perfectly perpendicular to the wood."—**Arden Cogar Jr., third-generation lumberjack and four-time Stihl Timbersports champion**

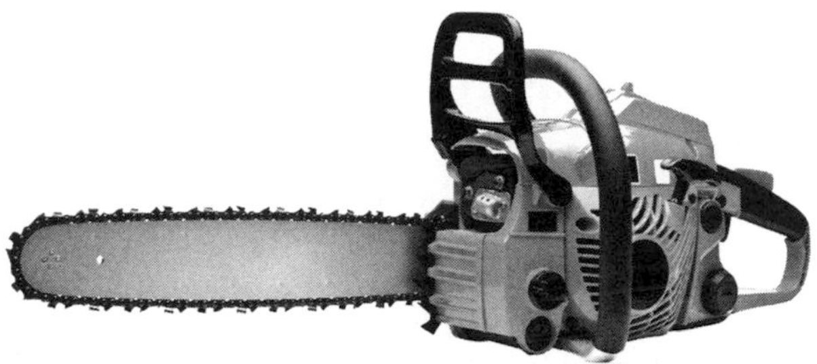

Handle a Chain Saw

Cut wood, not your appendages. Curtis Ingvoldstad, a champion chain saw artist, breaks it down.

Fight Your Testosterone

In the tool aisle, look for balance, not horsepower. For smaller branches, a 30 cc saw with a 12-inch bar (the cutting part) is fine. For thicker limbs (10 to 16 inches in diameter), buy a 40 to 50 cc model with a 16- to 18-inch bar.

Suit Up

Put on safety chaps, hearing protection, steel-toed boots (chain saw whiplash could slice your toes), and safety glasses. They'll keep you out of the ER.

Stand Sturdy

Stand with your feet shoulder width apart and bend your knees. Next, move your torso behind and in line with the bar. Angle your head away from the chain and operate the saw below your waist or you run the risk of serious injury.

Guide, Don't Gouge

While cutting, keep both hands on the saw and lead it with your front hip, directing the bottom third of the chain through the wood. If you cut with the tip, you risk kickback. Don't push with your arms—the blade will do the work.

Amputate a Limb

Remove problem branches right.

Time Your Cut

Prune during the dormant season, when the tree isn't leafy or flowering; for most trees, that's winter or very early spring. That way you limit the tree's exposure to sap-hungry, disease-carrying insects.

Find Your Entry Point

Look to remove branches that intersect in a V (as opposed to a U); these intersections are more likely to fail in snowy or windy conditions. Cut the branch half an inch from where it connects to the trunk or another branch.

Lop in Stages

A sturdy handsaw is your best bet for limb cutting. Saw the branch off in sections to keep it from tearing away at the joint, unnecessarily exposing more of the tree's flesh.

Let It Bleed

Unless the tree is an oak or elm that's wounded during a critical time of year, don't do anything to the exposed wound. Applying synthetic paint, a common wound dressing, could interfere with the healing process.

RULE # 3

Wear gloves when using brush tools like rakes, clippers, and shovels, even when you haven't touched them since last summer. Urushiol oil from poison ivy, oak, and sumac can stay active on tools and clothes for up to 5 years. It takes just 1 nanogram (billionth of a gram) to cause a rash.

RULE # 4

Let your grass grow. Taller grass (over 2½ inches) grows more slowly and maintains its health better (and keeps weeds down).

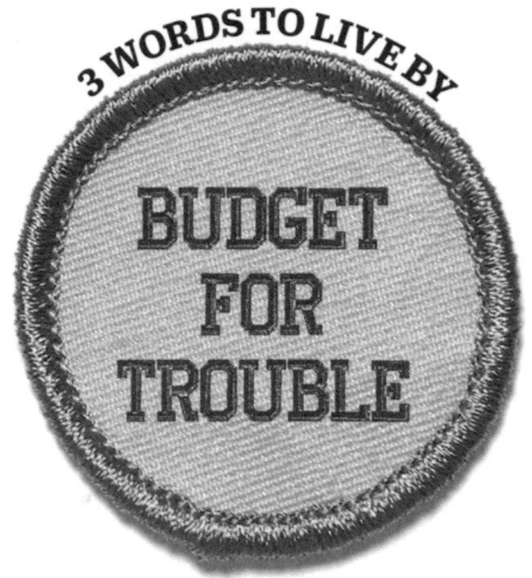
3 WORDS TO LIVE BY
BUDGET
FOR
TROUBLE

Dodge DIY Disaster

Painting a wall or laying tile can be a risky proposition. You can't just hit "undo" if you don't like the way it turns out. So before you start, make a half dozen photocopies of the tile pattern or paint color and tape them to the wall; this will give you a feel for the end result. **Bonus:** The copies can also help you figure out the best patterns for tile work.

Stack a Rock-Solid Woodpile

Season wood, save money, and avoid a midwinter collapse.

Step 1: Choose Your Trees

Buy mixed hardwoods, like maple, birch, and oak. (Find a dealer at firewood.com.) When hardwoods like these are seasoned properly, they yield more heat because the dry wood burns more efficiently than damp wood.

Step 2: Keep It Dry

Water is firewood's greatest enemy. Select a spot on stone or concrete so the wood won't draw moisture from the ground. Then, for maximum dryness, pick up some wooden pallets from a lumber dealer or hardware store to line the length of the pile and serve as a base. Don't have a sheltered spot for your pile? Protect the wood with a tarp, staked down a few feet from the woodpile to allow air to circulate.

Step 3: Create Your Supports

Make end pillars by stacking layers of wood in alternating three-piece rows—like a Jenga tower—about 4 feet high. The wood within the tower will be able to breathe, preventing dry rot, and alternating the layers creates a strong support structure. For stable columns, make sure each piece is roughly the same height and shape. Leave a few inches of space between pieces.

Step 4: Fill the Gap

Pile your remaining firewood between the support pillars. Forget about making neat rows: Random stacking is more likely to fill in cracks and gaps, making for a more stable woodpile.

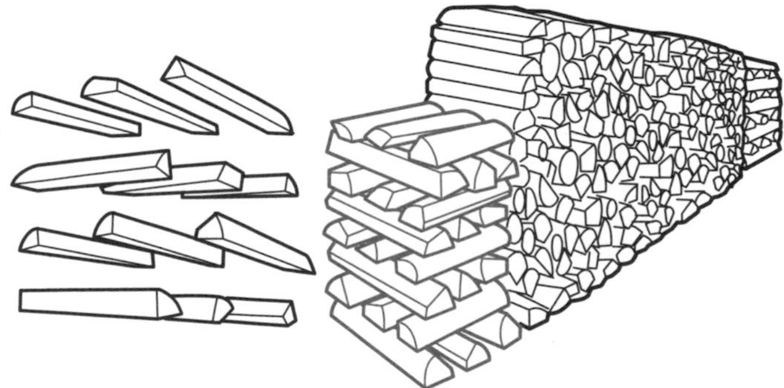

Craft Your Own Kegerator

Somewhere inside every fridge lies a keg just waiting to be tapped. What if you could combine the best of the bar (beer on tap) with the best of home (no line at the bathroom)? You'd be a genius. All right, genius, here's the plan.

WHAT YOU'LL NEED
One old (but operational) single-door refrigerator
1"-diameter wall spacer
5" beer shank
Stainless-steel faucet head
CO_2 regulator
5-lb CO_2 tank
Keg coupler
5 feet of 3/16" beer line and connectors
4 feet of 1/4" air tubing with clamps
Drip tray
Assorted tools

If your town hasn't seen a home brewery supply store since Prohibition, you can still order everything you need from kegerator.com or Beveragefactory.com.

RULE # 5

Wash mousetraps well between exterminations, because a mouse's nose is sensitive enough to detect the odor of a departed cousin. For a better mousetrap, bait it with after-dinner mints; the scent is a strong lure. Peanut butter works better than cheese, too.

HOW TO BUILD IT

You can download far more detailed instructions for converting an old fridge into a beer keg tap, but these are the general steps for motivation.

1. Unplug the fridge. Remove the plastic shelving from the door. At a spot 4 feet up the door, drill a 1-inch hole.
2. Insert the wall spacer and cut to fit with a hacksaw.
3. Remove the nut from the shank and slide it into the hole. Screw the nut back on and tighten. Screw the faucet onto the other end.
4. Cut a scrap of plywood to the dimensions of the fridge floor and drop it into place.
5. Screw the CO_2 regulator onto the CO_2 tank and place it in the corner of the fridge.
6. Join the keg coupler and the shank with the beer line, and the regulator and the keg coupler with the air line. Secure everything with hose clamps.
7. Install the drip tray 10 inches below the faucet.
8. Plug in the fridge.
9. Introduce keg to fridge and then tap the sucker. Loosen the regulator screw and open the CO_2 tank. Set the pressure to about 12 psi. Check for leaks.
10. Ask yourself what you'll have and then draw a pint.

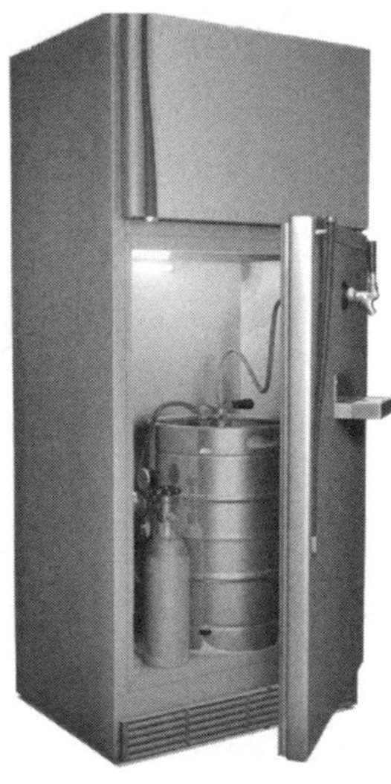

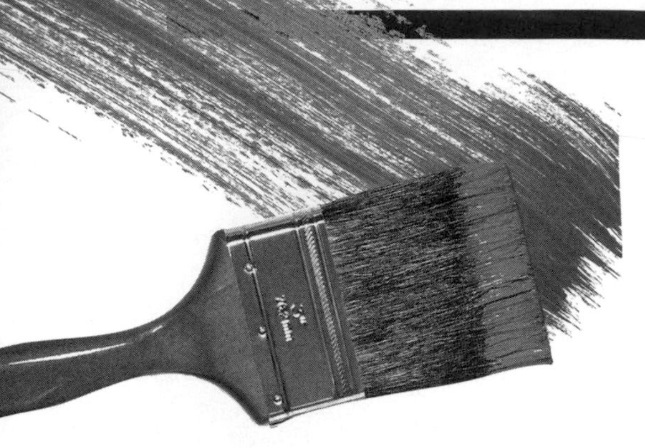

Repaint a Room in *Record Time*

1. Pick Your Paint

Buy a high-quality, premium paint for the best, most even finish. We like Olympic Premium Interior Paint (olympic.com). And for faster coverage, use a primer that's been tinted to the paint's color.

2. Prep the Room

After clearing out as much as you can from the room, move everything else to the center and cover the pile with old sheets. Then remove any grime on the walls by wiping them down with a wet dish towel or painter's cloth, neither of which will leave lint behind. As the walls dry, apply painter's tape to the edges of baseboards and trim, pressing the tape with a 5-in-1 tool or credit card to seal its edges.

3. Set Up a Paint Station

The ideal spot is in front of a window, where you won't spend much time painting. Don't put paint cans near the center of the room—that's where you're most likely to back into them.

4. Brandish the Brush and Rollers

Throw a tarp on the floor, put on painters' gloves, and start applying primer to the trim with a 3-inch acrylic brush. Keep a steady hand: Hold the brush near the bristles (not on the handle) with your thumb on one side and fingers on the other. Brush at a 45-degree angle so the bristles splay evenly. Then use a roller to paint the walls in an M or W pattern; this distributes paint better. Let the primer dry, and apply paint.

5. Peel Back the Tape

When the last coat is almost dry, gently remove the tape at a 45-degree angle. If you do pull off some paint, use a 1-inch brush to touch up the spot. Show your wife; earn points.

Keep Paint from Dripping on Your Floor

Roll a piece of masking tape to make it double-sided sticky and stick it to the middle of a paper plate. Now place your paint can on top of the tape. The paper plate will stick to the bottom of your paint can even if you move it, and it will catch all the drips. And now you have a handy place to rest your brush.

Find That Small Widget You Dropped

Screws, contact lenses, fingernails that flew off the clippers—they hit the floor and seem to disappear. So make them bigger: Turn on a flashlight and lay it on the floor. Small objects cast big shadows.

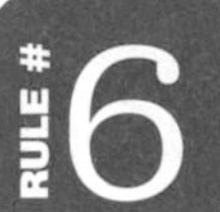

Measure twice, cut once.

Replace a Busted Door

Replace a dated or busted interior door with this step-by-step guide from James Carey, cohost of the home-improvement radio show *On the House*.

What you'll need: A prebored door (that has the same dimensions as the old one), nail punch, hammer, pliers, towel, screwdriver, tape measure, pencil, utility knife, chisel, drill, and sawhorses or a workbench.

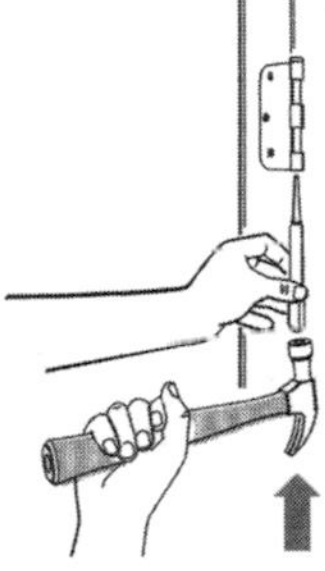

1. Remove the Hinge Pins

Close the old door and place the tip of a nail punch on the underside of the bottom hinge pin. Tap the punch with a hammer until the pin is almost out of the hinge knuckles. Pull it out with pliers and set it on a towel. Repeat with the remaining hinges, top hinge last.

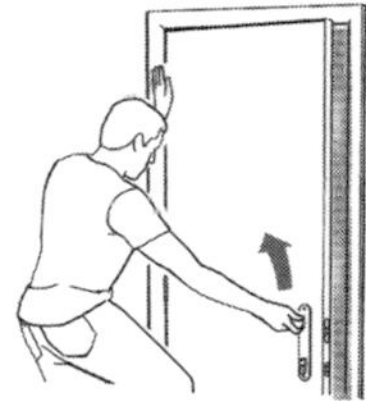

2. Ditch the Door

Hold the doorknob with one hand and steady the door with your other. Jiggle the door and pull it toward you; once it's loose, rest it against a wall. Unscrew the lock set and measure from the bottom of the door to the bottom of each hinge. Jot down the numbers—you'll need them later.

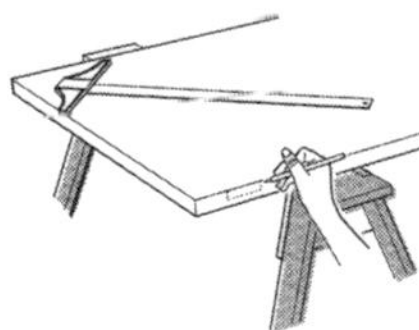

3. Mark the Spots

Rest the new door on sawhorses or a workbench. You'll install the hinges on the side opposite the prebored hole for the door handle. Pencil those hinge measurements on this side.

4. Carve Some Space

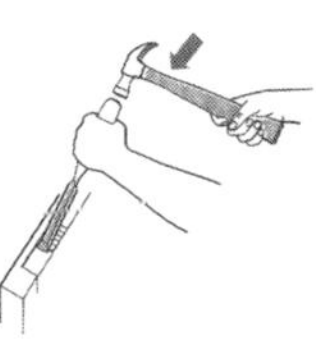

Unscrew the old door's hinge plates. Align the bottom of a plate with one of the pencil marks, pencil the plate's outline, and score this outline with a utility knife three times to break up the wood fibers. Use a hammer and chisel to carefully gouge the outline so the plate will be flush with the door. Set the plate in your gouged-out spot and mark the screw holes. Then tap the nail punch on each mark to make a divot so the drill bit won't skip. Repeat these steps for the other hinge plates.

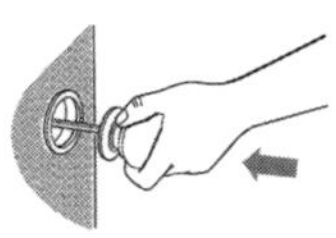

5. Install the Hardware

Drill pilot holes using a drill bit that's smaller than the screws. Then, with the plate in place, drive in the screws; repeat with the other hinges. Now ask a helper to hold the door in place as you align the hinge knuckles. Slide a pin into the top hinge and tap it with a hammer until it's secure. Repeat with the remaining hinges. Hold the latch faceplate to the latch hole and trace the outline using a pencil and then a utility knife. Gouge out the area so the plate sits flush. Insert the latch set through the latch hole. Mark the screw locations, drill pilot holes, and drive in the screws. Slide the exterior doorknob into place. Mark holes for the screws, drill pilot holes, and drive in the screws. Repeat with the interior doorknob.

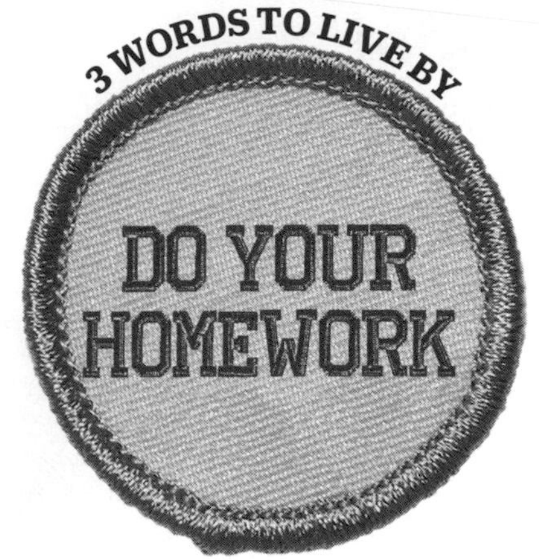
3 WORDS TO LIVE BY
DO YOUR HOMEWORK

Let Nature Clean Your BBQ

Hold the elbow grease. Remove your grates from the grill and place them top-down on an inconspicuous patch of lawn to sit out on a clear night. Overnight, the dew will loosen the crud, making it easier to wipe off using paper towels.

Get a Slug DRUNK

If slugs and snails are chowing down on your garden, buy 'em a beer. (Make it cheap stuff; no uppity craft brew.) Bury a few empty jars or used beer cans so their tops are flush with the soil in your vegetable garden. Now fill them with beer. See, like you, slugs find some of the compounds created during beer fermentation pretty great. And when they go in for a sip, they'll slip and drown.

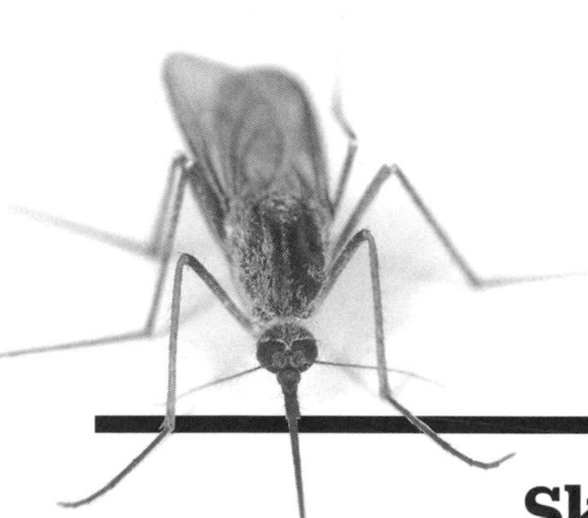

Skeeter Beaters

Biting insects can be a barbecue buzzkill. Joseph Conlon, technical advisor to the American Mosquito Control Association, and Daniel Kline, PhD, a research entomologist with the USDA, offer some planet-friendly tactics to ward off pests.

1. Stage a Drought

Even a bottle cap filled with water can be a mosquito breeding spot. Wipe down tables and your grill after a rain, and keep an eye out for stagnant water in random places—that tarp on the woodpile, a planter tray, a cup or bottle left outside. For your trash can and recycling bin, use a drill with a ¼-inch bit to add drainage holes in the bottom.

2. Smoke Out Trouble

Mosquitoes hate citronella, but most candles can't protect past a 5-foot radius. Scented torches are better because they give off more smoke, another pest peeve, for a few more feet of coverage. If you just can't stand the smell, then go with a portable Thermacell outdoor lantern ($32, thermacell.com). It releases allethrin, an odor-free bug blocker.

3. Blow 'Em Away!

Many pests are weak fliers, so point a floor fan toward the area where your guests will gather to create turbulent air space.

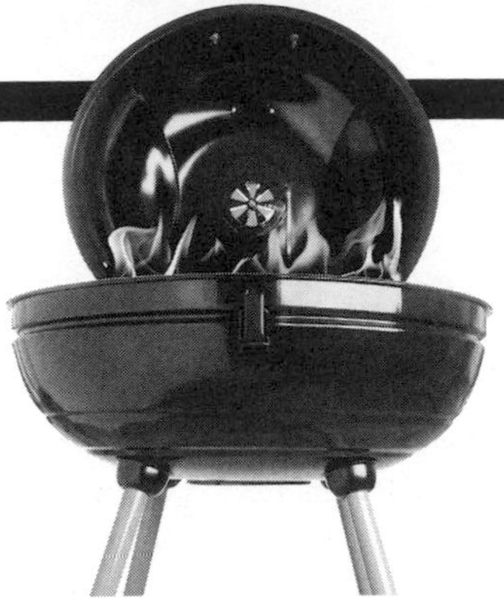

Grill Your Salsa!

Char an onion, a jalapeño, and two large tomatoes on all sides over direct heat, about 10 minutes. Remove the vegetables to a plate to cool. Peel, seed, and dice. Mix with cilantro, lime juice, garlic, and salt to taste.

Silence a Floor Squeak

Sprinkle talcum powder or foot powder between the floor boards and work it into the cracks with a cloth or brush. Squeaks happen when boards rub against one another or against a nail. The powder will help lubricate and silence those boards. (You might need to do this a few times.)

SHOVEL SNOW WITHOUT *Killing Your Back*

Test a shovel in the store by holding it as you would if you were pushing snow. Note where the handle rests—it should be near your belt buckle. If it rests above that, you'll work harder; if it's below, you'll hunch more.

Take a minute before heading outside to stretch your lower back and hamstrings. (A few jumping jacks aren't a bad idea, either.) Be sure to dress appropriately for the weather.

If you can, push the snow instead of shoveling it. Your arms and legs, not your back, will do the work. If the snow is too deep or heavy to push, think wall squat: Set your feet shoulder width apart, keep your lower back and core set, and lift with your legs and butt.

Fix a Drywall Ceiling

With your very own, make another pair of hands—a deadman brace.

Hanging drywall is typically a two-person job, especially when installing panels on ceilings. But you can install ceiling drywall yourself (or easily with another person) if you use a brilliant device called a deadman brace. A deadman is nothing more than a T-shaped brace made from scrap 2 × 4s and a wall stud; use it to hold a drywall panel against the ceiling while you fasten the sheet to the joists. Here's how to make one:

What You'll Need: Scrap 2 × 4-inch lumber; wall stud; measuring tape; saw; nails or wood screws; hammer or drill with screw-driver bit

Step 1. Cut two 36-inch pieces from the 2 × 4s. These will be the top and bottom cross braces. Nail or screw the middle of these brace pieces to the ends of the stud. Use a measuring tape to ensure that the whole brace is 1 inch shorter than the distance from the floor to ceiling to allow for the thickness of the drywall.

Step 2. Cut and install 2 × 4 braces between the stud and cross braces at 45-degree angles for support. Be certain the cross braces and stud are perpendicular.

Step 3. Nail a 6-inch scrap wood "cleat" near the top of one of the middle wall studs in the room to create a holder over which to slide one end of the drywall. While holding the sheet over the cleat and against the ceiling with one hand, slide the deadman under the free end of the panel. Straighten the brace to secure the sheet. Get a ladder and screw or nail the drywall to the ceiling joists.

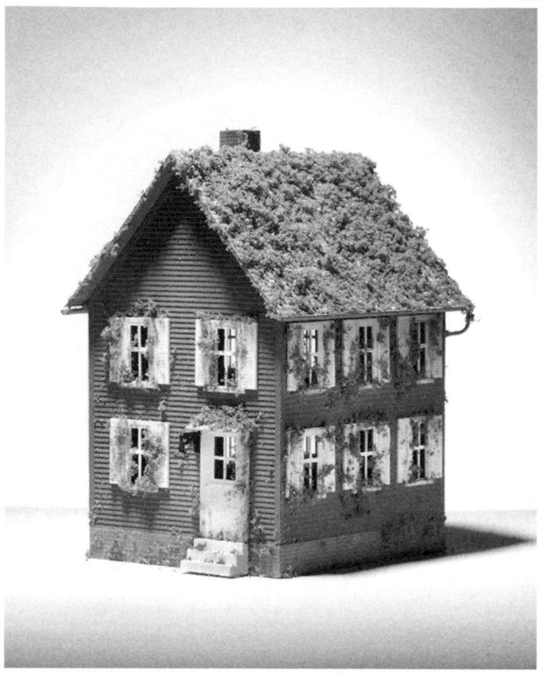

This Mold House

Fungus among us? One leak under your kitchen sink can start a colony of *Stachybotrys chartarum*. The greenish-black mold festers on fiberboard and dust particles when there's extra moisture. Clean it up by finding the leak first. Then spray a 1:16 mix of bleach and water on the spots. After 1 hour, scrub. Let it dry, then keep it that way with moisture-sucking crystals like DampRid.

De-Ice Your Driveway

Put down the pickax. There's an easier (and safer) way to thaw a sidewalk or driveway.

Add Water

For smaller areas, shovel off any snow and pour warm water on the exposed ice. When you eventually throw on rock salt, you'll create a brine, which should melt the ice faster.

Harness the Sun

Coat the ice with a dark-colored abrasive material, such as coal ash or dark sand. The dark color can then absorb heat from the sun and help melt the ice, as well as provide traction for walking and driving.

Shake On the Salt

Rock salt lowers the freezing point of water, so when it's added to ice, it speeds the melting process. Be wary: Salt can damage concrete and plants if you let it collect, so when the ice is gone, sweep it up and toss it.

Blow Out a Sink Clog

Unclog your sink quickly with help from *This Old House* plumbing expert Richard Trethewey. Fill a milk jug or empty 2-liter soda bottle with water. Cover the overflow drain of the sink with a piece of duct tape—this cuts off the air's escape route. In one quick motion, jam the top of the bottle into the drain and squeeze the bottle hard to send a jet of water into the drain. Take off the tape and run the water to see if the clog's gone. Didn't work? Repeat the steps again, but if three tries don't work, call a plumber.

If your plunger can't budge a clog from a drain, stuff a wet towel in the basin's overflow port and try again. This will boost pressure in the pipe.

How to Hang Out

Derek Hansen, author of *The Ultimate Hang: An Illustrated Guide to Hammock Camping*, explains how to rig the perfect napper's paradise.

What you'll need: 1 polyester or parachute-nylon outdoor hammock (about 10' × 5'); 2 polyester or polypropylene webbing straps (each 4' long with stitched eye loops on either end); 2 climbing-rated carabiners; travel pillow; towel

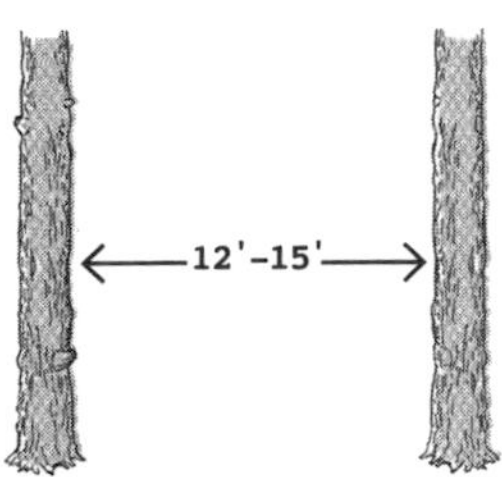

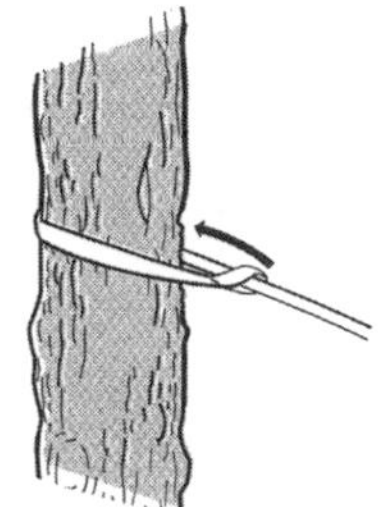

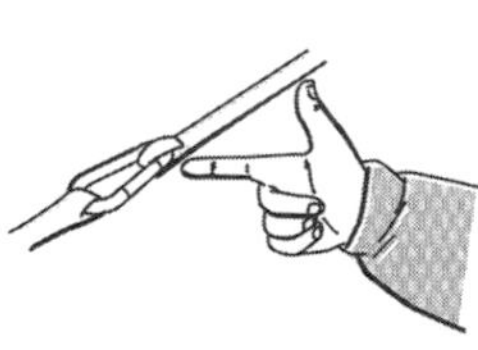

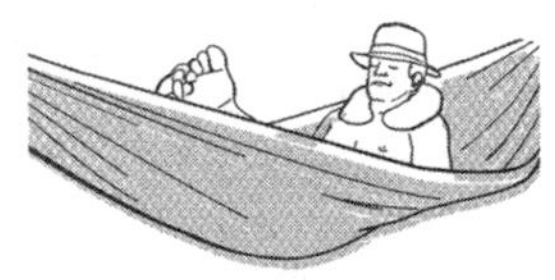

1. Seek Shade

Locate two trees with sturdy trunks that are at least 6 inches in diameter. They should be 12 feet to 15 feet apart; for most guys, that distance is about five comfortable steps. Check overhead for dead limbs or broken branches that could fall on you. You want sleep, not a dirt nap.

2. Rig Ropes

Wrap each webbing strap around a tree at about head height to create an anchor point: Feed one end through the opposite eye loop and then pull the strap tight to secure it. Now use the carabiners to clip the hammock to the loops. It should hang 20 inches off the ground.

3. Control Comfort

Your hammock should slope downward at a 30-degree angle from each tree. To test the angle, form a "finger gun" with your thumb parallel to the tree. Your thumb and index finger should both touch the strap. If the angle is too steep, unhook the strap, twist it, and reconnect.

4. Recline Right

Don't just lie in the center of the hammock. Drape your body across it diagonally with your head on one side and your feet on the other. It'll help you keep your back straighter, easing pressure. Break out the pillow and put a rolled-up towel under your knees. Nap-test often.

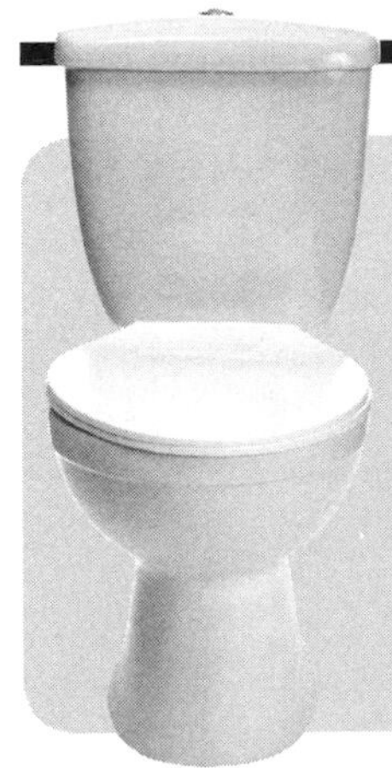

Tidy Up Your Bowl

Got to swab the loo? Don't bother with store-bought bowl cleaner. Go with vinegar and baking soda, which combine for a gunk-busting reaction, says Martin Mulvihill, PhD, a researcher of green chemistry at UC-Berkeley. Sprinkle ½ cup baking soda around the inside of the bowl, add ½ cup vinegar, and scrub while the effervescence does the work.

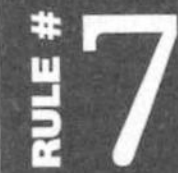

RULE # 7

For every roach you see, there are 800 more in your kitchen.

Build a Tree House

No tree? No problem. Put the house on stilts and trick it out with add-ons. We asked David Stiles (stilesdesign.com), author of the book *Forts for Kids*, to create a customized, *Men's Health*–approved stilt house that does not damage trees. Start sawing, and make your kid the neighborhood hero (though the other dads may hate you).

What You'll Need

PART	QUANTITY	PURPOSE
4 x 4 ACQ pressure-treated posts	10'	4 support posts
2 x 6 #2 fir	8'	7 floor joists
2 x 4 cedar	12'	2 knee braces
concrete mix	(80-lb bag)	4 post footings
5⁄8" x 6" cedar decking	8'	6 deck floor
3⁄4" exterior plywood	4' x 8'	1 interior floor
2 x 3 spruce	8'	14 framing posts

PART	QUANTITY	PURPOSE
2 x 4 fir	8'	1 ridge beam
5⁄8" exterior grooved plywood	4' x 8'	4 roof, front & back sides
4 x 4 cedar	16'	1 railing post
2 x 6 cedar	8'	2 railing posts
plastic-coated wire fencing	50'	1 railing enclosure
3" galvanized butt hinges	4	windows
1⁄2" x 5" lag screws,	36 corners	knee braces
1 box each of 2" and 3" epoxy-coated square-drive screws		

Raise Your Kids Right

Structures built in trees can damage limbs and vice versa. So build your fort on posts near a tree for a similar but safer effect. This A-frame design is easy and inexpensive to build. Start your planning here, and then head over to MensHealth.com/treehouse for the expanded instructions.

Accessorize

Build a removable periscope to scan for spies. (See our instructions online.) To use the periscope, poke it up through a hole in the roof and rest its support shaft on the floor. Another cool add-on: a pulley system at the end of the ridge beam.

1. Check the Codes

Ask your municipality if you need a permit to build. Make sure no pipes or cables are buried in the area where you plan to dig.

2. Go Shopping (Est. Cost: $500)

See list of materials above.

3. Set Up Your Support Posts

Mark out an 89 1⁄2 × 66 3⁄4-inch cleared area with string to show where the centers of the four support posts should be. At those corners, dig four holes, each 12 inches in diameter and 3 feet deep; place the 4 × 4 posts loosely in the holes. Temporarily brace the posts, but don't backfill the holes until the platform is in place.

4. Build the Platform

On the ground, build the floor frame with the joists, using epoxy-coated 2-inch square-head screws. (See illustration A on page 242 for measurements.) Then have four friends lift it over the posts. Level it and attach it at the 6-foot-high mark. Cut and add the eight 2 × 4 cedar braces to the posts and frame on each side. Make sure everything is plumb and level, and then partially fill the holes with soil, tamping the dirt with a 2 × 4 as you work. Mix the concrete and fill the top 10 inches of the hole; let the concrete cure for at least 24 hours.

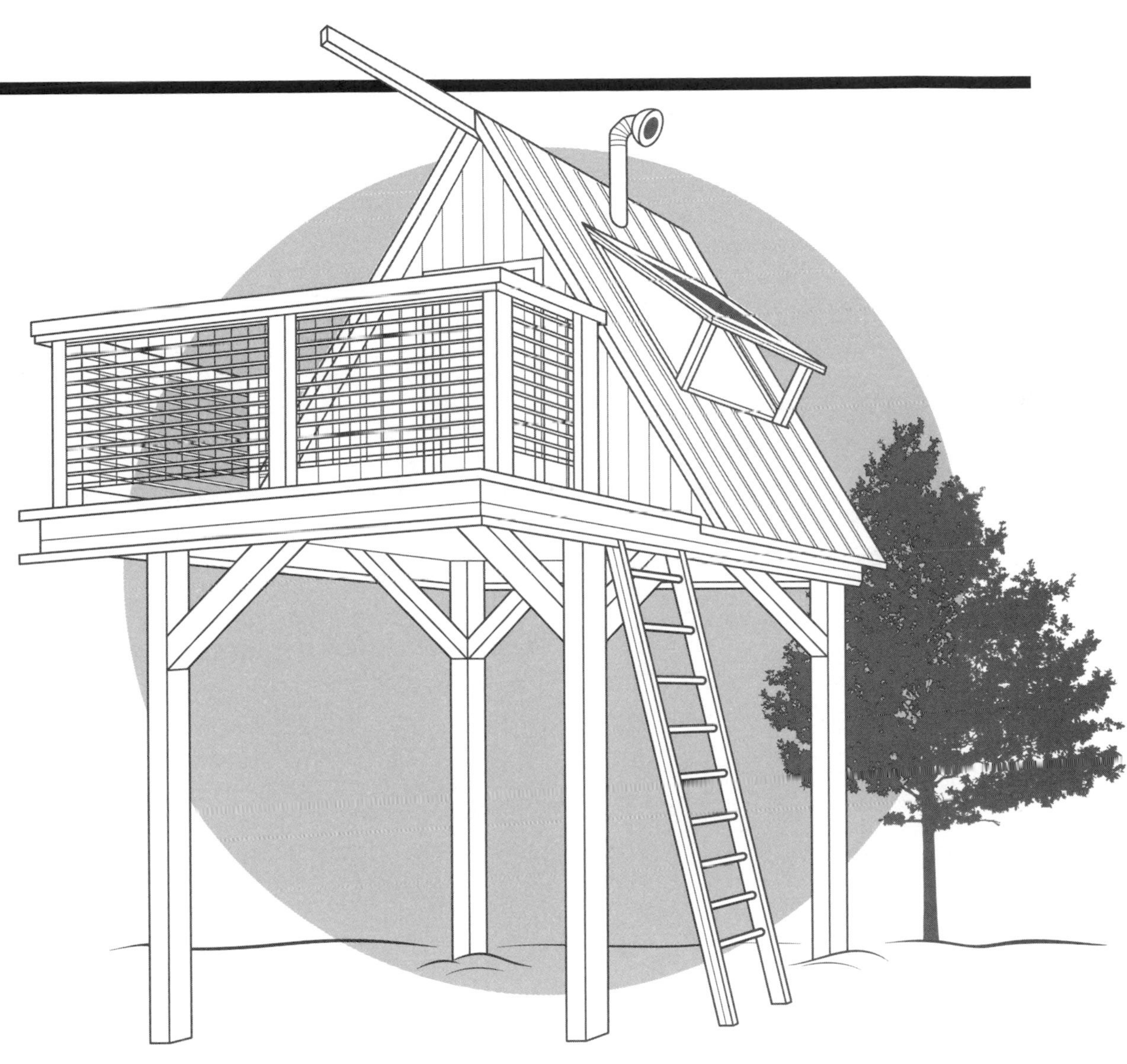

5. Construct Your A-Frame

Use five 4 × 6 deck boards for the front deck, and plywood for the interior floor. Build up your A-frame and sheathe it in plywood. (See illustration B on page 242.) Build the railing with the cedar 4 × 4s and 2 × 6s, leaving at least a 20-inch gap on one side for access. Use the fencing to enclose the railing. Cut out the window and secure it with the hinges. Attach a rope or wooden ladder at the opening. Now stand back and graciously accept applause from your kids.

(Continued on next page.)

(Continued from previous page.)

A. Platform Floor Plan

Attach the platform to the posts using lag screws. Cut the 3-foot knee braces from 2 x 4s. Use lag screws to attach the tops to the inside of the floor frame and the bottoms to the support posts.

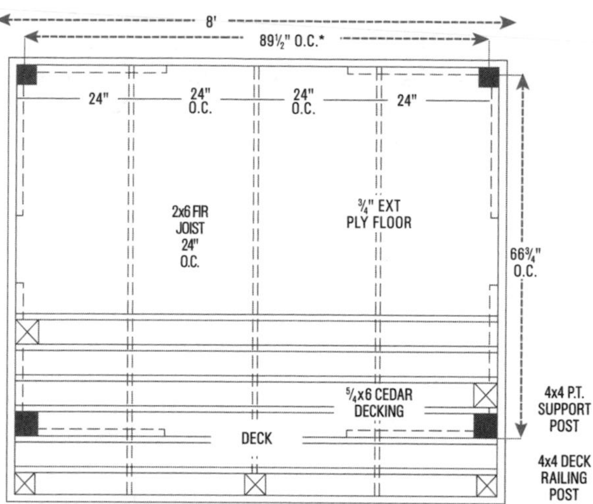

B. A-Frame Plan

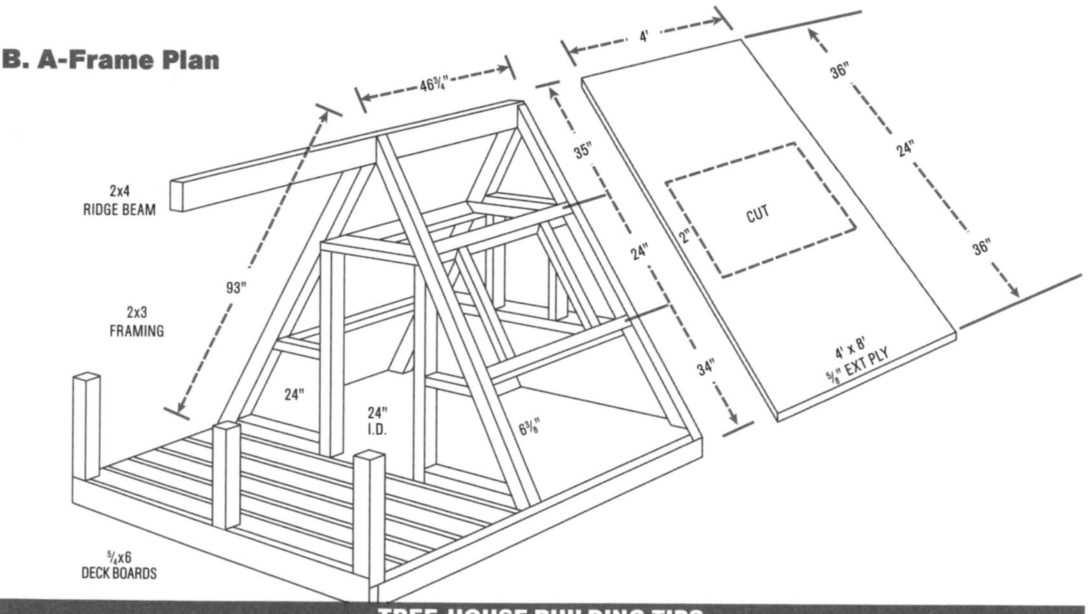

TREE-HOUSE BUILDING TIPS

1. If you decide to build in a tree, search for plans online that minimize damage to the tree. Never cut pieces out of the tree for support, as it exposes living tissue, and keep damage to bark to a minimum to reduce infection.
2. Don't climb ladders or trees with tools in your hand—for safety reasons. Instead "bucket your tools." Place them in a bucket and tie a long rope to the handle so you can pull up.
3. Build cool additions: a clothesline pulley with a bucket between the tree house and kitchen so you can snag snacks, zip line, rope swing, rope bridge, water cannon and solar-powered lights. For more ideas, visit relaxshacks.com, nelsontreehousesupply.com and treelesstreehouse.com.

BE A HANDY MAN

Save money and earn bragging rights with these quick fixes for domestic snafus.

PULL A STRIPPED SCREW. Using a chisel, cut a deep horizontal groove across the head of the screw. Now use a flathead screwdriver to back out the screw.

FIX A HOLE IN DRYWALL. 1. Cut a square or rectangle around the hole with a utility knife. Be sure to expose half the width of the closest stud. 2. Cut a new square of drywall to fit. Screw the patch into the stud and cover the cracks with a piece of joint tape. Coat the work area with a thin sheet of joint compound. 3. When dry, sand the area with a fine-grit sandpaper and apply paint primer over the patch.

UNJAM A GARBAGE DISPOSAL. Most disposals have hex-wrench holes at the bottom. Insert your wrench and reverse the blades, freeing the jammed item. Reach in and yank it out.

REMOVE THE BASE OF A SMASHED LIGHT BULB. Make sure the lamp is unplugged or, if it's hardwired, flip off the circuit breaker. Clean over the bigger shards from the base, then press the cut side of a half potato down on it. Turn it counterclockwise.

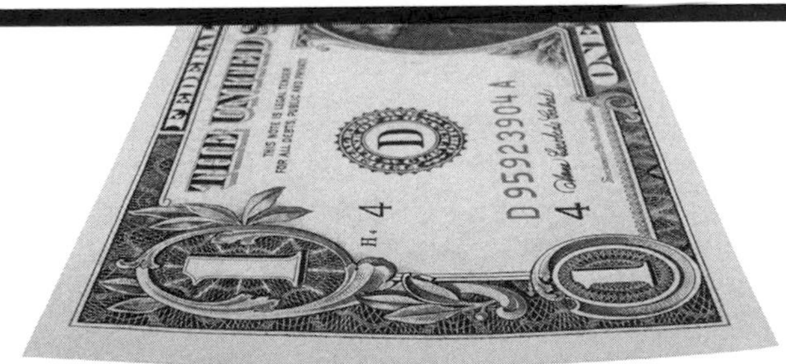

Measure with Money

Can't find a ruler or tape measure? Throw money at your problem. For small measurements, use a penny, which is exactly three-quarters of an inch across. For bigger measures, use any US paper currency, which is 6½ inches long.

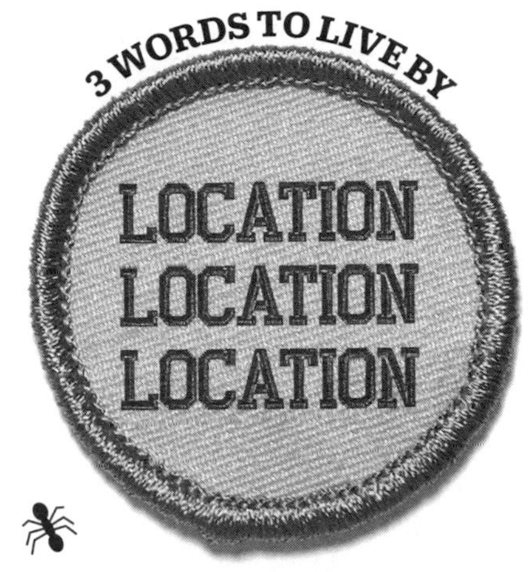
3 WORDS TO LIVE BY
LOCATION
LOCATION
LOCATION

Q I have ants. What's the best way to get rid of the buggers?

A. Avoid those aerosol cans of ant killer, because they won't work: When you spray an insecticide, you annihilate only the ants you can see, which is just 10 percent of the nest, says Peggy Powell, PhD, an entomologist with the West Virginia Department of Agriculture. The smarter salvo? Baits. Try the Advance 360A Dual Choice ($10, epestsupply.com), which uses a poisonous protein-and-sugar-based goop that ants scramble to take to their colony. Place the bait stations near where you think your invaders are entering. And remember: Since their main goal is to haul back as much grub as they can to feed their queen and crew, be sure to clean up every last food crumb in your home. Once the ants' supply of snacks is gone, they'll go straight for the bait, aka their last meal.

Spiff Up Your Deck

Add luster and life expectancy to your wood deck with these simple staining steps.

Got Wood?

First, decode your deck's material. If you live anywhere from the East Coast to Denver, chances are you have pressure-treated southern yellow pine. West Coast folks are likely to have western red cedar decks. Don't think it's either? You could be looking at an exotic hardwood. Scrape the wood with your fingernail. If your nail leaves a groove, the wood is cedar. Only a light scratch? It's yellow pine. Dense, exotic hardwoods, such as ironwood and Brazilian walnut, show no marks when scratched.

Scrub Down

To wash away 99 percent of the dirt on bare wood, use a detergent that contains carbonate, such as OxiClean Versatile Stain Remover Powder or Tide powder without bleach. Fill a bucket with hot water and add a quarter cup of the cleaner per gallon, letting it dissolve for 15 minutes. Hose down the deck and apply the solution using a pump sprayer, then use a push broom to scrub the dirt away. Hose the deck once more to rinse.

Stain It Up

Choose a semitransparent stain with microreflectors, or a full-body stain with added color. These stains prevent cracks and blisters and block damaging UV rays. Apply the stain with a 6-inch microfiber brush, coating a single board at a time to avoid an overlapping, streaky pattern.

Wait It Out

Once you've finished, allow the stain to dry anywhere from overnight to 72 hours before busting out the grilling gear. Read the manufacturer's label to determine whether a second coat is needed and, if so, whether it should be applied while the first stain is still wet or after it has dried.

Most of what you want in life may be found in a hardware store, not counting sex.

Clean Your Second-Story Windows on the Cheap

Sure, you could buy a squeegee on a stick. But DIY expert Spike Carlsen has a plan that's more fun.

1. Mix 2 cups water with 1/4 cup vinegar and 1/2 teaspoon liquid detergent.
2. Pour it into a Super Soaker and shoot your windows from outside.
3. Reload with fresh water and rinse. It's best to do this on an overcast day so the solution won't dry and cause water spots before you can rinse.

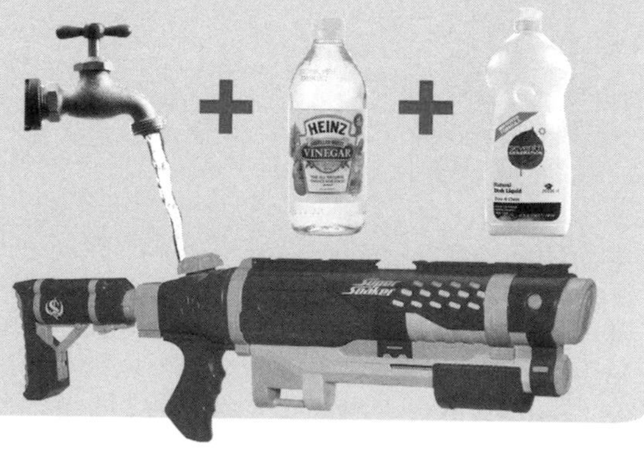

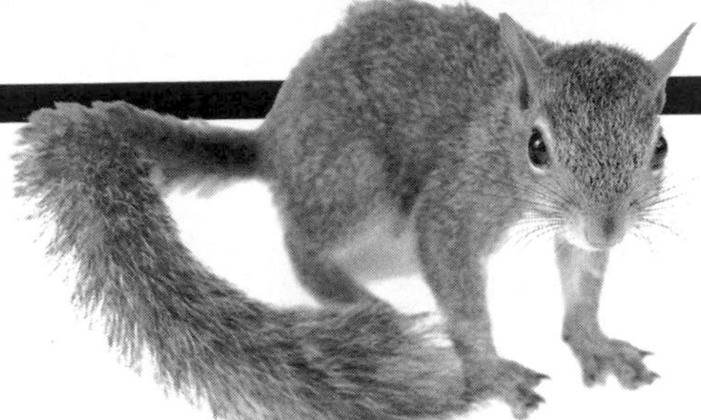

Evict a *Critter* from Your Home

Defcon 1: Squirrel

It can bite. So try to corral the little nut muncher in a room that has an open door or window. Squirrels are drawn to light, so try to make the room dark except where you'd like it to go. Eventually it'll find its way outside.

Defcon 2: Bird

Try the squirrel tactic first. If that doesn't work, close the drapes, darken the room, and cover any windows. When the bird settles in one spot, place a towel over it (use a hand towel for a tiny bird) and carefully scoop it up. Release the bird outside near a tree or shrubbery.

Defcon 3: Bat

Wait until Dracula lands on a wall. Open a window, close any doors, and let the bat escape at night. No dice? Quietly approach the bat and cover it with an open shoebox. (Wear gloves.) Slide a piece of cardboard under the box to gently detach the bat so it falls into the box. Release the bat outside, holding the box away from your face.

Snuff Out a Small Fire

It's always better to let the pros handle a fire. But if you insist on fighting it any way, at least arm yourself with the right weapons and technique (below). Buy a UL-listed multipurpose ABC extinguisher, like the Kidde Full Home ($47, homedepot.com), for each floor.

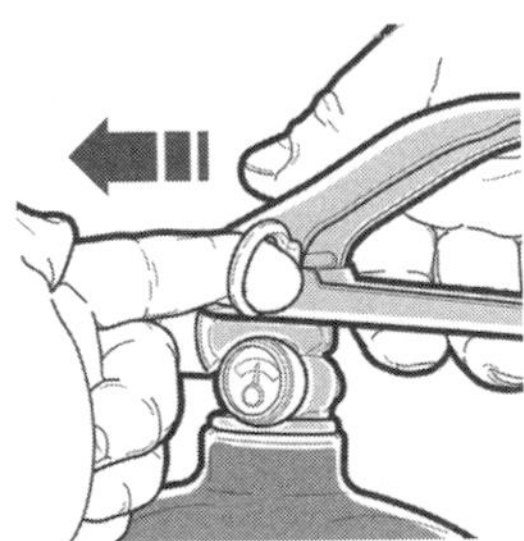

Pull the Pin

Remove the safety pin from the extinguisher to unlock the trigger. Stand about 8 feet away from the fire; keep your back to a clear exit route at all times.

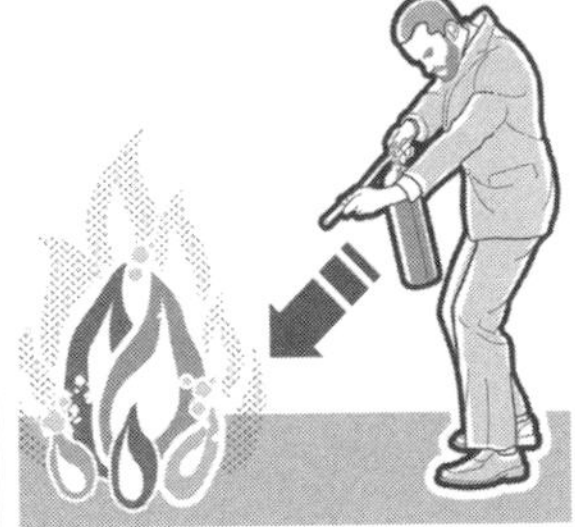

Hit the Floor

Aim at the base of the fire and squeeze the trigger. Don't blast straight at the flames; you won't put out the fire, but you will waste extinguishing agent.

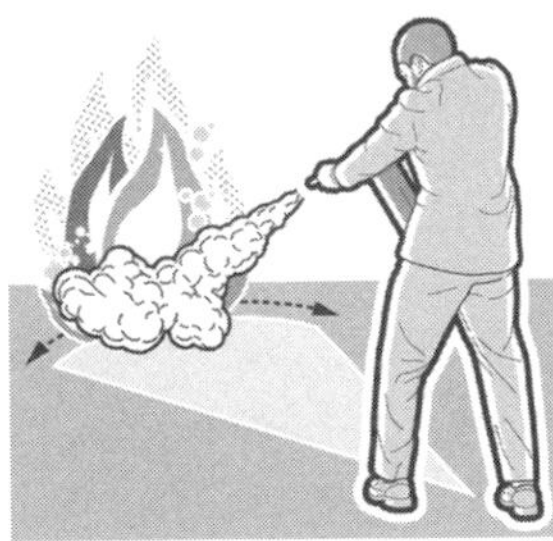

Tame the Flames

Sweep the nozzle back and forth. Don't stop until either the fire is out or the extinguisher is empty. If the fire is still burning or smoking, exit the area and call 911.

Catch a Mouse—Alive!

Yeah, you could just buy a trap and kill the bugger. But that can turn messy. And it's mean. This way, the mouse is gone and your girlfriend/wife/kids aren't grossed out.

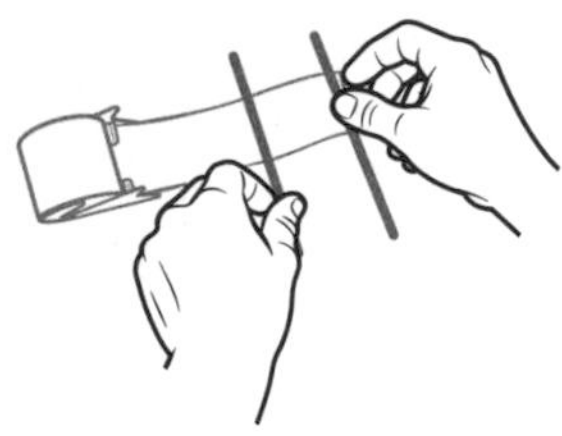

Step 1.

Tear off a piece of wide packaging tape. Place two sticks or pencils on the tape an inch apart and about two-thirds of the way up.

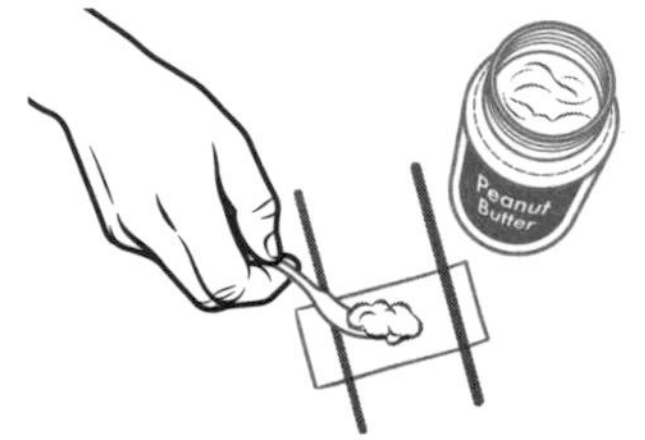

Step 2.

Attach bait to the tape. Peanut butter or potato chips work great.

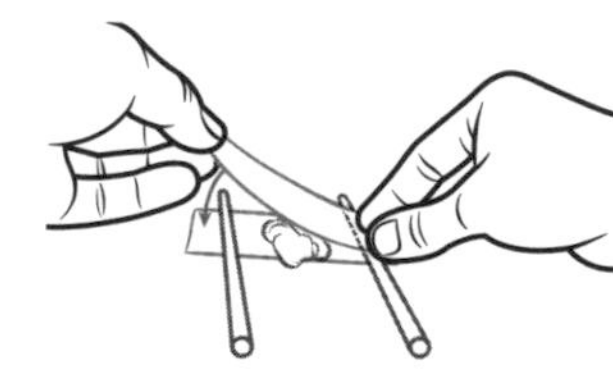

Step 3.

Use a second piece of tape to keep the bait in place, but leave some food exposed.

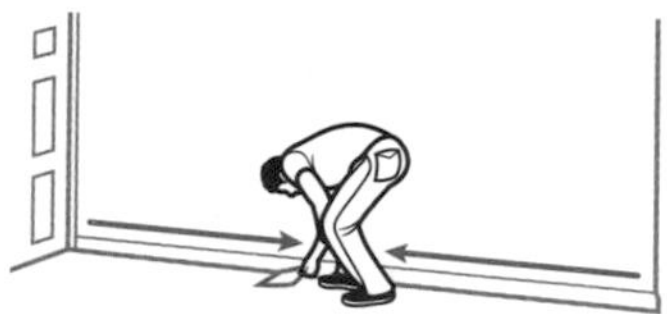

Step 4.

Mice scurry along the edges of rooms, so pick a spot along a wall about halfway between two corners. Put a piece of cardboard on the floor.

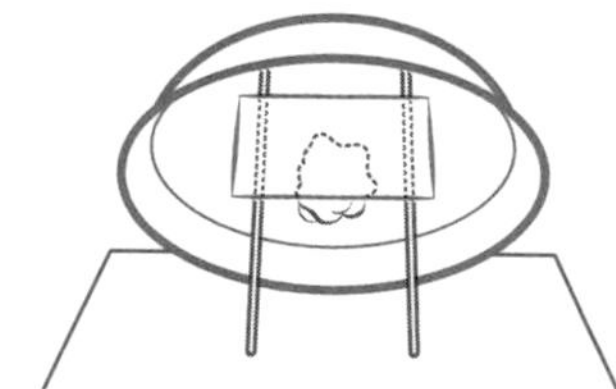

Step 5.

Stand the sticks up on the cardboard and use them to prop up a semitransparent bowl, with room for the mouse to crawl under.

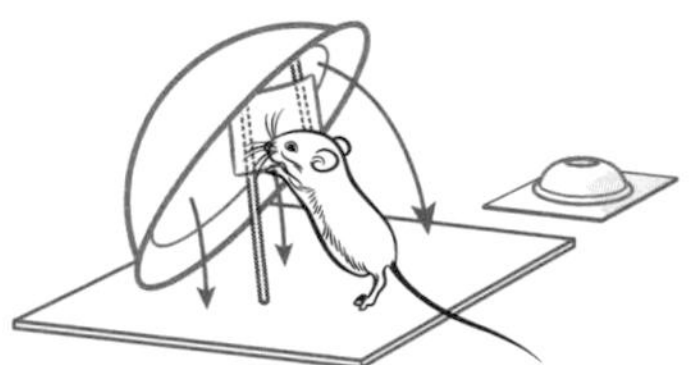

Step 6.

When the mouse reaches for the bait, it'll push the sticks over and trap itself. Check your trap regularly.

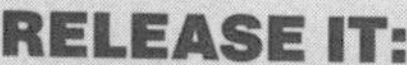
RELEASE IT:

Pick up the cardboard and bowl and take the mouse at least 100 feet away from your place so it doesn't come back. Clean and disinfect any areas where the mouse may have been, using a bleach solution or disinfectant. Patch up any holes in your walls that mice might crawl through—they can fit through a space as small as a dime.

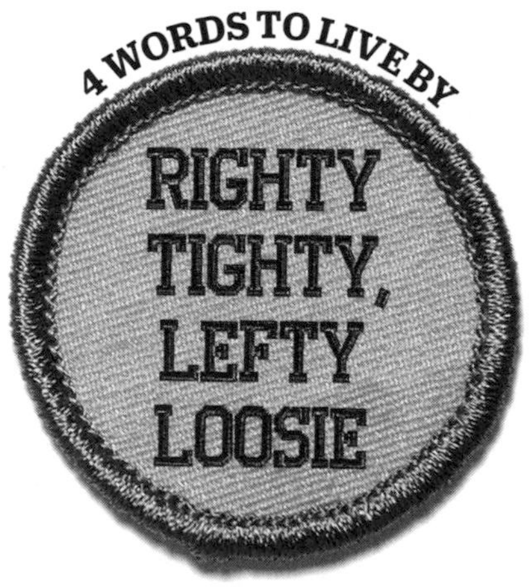
4 WORDS TO LIVE BY
RIGHTY TIGHTY, LEFTY LOOSIE

Build a Canine Crib

Jason Cameron, host of DIY Network's *Man Caves,* shows how to shelter your best friend.

WHAT YOU NEED:	
1 bag crushed stone	8-12 batts mineral wool insulation
4 concrete pier blocks	2-4 cans (24 oz each) spray foam
3 pressure-treated 2 × 4 × 8s	2 sheets ¾" T1-11 plywood siding, 4 × 8
4 sheets ½" plywood, 4 × 8	1 small roll #15 felt paper
8-12 tubes (10 oz each) Liquid Nails heavy-duty construction adhesive	1 bundle asphalt shingles
2 boxes (1 lb each) #9 × 3¼" stainless steel nails	2 boxes (1 lb each) #11 × 1¼" roofing nails
12 Douglas fir 2 × 4 × 8s	

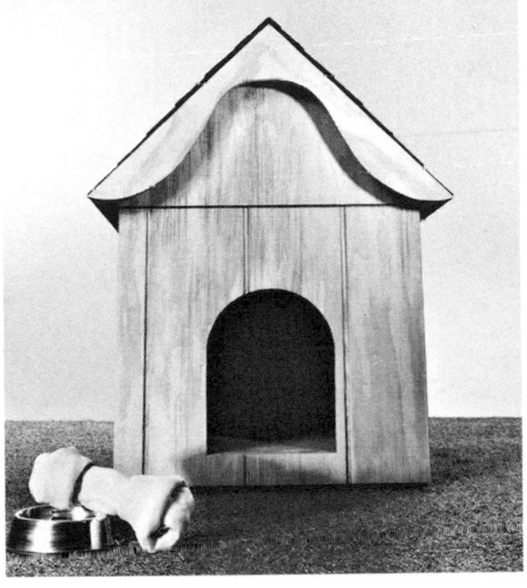

Step 1: Measure the Beast

A big house means a cold dog. Map these interior dimensions. Length: dog's hind end to tip of nose + 12 inches. Width: dog's shoulders + 18 inches. Height: dog's height (floor to top of head as he sits upright on hind legs) + 3 inches. Door opening: for width, dog's width + 2 inches; for height, dog's shoulder height + 2 inches.

Step 2: Lay the Groundwork

Make a foundation of crushed stone, raking it out evenly. Place a pier block at each corner and use a level to align the height of the blocks.

Step 3: Build the Base

Nail together pressure-treated 2 × 4s for a base frame. (Add 8 inches to length and width to fit the interior specs.) Cover the frame with ½-inch plywood, "A" side up. Glue it to the frame before nailing (corners first, then down the center of each 2 × 4).

Step 4: Frame Up the Walls

Using Douglas fir 2 × 4s, frame all four walls flat on the ground. Nail center studs in the back and side walls. (Keep the back wall stud 2 inches off center for the roof strut.) Glue and nail ½-inch plywood to the interior of the back and side walls and add insulation. Cover the walls with ¾-inch plywood. Mark and cut out the door. Stand the walls on the base and nail them to the base and each other. Toenail each corner. Spray foam into seams.

Step 5: Raise the Roof

Nail a 2 × 4 support (24 inches high) at the midpoint of the front wall top plate; do the same on the back wall. Cut a ridge board the length of the house and nail to the top supports. To make each of the eight rafters (four per side), cut one end of a 2 × 4 at an angle to meet the ridge; then cut a notch in the other end so it'll sit flat on the top plate. Nail the rafters into place. Sheathe the roof with ½-inch plywood (making sure there's overhang); cover the gables with plywood triangles. Then apply felt paper and shingles to the roof.

For complete plans on how to build this pooch palace, head to MensHealth.com/doghouse.

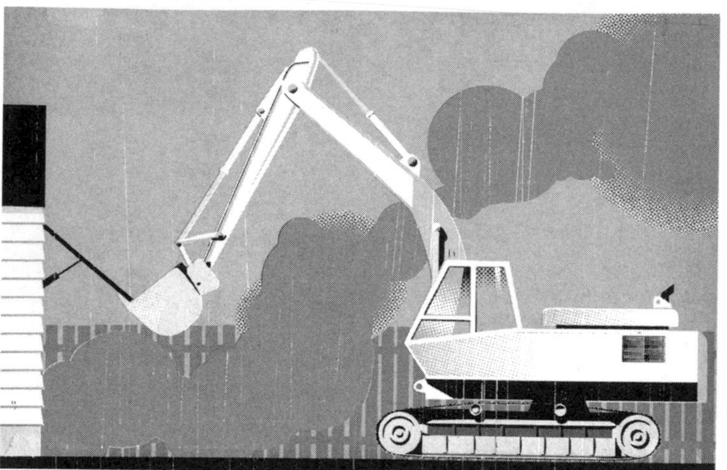

Organize Your Garage

Assess the Mess

Pick a sunny morning to pull everything out of the garage and take inventory; you'll immediately see what you no longer need. Make a yard-sale pile for duplicates or items you haven't used in at least 3 years. Make a separate pile for toxic or recyclable stuff—car batteries, old mower gas—and dispose of them responsibly. (Visit earth911.com for recycling advice and resources.)

Zone Your Space

With the garage clear, try to visualize where the big things (workbench, mower) might fit. Also, designate areas for specific items you need regular access to—yard tools, for instance.

Freshen Up

Hang pegboard for small tools, and metal reels for hoses and cords. Treat the floor with an epoxy coating, such as gray UCoat It (ucoatit.com), which takes 4 to 12 hours to dry. This finish prevents spill absorption and makes cleanups easier.

Mobilize Your Gear

Pull out a black marker and make a label for any box or bin with contents that are not immediately apparent. Place large items (cabinets, plastic bins) on plywood moving dollies. Mobility allows you to easily adjust the layout of the space if you need to. Now invite your pals over to show off.

Spring-Clean Your Car

Baby your ride to a showroom finish with custom car designer Stacey David, host of *Gearz* on the Speed Channel.

Scout the Facility

Skip the drive-thru joint; those giant spinning brushes may damage your car's paint job. Instead, seek out a human-operated car wash or detailer that uses microfiber towels, auto soap such as Mothers or Meguiar's, and compounds for polishing. The TLC should involve four steps: washing, cleaning, polishing, and waxing.

Order Smart

Many full-service car washes boost their profits with bell-and-whistle extras. Keep it simple: a base wash to blast off the dirt, a clay bar to remove grime, and a polishing compound or buff to bring out the shine. Finally, finish with a wax to seal and protect.

Spot-Clean

Keep your car's paint job in good shape by treating it to a full wash every 2 or 3 weeks, a wax every 2 or 3 months, and a spot-clean each week if needed. (Bird droppings and splattered bugs can alter the finish and color of your car.)

Clean Your Wheels

The metallic particles in brake dust will corrode expensive wheels—unless you keep them clean.

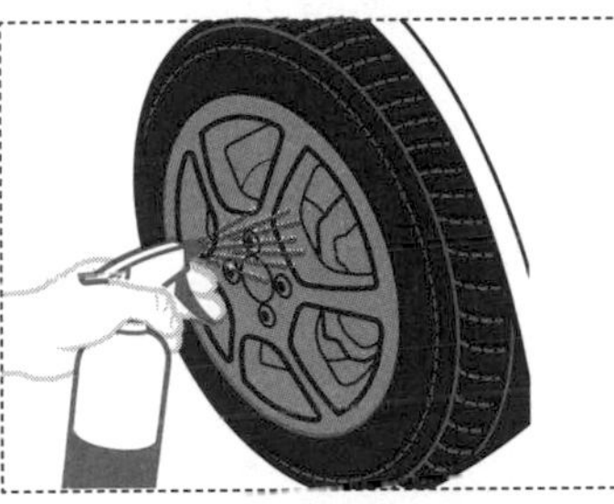

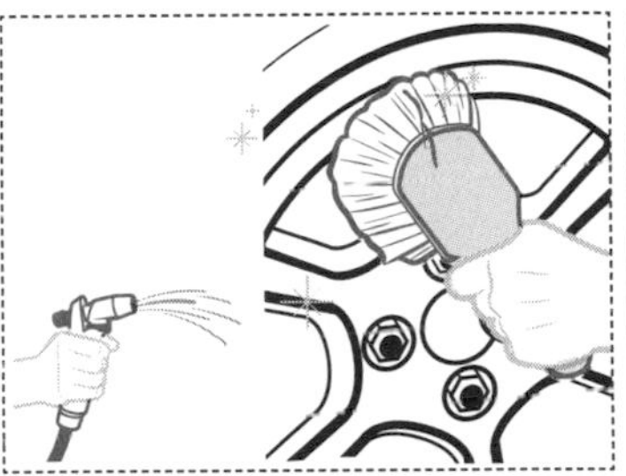

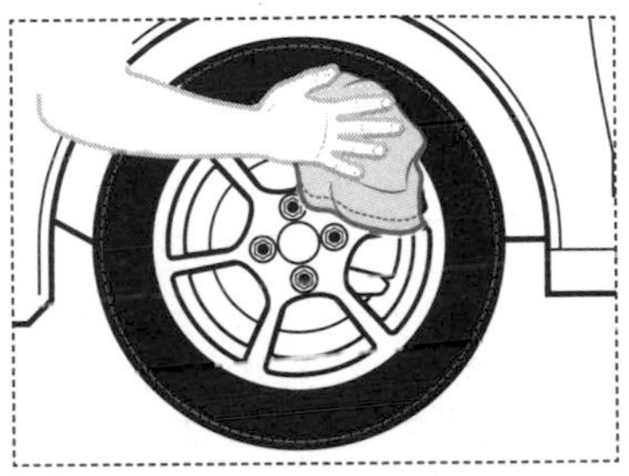

Apply

Spray on a mild, pH-balanced wheel cleaner and let it work to lift the particles off the wheel metal, following the bottle's directions. (Strong acids in old-school cleaners can damage the finish on today's wheels.)

Remove

Rinse the wheel. Scrub it with a microfiber wheel brush to remove lingering dirt. Dry with a microfiber towel; repeat the process for stubborn stains. Clean wheels individually so the cleaner doesn't dry on them.

Polish

Apply a high-quality wheel polish to your wheels with a clean, dry microfiber towel. Let the polish dry and then wipe it off with a regular cloth. This seals your wheel and helps protect it from debris.

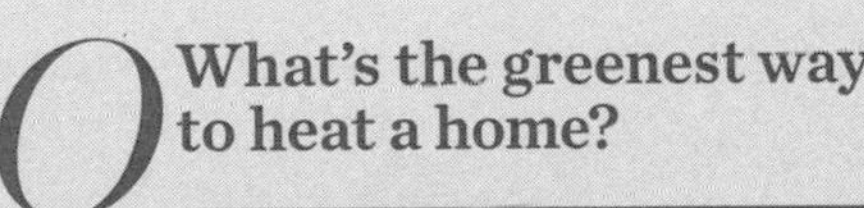

Q. What's the greenest way to heat a home?

A. Tap the well of warmth beneath your feet with a geothermal heat pump. They draw heat through looped pipes that run deep underground, where the earth's temperature stays more consistent. Geothermal heat pumps earn the highest possible LEED certification and produce fewer carbon dioxide emissions than other systems. It all comes at a hefty price—about $25,000—but in the long run, the extra efficiency means you'll save green by going green, says Max Sherman, PhD, a senior scientist at the Lawrence Berkeley National Laboratory. To find an accredited installer, check the "business directory" link at igshpa.okstate.edu.

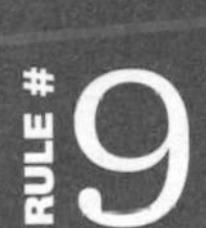

RULE # 9

If footprints remain in your lawn after walking on it, you need to water the grass.

Conquer Weeds with Water

Traditional weed killers can harm the environment and crawling kids. If your patio is becoming a weedy mess, try sticking a flat-head screwdriver in between the pavers or sidewalk slabs to excavate and destroy the weeds' root systems. If that fails, go full boil: Fill a kettle with water, bring it to a boil, and pour it on any weeds you want to die.

Patch a Hole in the Wall

Wild party last night? Fix a small hole with this fast, easy "blowout patch" technique from contractor John DeSilvia of DIY Network's *Rescue My Renovation*. No power tools or f-bombs needed.

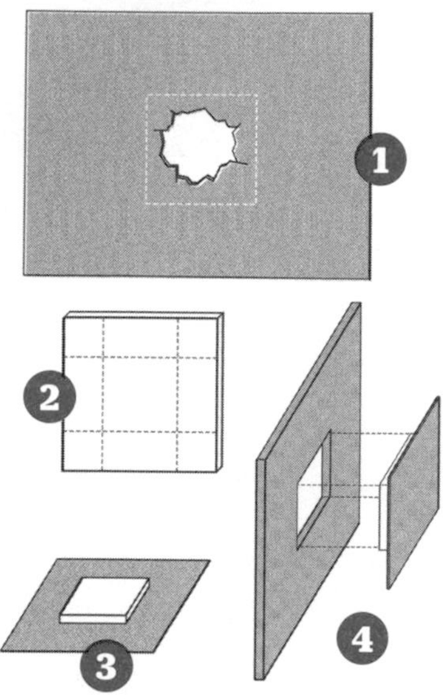

1. Prepare Your Patch

With a drywall knife, trim the hole to form a square (1). Cut a spare piece of drywall 2 inches larger than the hole on all sides. Then use the knife to score a border around the back of the piece, 2 inches in from the perimeter (2). Peel off the paper backing from this border; the result should be a hole-size piece of drywall with 2-inch flaps of paper on all sides (3). Set the blowout patch aside.

2. Cover the Hole

Spread an even layer of joint compound around the hole and place the blowout patch over the hole (4). As you apply pressure to the patch, those 2-inch flaps should adhere to the compound. Use a 9-inch taping knife to push out excess compound and scrape it away from the drywall, leaving a smooth, even surface.

3. Conceal the Evidence

Allow the joint compound to dry before applying another coat. After the second coat dries, sand the area smooth so the patch is flush with the wall. Now it's ready to paint. Hole? What hole?

Hang a Picture on a Brick Wall

WHAT YOU'LL NEED
Drill
$^1/_4$" masonry drill bit (used specifically for stone, brick, concrete); plastic anchor sleeves (which usually come in a kit with screws)
Hammer

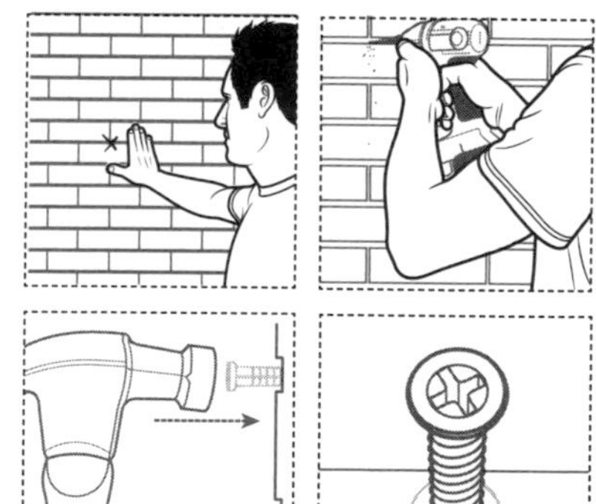

1. Don't drill into brick by a fireplace or near any type of flue—you may damage the flue pipe. If you're not sure what's behind there, don't drill.
2. Drill a 1-inch-deep hole into the mortar. Don't touch the brick. Mortar is easier to drill into—but it's also strong.
3. Blow the dust out and insert the sleeve into the hole, gently hammering it into place. Then twist in the screw that came with the sleeve, leaving its head sticking out $^1/_4$ inch.
4. Hang your art and enjoy.

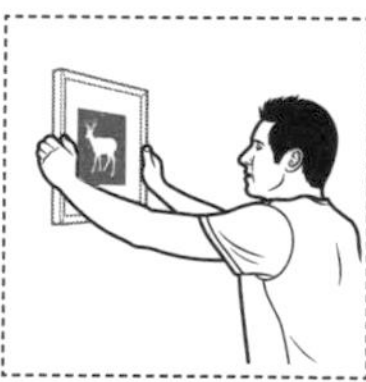

Move Furniture like a PROFESSIONAL

No sofa on earth will overpower you with these expert tips.

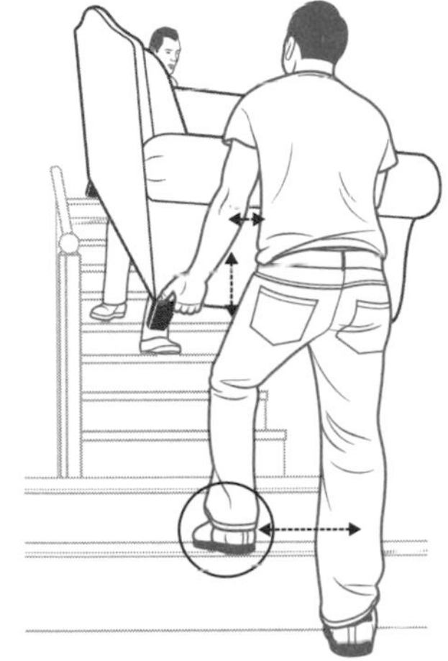

UP A FLIGHT OF STAIRS

1. The person moving backward up the stairs endures the most back and core stress. Put the stronger person there.
2. You both must grip the object's ends at similar points for stability. Keep your arms above your thighs and your elbows tucked into your body to prevent back strain.
3. Walk with a wide stance to support the weight. The top person controls the pace—left foot, right, left, right. Break on landings: It's safer than midflight.

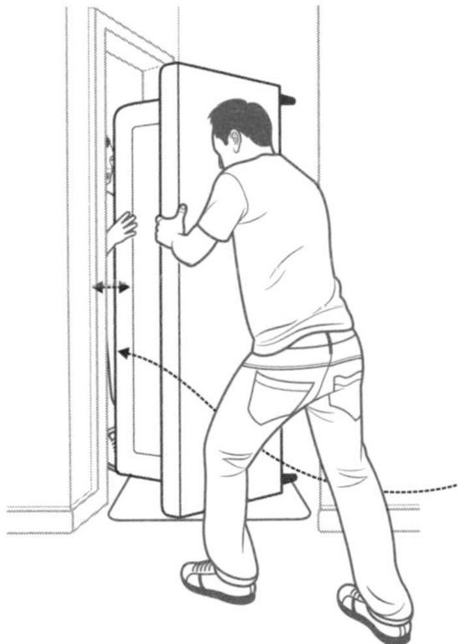

AROUND A TIGHT CORNER

1. Most people try to rest a couch on two legs and push it around at an angle. But that much stress on the legs may damage them. Movers prefer going vertical.
2. Stand the couch on end and push it around the corner. Make sure the sitting surface faces the inside of the corner you're trying to navigate; otherwise you might run the couch into the wall and cause damage.

RULE # 10

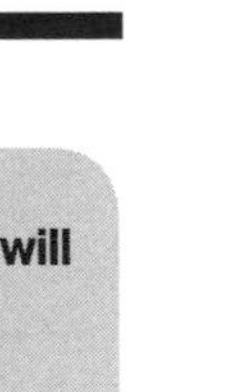

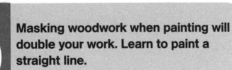

Masking woodwork when painting will double your work. Learn to paint a straight line.

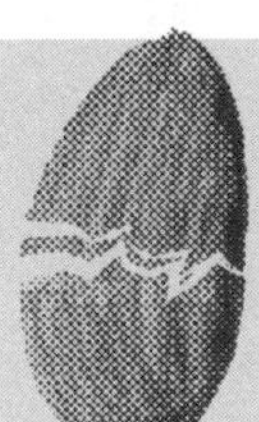

Cover Up Postparty Wood Scratches

Bite an almond in half. Rub the inside of the almond into the damage. The oil from the nut will help hide small scratches.

Clean Up a Grime Scene

Randy Gaines, vice president of engineering, housekeeping, and laundry operations for Hilton Worldwide, shows you how to polish your bathtub to five-star perfection.

1. Diagnose the Dirt

Save time and money by targeting specific tub stains with safe cleaners.

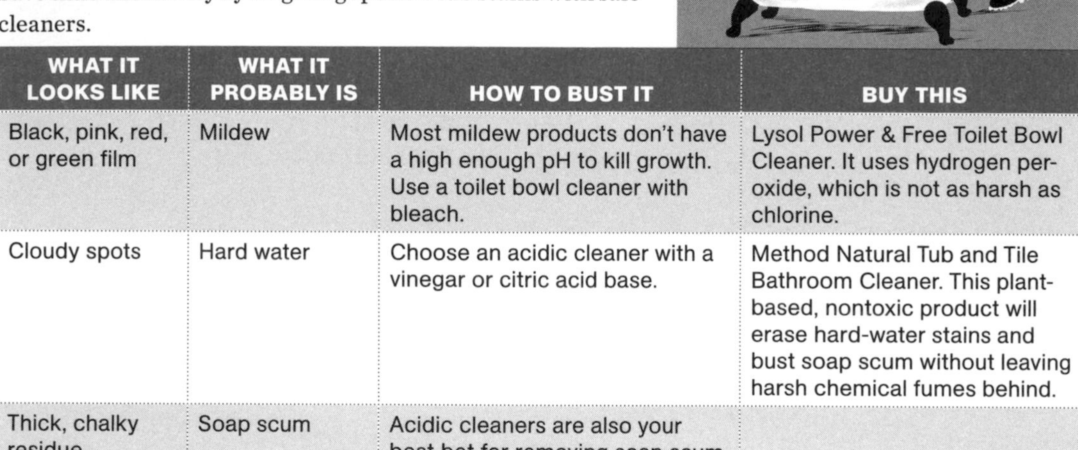

WHAT IT LOOKS LIKE	WHAT IT PROBABLY IS	HOW TO BUST IT	BUY THIS
Black, pink, red, or green film	Mildew	Most mildew products don't have a high enough pH to kill growth. Use a toilet bowl cleaner with bleach.	Lysol Power & Free Toilet Bowl Cleaner. It uses hydrogen peroxide, which is not as harsh as chlorine.
Cloudy spots	Hard water	Choose an acidic cleaner with a vinegar or citric acid base.	Method Natural Tub and Tile Bathroom Cleaner. This plant-based, nontoxic product will erase hard-water stains and bust soap scum without leaving harsh chemical fumes behind.
Thick, chalky residue	Soap scum	Acidic cleaners are also your best bet for removing soap scum.	

2. Blast the Crud

Spray the cleaner and wait at least 10 minutes for the active ingredients to penetrate the dirt. Using a nonabrasive brush or sponge, clean all surfaces, paying close attention to the area an inch or two above the tub base. That's where the most gunk tends to settle.

3. Achieve the Gleam

Rinse the tub until it shines. If it looks dull, then cleaner residue remains. Use a microfiber cloth to dry it. (Regular towels shed lint.) To make metal surfaces sparkle and guard against hard-water stains, use a tissue to apply a thin layer of petroleum jelly.

DESTINK YOUR FRIDGE

Place an open bowl of ground coffee on the bottom shelf. Within a week, the coffee will absorb all the foul odors—and leave behind the pleasing aroma of extra-bold Sumatra.

Keep Your Lawn Green

To avoid brown patches, don't mow short. Taller grass holds more moisture. If you live in the South, raise your mower deck to $1\frac{1}{2}$ inches; in the North, make it 3. And don't water after work; the best time of day for moisture retention is 2 a.m. to 6 a.m. Set a timer.

Thief-Proof Your Palace

Foil an intruder and stay safe with these tips from Chris McGoey, a security consultant with 40-plus years of experience, and Jesse Martinez, a senior police officer in Houston.

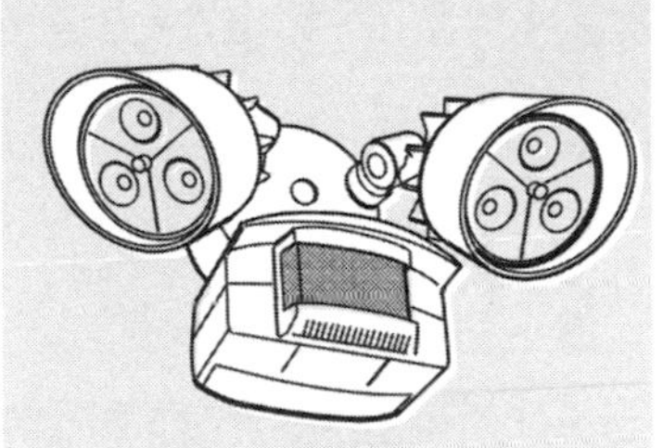

1. Secure the Perimeter

Rig a motion-sensor-activated light like this Lithonia Lighting floodlight ($120, homedepot.com) over each door. Trim shrubs so entries are visible from the street and police or neighbors can spot danger. Replace any half-inch deadbolt locks with ones that extend an inch or more into the door frame.

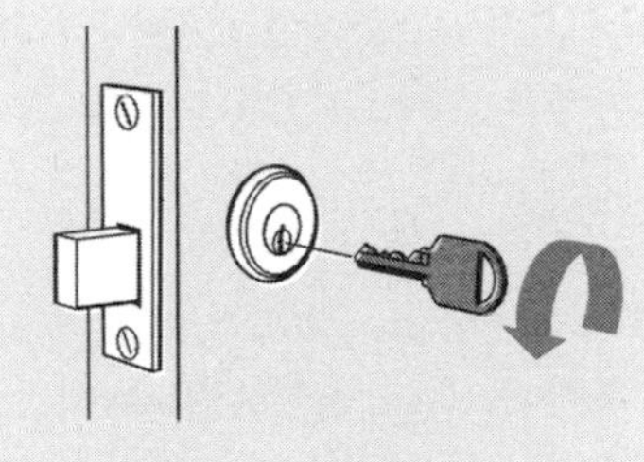

2. Round the Troops

Intruders want to catch you scared, so turn the tables. Add an exterior-door deadbolt to a bedroom door. If a break-in occurs, hide in that room with your family. Surprise the crooks with lighting that's iPhone- or iPad-controlled, like the Philips Hue Wi-Fi-enabled LED lightbulbs ($200 for three, apple.com).

3. Call for Backup

If possible, call 911 from a landline so your name and address display automatically. (Cell phones ping the closest tower; a dispatcher may have trouble determining where to send the police.) No landline? Try a smartphone app like LifeLine Response ($7 to $9, plus $7 to $8 yearly fee, iPhone and Android).

RULE # 11

To be safe, a leaning ladder should be 1 foot away from the wall for every 4 feet that the ladder rises. So if your ladder touches the outside of your house 16 feet above the ground, the feet of the ladder should be 4 feet from the wall.

SAVE THE PLANET— PLANT A TREE

The average mature tree sucks up 48 pounds of carbon dioxide a year and releases enough oxygen to sustain two people. Need more incentive to grab a shovel? A few 25-foot sunblocking deciduous trees on the south and west sides of your home can reduce your cooling costs by 25 percent. Check out the National Arbor Day Foundation (arborday.org) for a great deal on seedlings and instructions on how to plant them right.

THIS **SOLD** HOUSE

How to get more for your home.

Besides putting a bowl of McIntosh apples on the kitchen counter, there's much more you can do to make your place more appealing to prospective home buyers—and get better offers.

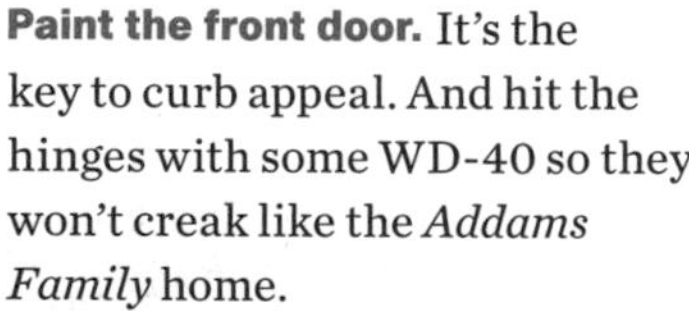

Paint the front door. It's the key to curb appeal. And hit the hinges with some WD-40 so they won't creak like the *Addams Family* home.

Purge your closets. Box up half the clothing in the closet and leave it with a friend or in a storage unit. You want to sell the notion of ample storage space. Do the same with kitchen cabinets. Buyers will open every cupboard and drawer.

Plant some colorful flowers in pots or in the ground out front. Again, think curb appeal. You want buyers to start forming a positive impression as soon as they pull up.

Don't bother painting rooms. Buyers will expect to do that, since it's likely they won't like the color you've chosen. However, do take a wet cloth and dust off the baseboards. If they look really nasty, give them a touchup.

Clean your bathrooms well. Don't paint or upgrade these rooms. Buyers often expect to do that. But dirty bathrooms, especially toilets, sinks, and showers, are a real turnoff.

Thaw a Frozen Water Pipe

On the coldest of nights, especially if you will be away from home, allow a tiny drip from faucets to prevent the pipes from freezing. If you end up with a frozen water pipe, thaw it before it bursts and causes water damage. Here's one way:

1. Open the faucets near the pipe, but don't force it. It may be frozen, too.
2. Get an old hand towel or bath towel and wrap the pipe with it. Secure the towel in place with a few wraps of duct tape.
3. Pour boiling water over the towel (be careful not to scald your hands).
4. Keep pouring hot water over the towel until the line clears of ice.

18

Percentage of men who have so much junk in the garage, the car won't fit.

Turn a Pallet Into a Patio Chair

MATT BLASHAW, HOST OF HGTV'S *VACATION HOUSE FOR FREE*, TRANSFORMS A SHIPPING PALLET INTO AN ADIRONDACK CHAIR.

WHAT YOU'LL NEED	
1 large shipping pallet with 2 center support beams (stringers)	Cordless drill with bit set and Phillips bit driver set
Circular saw, or reciprocating saw with bimetal blade	Hammer
	2 carriage bolts (5") with nuts and washers
Cat's-paw nail puller	Orbital sander
24 coated deck screws (2")	Exterior-grade solid stain, or primer and paint

1. Pick Your Pallet

Ask a furniture store or supermarket for a spare pallet. If the place lets you root around, find one without cracked or busted slats. Make sure the slats are evenly spaced and that all the nails are flush and unbroken.

2. Make Your Cuts

Using the saw, cut the slats along the inside edge of one center stringer. The skinnier section will be the seat.

3. Assemble the Pieces

Trim the slats on the larger section so it will fit inside the width of the seat to form the chair's back. Use the cat's-paw to remove the stringer from the scrap piece you just cut. Use deck screws to secure the stringer to the chair's back. Carefully hammer off all but five of the slats from the back and all but four from the seat.

4. Build the Chair

Form a V with the two pieces; drill holes where the stringers cross. Secure the seat on both sides using carriage bolts, washers, and nuts. Attach leftover slats to the seat for front legs. Trim back legs to adjust recline.

5. Do It Up in Style

Sand your chair with an orbital sander. Stain it with exterior-grade solid stain, or prime and paint it.

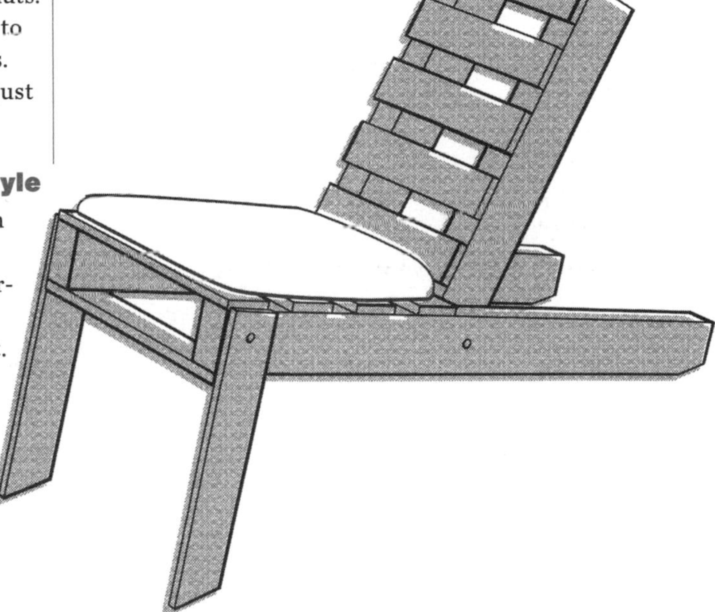

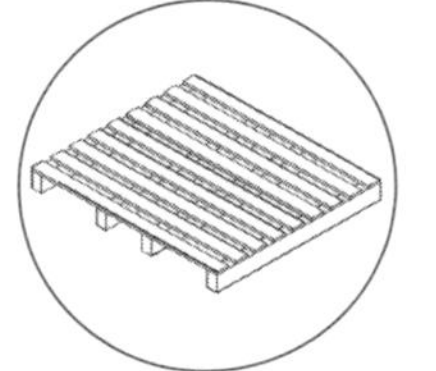
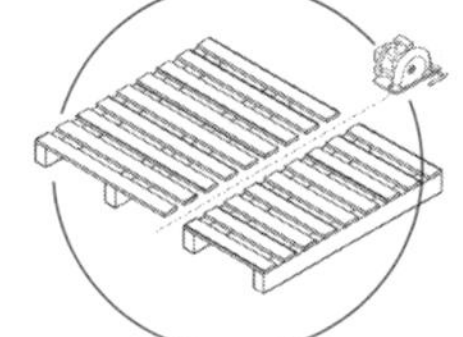
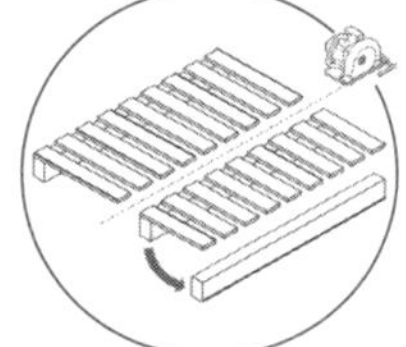
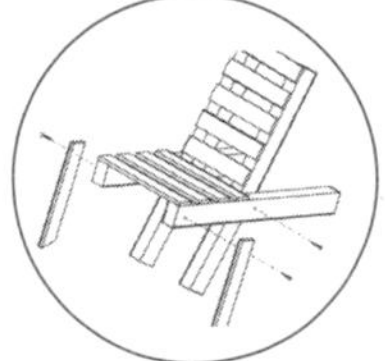
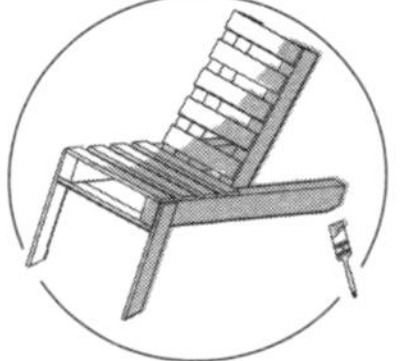

The Handy Man's Revolver

A battery-powered drill/driver is one of the most useful tools for a homeowner handyman. But it's useless without the right bits. Keep this ammo on hand in addition to normal wood bits.

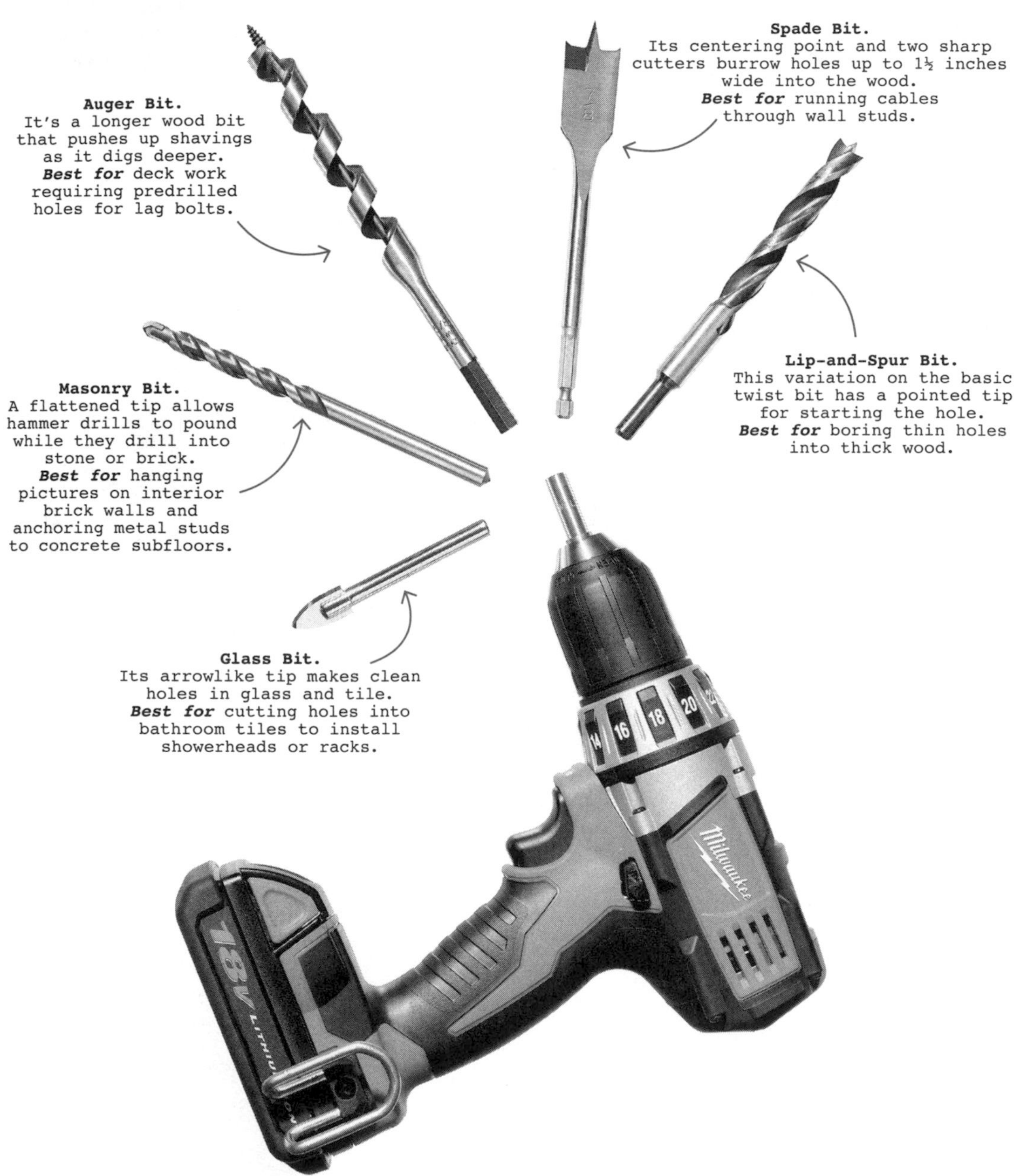

Spade Bit.
Its centering point and two sharp cutters burrow holes up to 1½ inches wide into the wood.
Best for running cables through wall studs.
Auger Bit.
It's a longer wood bit that pushes up shavings as it digs deeper.
Best for deck work requiring predrilled holes for lag bolts.
Lip-and-Spur Bit.
This variation on the basic twist bit has a pointed tip for starting the hole.
Best for boring thin holes into thick wood.
Masonry Bit.
A flattened tip allows hammer drills to pound while they drill into stone or brick.
Best for hanging pictures on interior brick walls and anchoring metal studs to concrete subfloors.
Glass Bit.
Its arrowlike tip makes clean holes in glass and tile.
Best for cutting holes into bathroom tiles to install showerheads or racks.
14
16
18
20
Milwaukee
18V

BUILD THE ULTIMATE HOME GYM

You can't beat the perks of a home gym: Parking's a snap, there's never a crowd, and it always plays music you like. Plus, the towel service is excellent, and you can grunt all you want. Best of all, it's convenient, meaning you're more likely to use it for the ultimate home construction project: your body.

Here are 10 essential pieces of equipment to help you create your basement body shop.

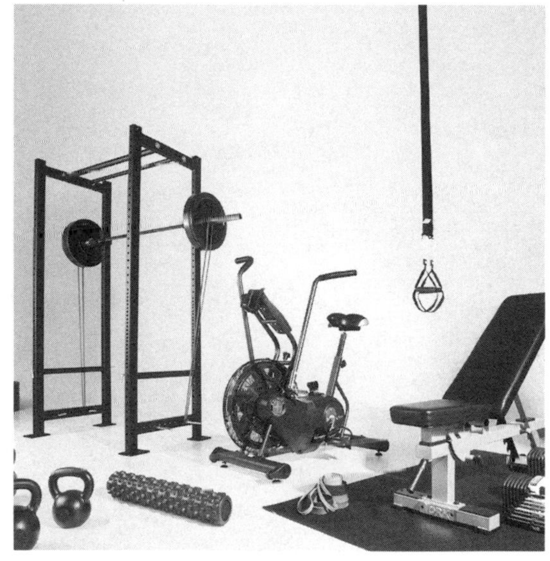

POWER RACK It provides a framework for everything from body-weight exercises to hardcore strength training. It's also an ideal anchor for suspension trainers and resistance bands.

OLYMPIC BAR AND BUMPER PLATES Unlike "standard" bars, which typically weigh less than 30 pounds, a 45-pound Olympic bar can handle heavy loads without permanent bending.

KETTLEBELLS Buy a few sizes to allow for different exercises—and your increases in strength.

FOAM ROLLER Use it before and after a workout to boost performance and accelerate muscle repair. Start with your calves and work your way up your body, front and back.

CARDIO MACHINE Unlike a Spin bike, an Airdyne uses a fan instead of a front wheel to generate air resistance, which is exponential—the harder you pedal, the harder pedaling becomes.

RESISTANCE BANDS Not only are bands great for mobility work, but you can also use them to make body-weight moves like pullups and pushups easier or harder. Looped around the ends of a barbell and the pins at the base of a power rack, they can also increase the intensity of heavy lifts, like squats and presses.

SUSPENSION TRAINER A comprehensive training tool in its own right, a suspension trainer is also the ultimate workout accessory. Attach one to your power rack to instantly accommodate 100 body-weight exercises of varying difficulty.

ADJUSTABLE BENCH Like the power rack, an adjustable bench sets the stage for hundreds of different lifts, from hip thrusts and supported rows to bench presses and stepups.

DUMBBELLS Use one at a time to develop stability, or grab a pair to build strength and power. Short on room? Save money and space with adjustable versions, which can replace an entire rack of conventional dumbbells for about half the price.

RUBBER FLOORING Rubber mats will help protect both floors and weights from damage and also deaden the sound of dropped weights.

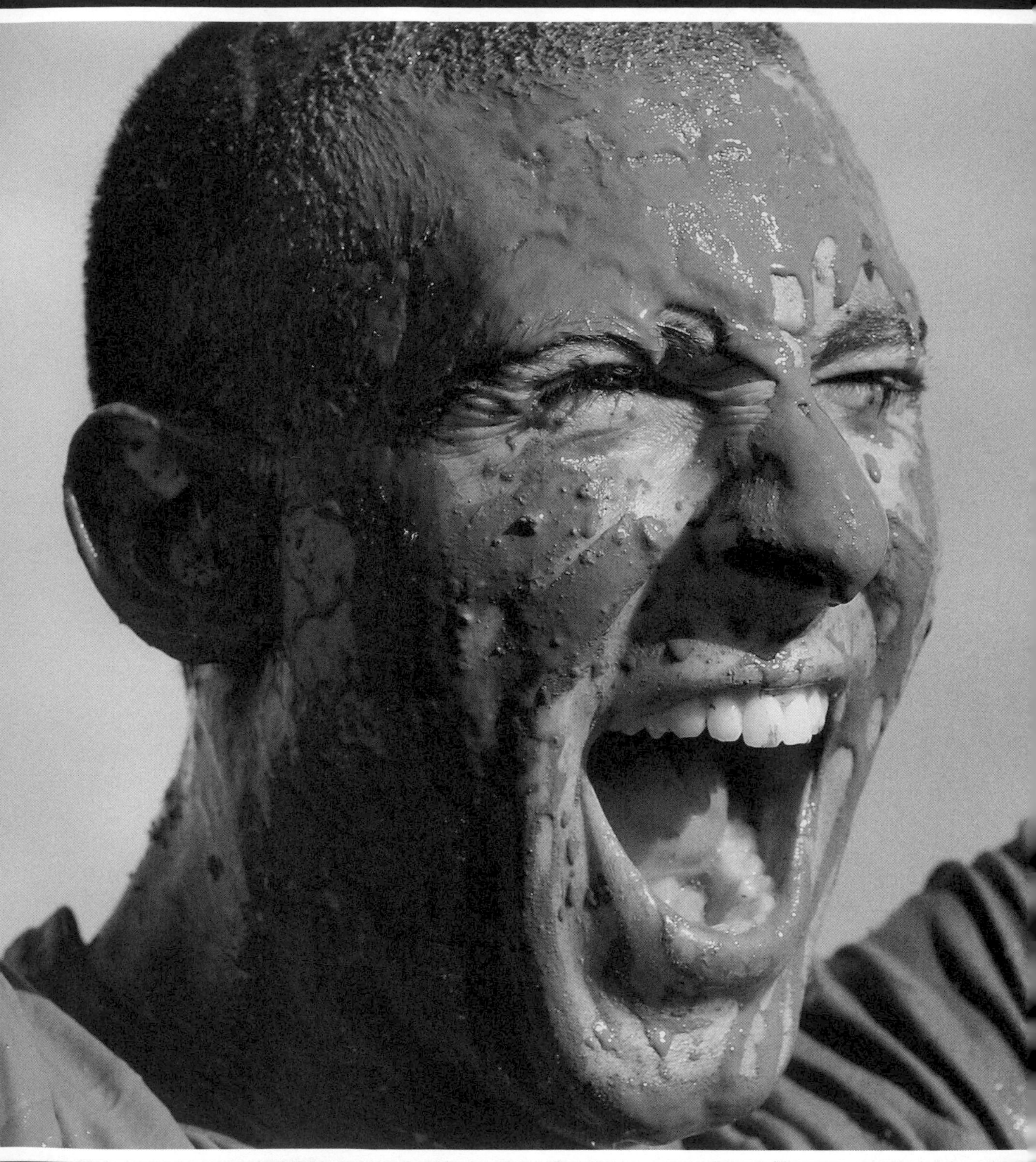

Big Fun

"Boredom Always Precedes a Period of Great Creativity."

—Robert M. Pirsig,
author of *Zen and the Art of Motorcycle Maintenance*

Life's too short to sit around trying to think up something to do on a long weekend. Put down that Weedwacker and pick up our list of uncommonly cool projects to make your life much sweeter. Here's a bucket list of homegrown fun:

Rig a Rope Swing	*pg. 260*
Build Your Own Water Park	*pg. 261*
Teach Your Dog to Fetch a Beer	*pg. 262*
Build Ladder Golf	*pg. 263*
Carve a Smashing Pumpkin	*pg. 264*
Fly a Stunt Kite	*pg. 265*
Host an Epic Poker Game	*pg. 268*
Build a Backyard Ice Rink	*pg. 269*
Scare the Bejesus out of Trick-or-Treaters	*pg. 270*
Throw an Outdoor Movie Party	*pg. 273*
Hightail it Outta Town	*pg. 275*
Dig a Legit Horseshoe Pit	*pg. 276*

. . . And much, much, more.

Rig a Rope Swing

Practice your jungle yell, Tarzan. You're about to make your yearly family picnic by the river way more interesting.

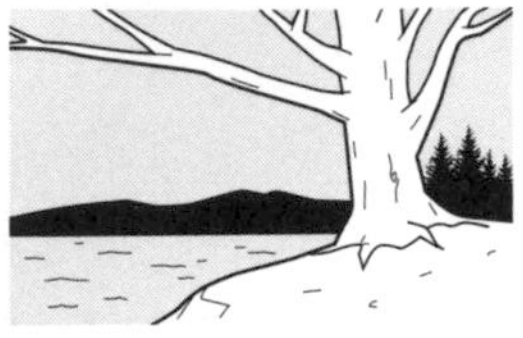

Locate a Limb

For safe swinging, find a thick, sturdy branch that's at least 8 inches in diameter and leans out over deep water—10 to 15 feet is ideal. Clear the launch spot, swing path, and landing area of fallen branches, sharp rocks, or any other objects.

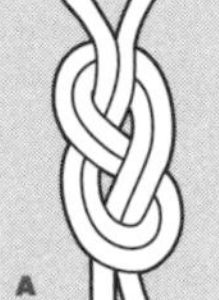

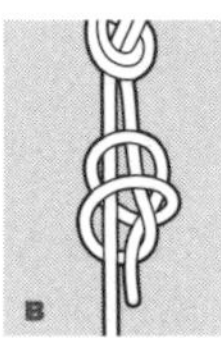

Gather Your Parts

- 24 to 32 feet of nylon rope that's at least 1 inch in diameter
- A clothesline or a narrow rope that's at least as long as the nylon rope
- A heavy object, such as a padlock

Prep Your Rope

Make a loop using the figure 8 knot (A) (find the steps at MensHealth.com/knots) and then secure the loop using a double stopper knot (B). Starting at the rope's other end, tie several double knots 2 feet apart for handholds and footholds.

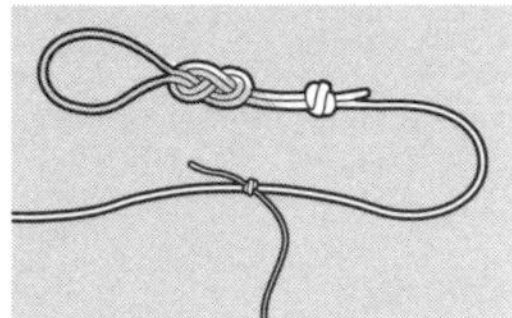

Add a Retrieval System

You need a way to get the rope back for your next swing. Tie the thinner line to the main rope about 3 feet below your loop. Make this retrieval line long enough to allow for a wide swing, and find a place to anchor it near the tree trunk.

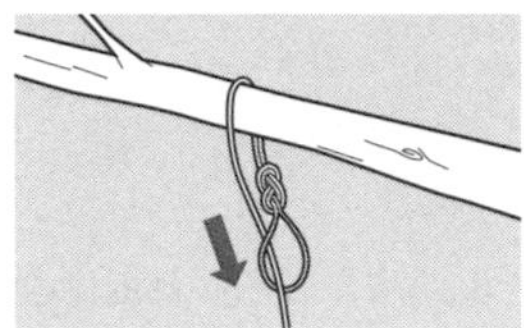

Secure the Swing

Weight the retrieval line and heave it over the branch. Pull the loop over the branch so you can thread the other end of the main rope through. Pull tight. Remove the weight from the retrieval line and anchor the line to the tree. Now start swinging!

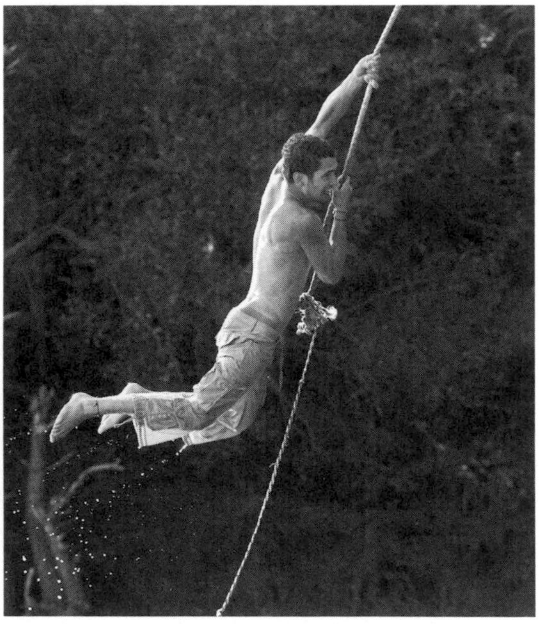

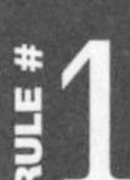

Take the day off after your boss's day off. He'll come back to a pile of work and will look for someone to unload it on like YOU unless you are out of the office.

Build Your Own *Water Park*

Leave the overpriced kit at the store—building a slide is easy. Ken Denmead, the author of *Geek Dad: Awesomely Geeky Projects and Activities for Dads and Kids to Share*, shows you how.

WHAT YOU'LL NEED	
Heavy plastic (6' × 25')	Hose (50') with sprinkler attachment
8 pool noodles (each 4' to 5' long)	3 wire loop stakes (each ½" to ⅝")
1 roll of sticky-back Velcro (¾" × 15')	1 bottle of baby wash (15 oz)
Scissors	Rope (½" diameter and 8' to 10' long)

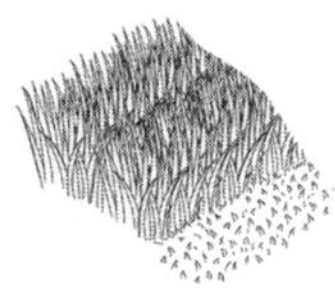

1. Pick Your Spot

Bypass the steep hills—you want a rush, not a wreck. Look for a gentle, grassy slope within hose length of your house. (Hint: Skip mowing the week before.) Leave at least a 5-foot clearance on all sides—that way you'll prevent painful wipeouts.

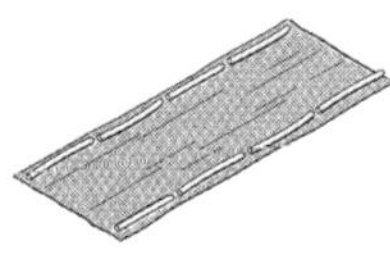

2. Use Your Noodles

Assemble the underside of the slide first. Unroll the plastic and arrange your pool noodles in a line along each long side. Keep a few inches between each noodle end and position them just a few inches from the tarp edge, like lane markers.

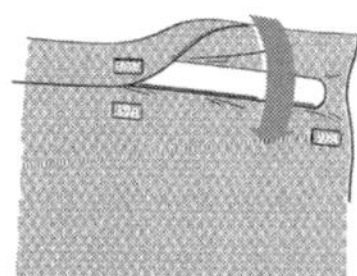

3. Fortify the Walls

Pull the plastic up and over the noodles, and place 2-inch Velcro strips at 6-inch intervals to keep the noodle casing in place. Roll each noodle over about a quarter turn more to secure the side walls. Flip the slide over completely. Now you have guardrails.

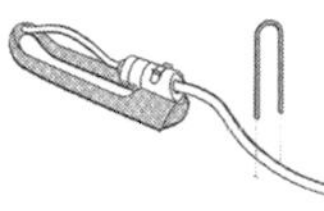

4. Make It Rain

Place your sprinkler a few feet from the side of the slide, about halfway down, and adjust the settings so the spray will hit the entire length of the plastic. Secure the hose with loop stakes so no one trips over it. Turn it on and soak the splash zone.

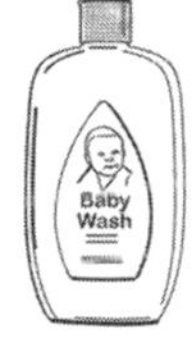

5. Lube the Runway

For a faster ride, dribble a line of baby wash down the middle of the slide. This will make the chute more slippery. Another idea for super speed: Have the slider hold the rope while another kid runs alongside the slide, towing the slider along.

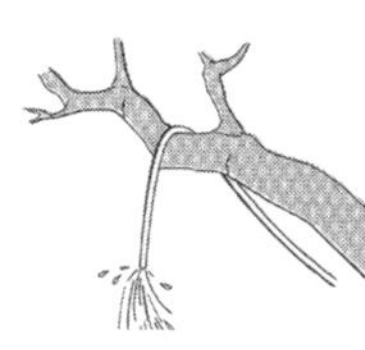

6. Rinse and Repeat

When you are finished, hang the hose on a nearby tree or fence to create an outdoor shower for rinsing off. Then don't clean up. Seriously. Do. Not. Bother. Leave the rest of the work for the morning. Plastic rolls up more easily when it's dry.

Teach Your Dog to Fetch a Beer

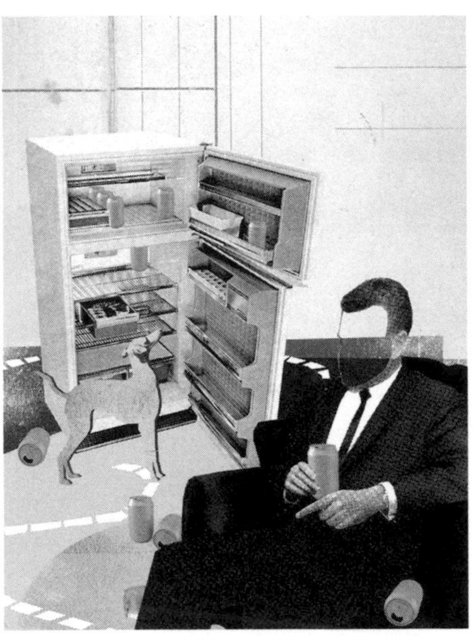

Open the Fridge

(1) Put a smelly treat inside a dish towel and tie the towel to the door handle. Wiggle the towel and reward your dog for touching it. **(2)** Wait for him to put his mouth on the towel, say "good!" and give him a treat. **(3)** Once your dog is biting the towel, reward him only when he pulls it. In the final stage, use "open" as your cue for him to pull hard and open the door.

Grab the Beer

(4) Empty a beer can. Play fetch with it. (A cozy will make the can easier for the dog to carry.) **(5)** Place the can on a low shelf in an open, uncluttered fridge and have your dog fetch it, using the command "fetch." Give him a treat.

Close the Fridge

(6) Open the door a few inches and hold a treat against the door at your dog's nose height. Encourage him to "Close. Get it!" When he shows interest in the treat, raise it higher against the door, just out of his reach. In an attempt to reach it, the dog will raise both front paws and slam the door closed. For best results, reward him when his paws are on the door. **(7)** Once your dog has the hang of the first step, try tapping the door to encourage him to push on it. Reward him for closing the door. **(8)** Finally, send him from a distance to "close" the door. Once your dog is comfortable with all three steps, start to phase out individual commands and use "Get me a beer" to represent it all.

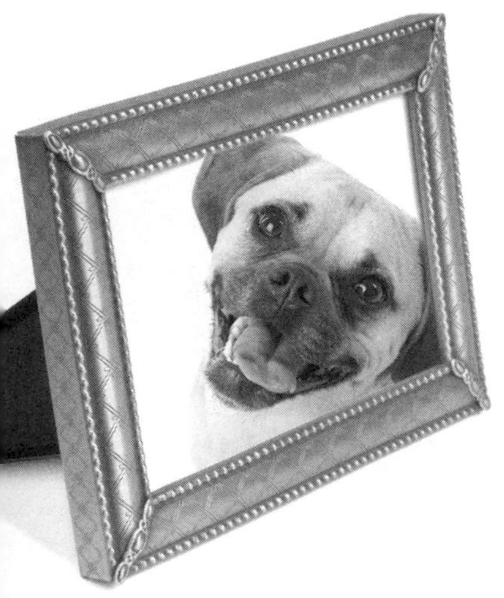

Snap the Perfect Pic of Your Pooch

Train with Treats

Long before your photo session, teach Spike the "watch me" trick. Before his dinnertime, take a prized treat (peanut butter or beef jerky, for example—something you don't normally give) and place it between your eyes. When the dog looks you in your eyes, say "watch me," and then give him the treat. Repeat until the dog looks you in the eyes when you say "watch me" even when you're not holding a treat.

Prephoto Exercise

Play chasing games or toss around a ball before setting up the shot. A panting dog will appear happier than a stoic one.

Snap the Picture

Once you've framed the shot, say "watch me" to have your dog look up. If it's a group photo, call Spike into the picture last so you don't exhaust his attention span.

Build Ladder Golf

Ladder golf—a game in which you toss golf-ball bolas at ladder rungs to score points and waste time—is the best new beer-in-one-hand backyard game since Jarts. But you don't have to buy the sporting-goods store version. Build the game yourself on a sunny morning with these instructions from Jason Cameron, host of DIY Network's *Man Caves*. Pals will show up spontaneously, with beer, when you finish.

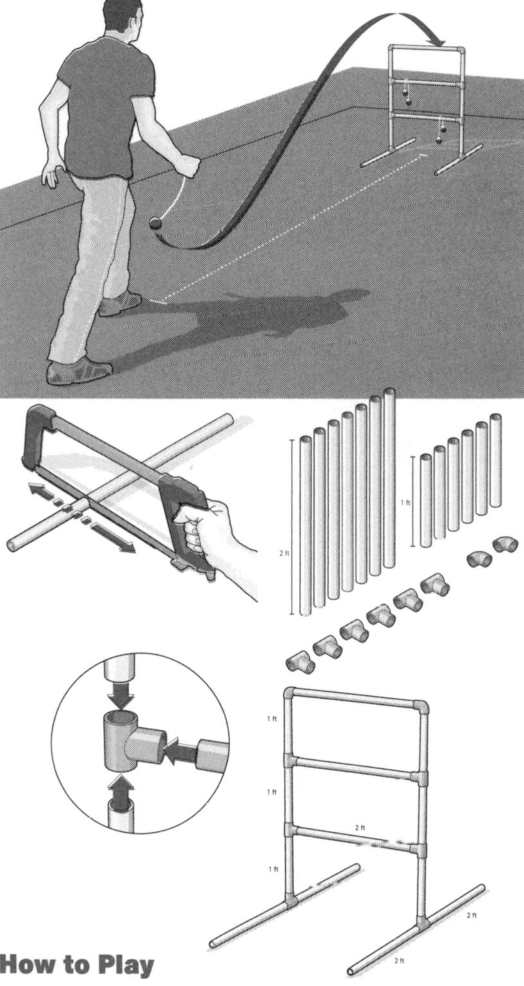

WHAT YOU'LL NEED	
4 10' lengths of 1" PVC pipe	Hacksaw
4 1" PVC elbow connectors	Drill (with ½" bit)
12 1" PVC "T" connectors	Heavy-duty scissors
9' ½" rope (six 18" lengths)	Vise (optional)
12 colored solid-core golf balls (6 each of 2 colors)	*This makes two ladders, enough for a full game.*

Step 1

Cut the pipe: Using a hacksaw, cut 14 pieces of 2-foot lengths and 12 pieces of 1-foot lengths.

Step 2

Build the ladders: Assemble the pipe lengths and joint connectors, starting with the leg supports and working up. For ease of assembly and transport, do not glue the joints together. Use the dimensions shown in the illustration.

Step 3

Make the bolas: Drill a ½-inch hole through the center of each golf ball. Thread a piece of rope through the hole in one of the balls, and knot the end. Secure the ball by making a second knot tightly against it. Measure 12 inchesof rope and create a third knot. Secure the second ball (same color) in place by tightly crafting a fourth knot. Trim the excess. Make five more bolas.

How to Play

Arrange: Place your ladders 25 feet apart. Each two-person team should have one member at each ladder.

Toss: Opponents stand to the sides of the ladders and take turns throwing bolas at the opposite ladder. Wrapping a bola around the top bar nets 3 points, the middle bar 2, and the bottom bar 1. Hit all three in one round and score 10.

Tally: Add up points at the end of each round. The team with the most points carries the difference to the next round. Example: If Team A scores 6 points and Team B scores 9 points, Team B keeps 3 points. The first to score 21 wins.

Carve a Smashing Pumpkin

One-up your neighbors' boring designs with help from Ray Villafane, a world-champion pumpkin carver.

Hit the Patch

Supermarket pumpkins are often too round and perfect to have much character. To find a patch near you, check out localharvest.org. Hunt for an oval-shaped pumpkin with a bright orange rind and no soft spot. A healthy pumpkin should feel heavy relative to its size. Also, look for an interesting stem, which can act as a creepy witch hat or nasty goblin wart.

Sculpt, Don't Carve

Using a knife to shape your jack-o'-lantern limits your ability to add detail. Pick up three sizes of clay loop tools from an art-supply store; these can carve contours into the pumpkin's rind. Start simply, carving a design like a skull, which has exaggerated features that provide some room for error. Use a printout reference image to help guide you.

Showcase Your Masterpiece

Instead of placing a candle inside the pumpkin, use an external spotlight to heighten the shadow effect. Spray the face of your jack-o'-lantern with lemon juice to preserve the exposed pulp. This trick helps keep the pumpkin fresh only about a day longer, so capture your creation with a camera. Turn the flash off for best results.

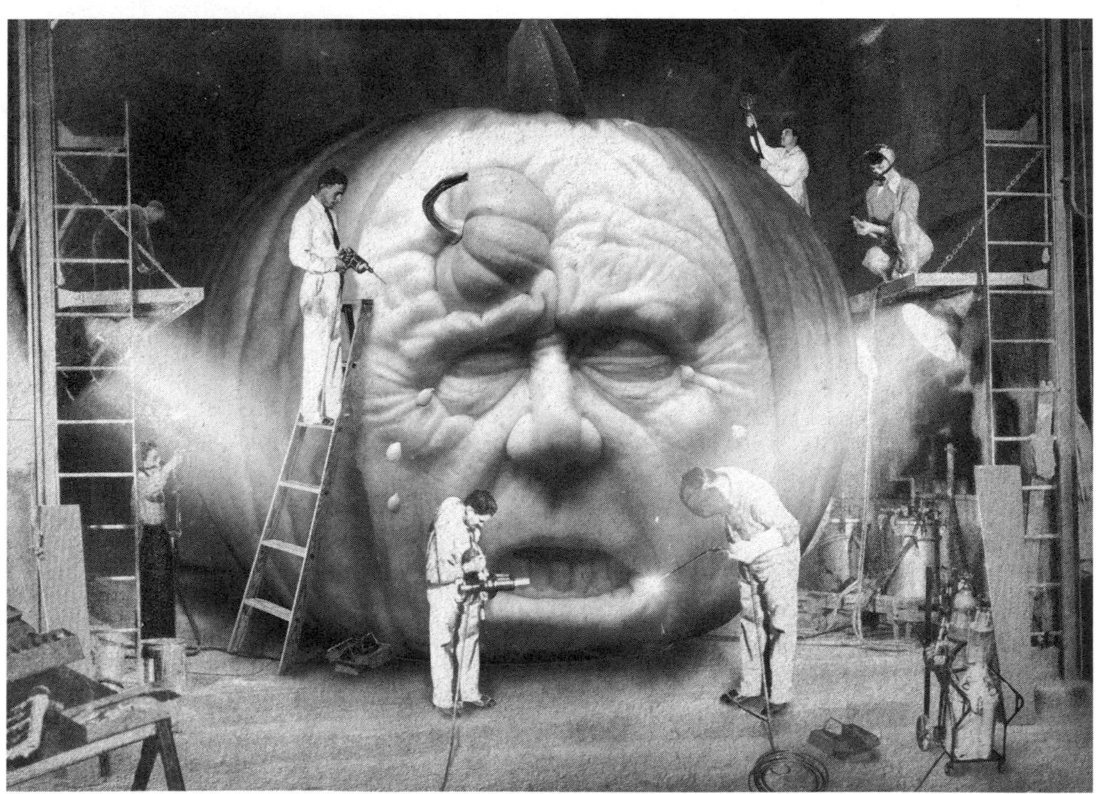

Fly a Stunt Kite

Take to the skies when the wind is right, and carve some awesome air with these tricks. (Ideal wind speed for kite flying: 6 to 18 mph.)

Gather Your Gear

Start with a basic two-line stunt kite, which costs $50 to $100. It's shaped like a stealth bomber and is the easiest type to control. Go with Dacron line, not Spectra line. (It'll say on the packaging.) Dacron stretches, giving you extra room for error as you pilot the kite.

Launch

Put your back to the wind and have a buddy hold the kite up. Walk away until you reel out all the line. With both lines taut, have your friend toss the kite straight up. Walk backward until the kite catches the wind. Keep your forearms parallel to the ground for better control.

Trick 1: 360

It's the easiest trick to start with. Just pull on one line and

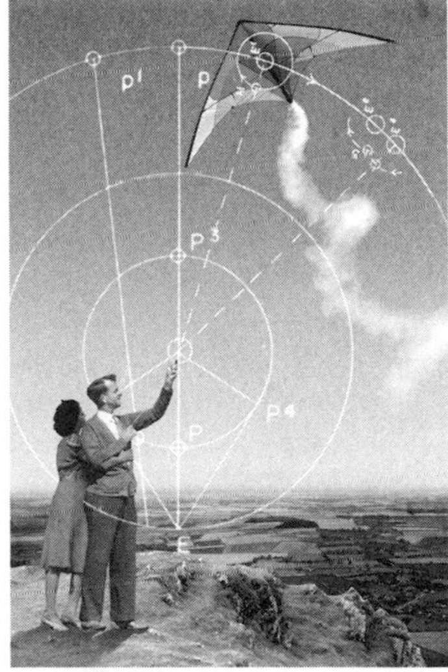

keep pulling as the kite makes a complete circle. Bring your hands level to each other to stop the 360.

Trick 2: Snap Stall

This trick makes a kite hover in midair. As your kite flies from left to right, jab your right hand forward as if you were delivering a kidney punch. Quickly take a big step toward the kite and push your left hand forward to match the extension of your right arm. This movement helps create that freeze-action look. Pull back to recover from the stall.

Land Softly

Don't start pulling the line in as if you're reeling in a fish with a fishing rod. The kite will fight back and could take a sudden nosedive. To bring it in gracefully, guide the kite down by flying it either to the left or right, and parallel to the ground. The kite will gradually descend until it reaches terra firma. Then go introduce yourself to the hordes of applauding onlookers who've gathered around you.

BASK IN BRAVERY

Summer is the best season for taking risks because your brain is primed for challenge. Exposure to summer sunlight triggers your pineal gland to produce more of the fear-fighting neurotransmitter serotonin than at any other time of year.

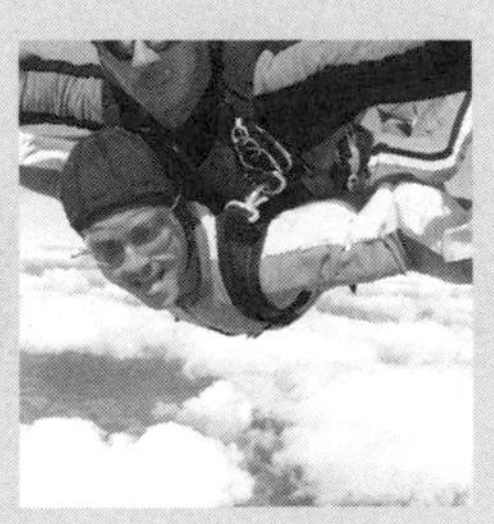

RULE #2

A sure way to avoid seasickness is to sit on the shady side of an old brick church in the country.

Life Is More Fun *with DOGS*

John Grogan, author of *Marley & Me: Life and Love with the World's Worst Dog*, offers this list of reasons you should really own a dog:

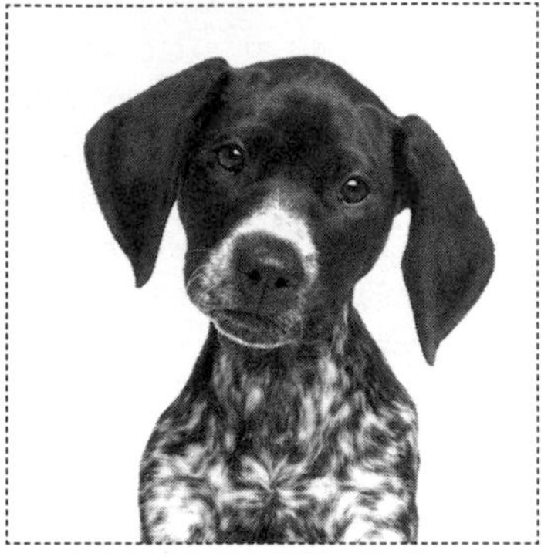

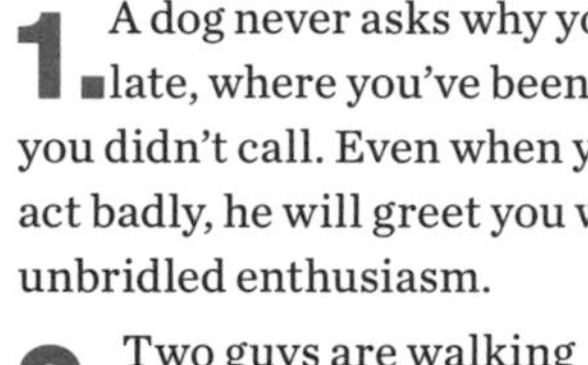

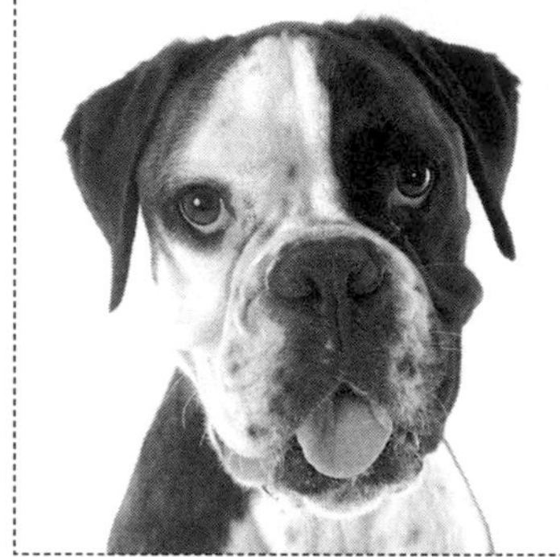

1. A dog never asks why you're late, where you've been, why you didn't call. Even when you act badly, he will greet you with unbridled enthusiasm.

2. Two guys are walking through a park. One is alone. One is with a dog. A beautiful woman approaches. Guess which guy she stops to talk with.

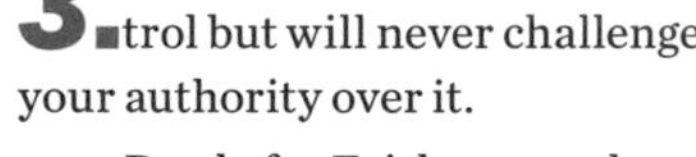

3. He may eat the remote control but will never challenge your authority over it.

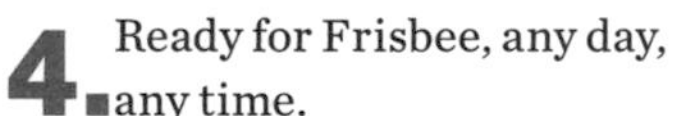

4. Ready for Frisbee, any day, any time.

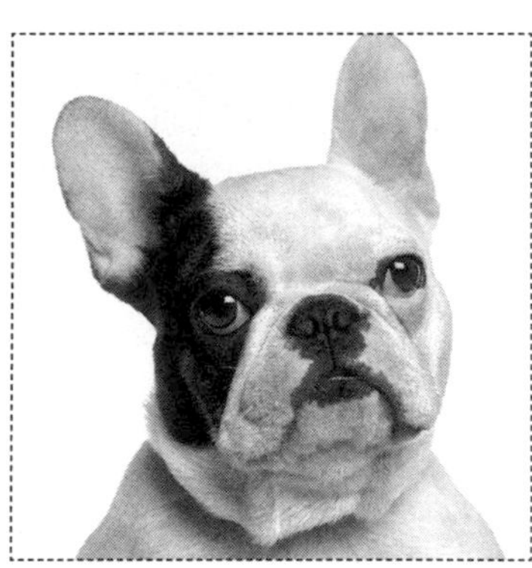

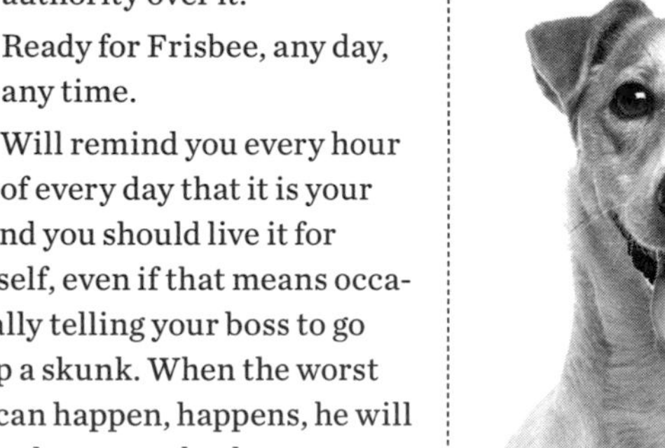

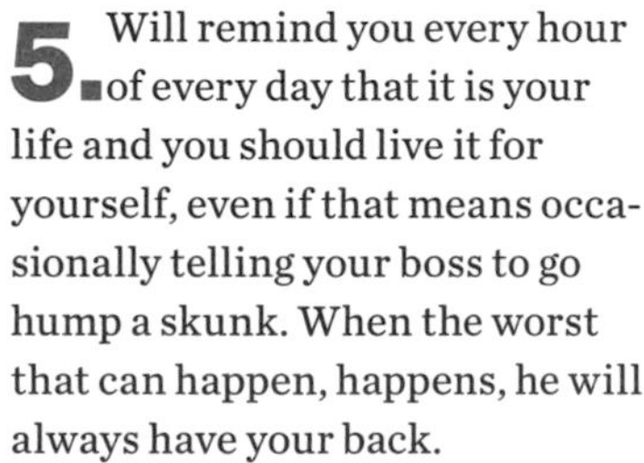

5. Will remind you every hour of every day that it is your life and you should live it for yourself, even if that means occasionally telling your boss to go hump a skunk. When the worst that can happen, happens, he will always have your back.

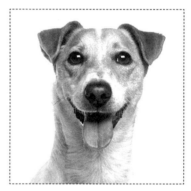

GO ON AN EPIC BIKE RIDE

"It's by riding a bicycle," wrote Ernest Hemingway, "that you learn the contours of a country best." Sculpt your calves and sense the ghosts at these historic sites.

California Gold Rush (easy). Jamestown, California, to Columbia State Historic Park is a trip of 13 miles and 150 years.

Lexington and Concord (medium). Go from Lexington Green to Concord Bridge, then take on the Minuteman Bike Trail, a 20-mile route.

The Oregon Trail (hard). It's a 12-day, 724-mile tour of what the pioneers did, but they didn't have to worry about flat tires.

The Erie Canal (hard). From Buffalo to Albany, it rolls through breathtaking scenery and impressive history with stops at breweries and wineries.

Teach Spot to Play Dead

Any dog can sit on command and proffer a paw. But will your best friend take an imaginary bullet for you? Teach any canine to do exactly that with this method from veterinarian and animal behaviorist Sophia Yin, DVM, author of *Perfect Puppy in 7 Days*. (Bonus: Train your kitty to keel over using the exact same steps!)

Trade the Treats

For incentives, use normal dog food, not snacks (and not human food!). Dog treats are typically high in calories and should not make up more than 10 percent of a dog's diet.

Move in Slow-Mo

First, instruct the hound to lie down and stay. Then slowly move a small handful of kibble behind his head so he shifts his weight onto his side. Reward him and then gradually move your hand with the food farther back; when he tips onto his side, immediately pull your treat hand away from him and back to your body. If he shifts his weight or stands up, he gets no kibble.

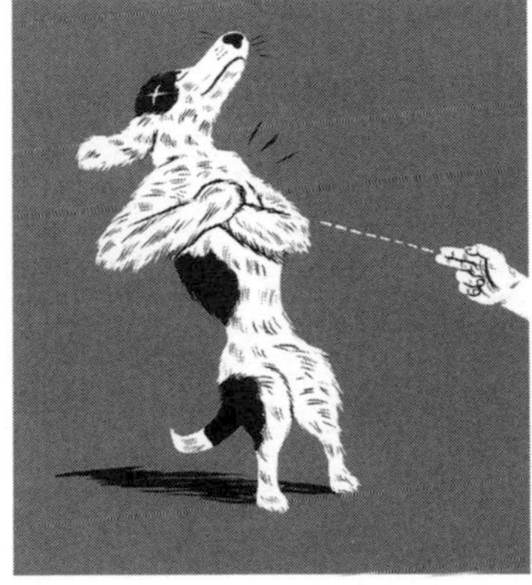

Pause for Effect

Once your dog is calmly resting on his side, feed him as his head rests on the floor. Little by little, prolong the time between rewards by pulling your treat hand away from him between treats. Work up to an interval of 10 seconds.

Ready, Aim . . .

After a few rounds of training over the course of several days, your dog should start lying on his side whenever he wants a snack. When he's about to go down, point and say. "Bang!" After repeating the routine over a few days, try it using the command to see if he'll play dead on cue.

HAVE MORE FUN ON A ROAD TRIP

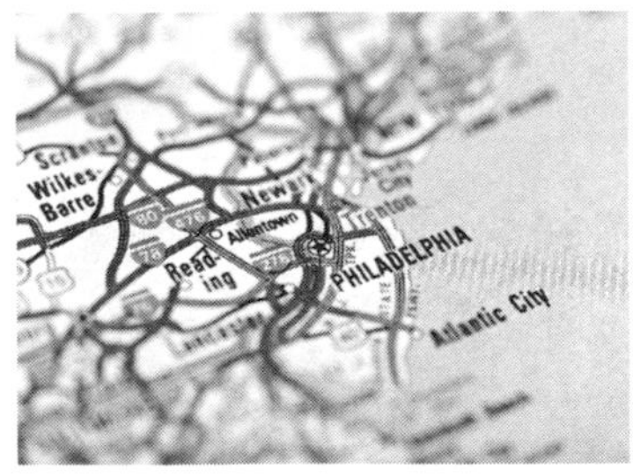

1. Give each person in the car a counting task: roadkill, Waffle Houses, speeding truckers, whatever. First to spot 10 wins.

2. Have the kids in the backseat scribble "Help! Killer bees are attacking this car!" (or something just as frightening) on a piece of paper and show it to passing drivers. They can sell it with some frenzied swatting.

3. First person to spot a horse pasture yells "Horses!" and tallies them up for his or her stable. Then the first person to spot a graveyard yells "Bury your horses!" and everyone else loses their horses. Owner of the largest herd wins. No farms on your route? Play biker convoys and state troopers.

Host an Epic Poker Game

Run a smoother, smarter tournament at your place and make everyone feel like a high roller.

Stack the Deck

Shoot for five to seven players. That's enough to bring action to every hand without being overwhelming. And choose a buy-in that's high enough to keep the game interesting, but not so high that it scares people away. Between $20 and $60 is ideal.

Stage like Vegas

Host the game in a private room—not the living room or kitchen, where there are distractions. Keep the lights low, and forgo the *SportsCenter* in the background in favor of some upbeat music. If players feel comfortable, they'll throw in more chips and have more fun. Hosting often? Elevate your game and pick up a specialized table at custompokertables.com.

Name the Game

Play Texas Hold 'em (for rules, go to pokertips.org/rules/texas.php). The buy-in should give players 40 to 60 chips. Allow rebuys once after an hour of play (at the same dollar value of the buy-in), and up the blinds every 30 minutes to keep the game moving. An app like PokerTimer (free, iTunes) can help you keep track of the game.

Maintain Focus

Distractions make for sloppy poker. Take down clocks so no one worries about the time. Stock a side table with beer and snacks and distance it about 15 feet from the poker table to prevent mindless eating. Discourage cell phone use.

Bet on the Side

Consider running a 7/2 pool: Guys who want to participate kick in $5 each. If you win a hand after being dealt a 7 and a 2 (the worst duo you can get in Texas Hold 'em), you win the pot.

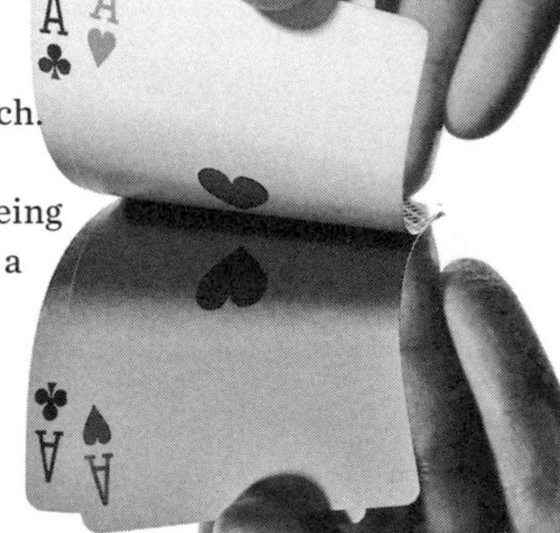

RULE # 3

A man derives great satisfaction from group work. If you've lost your social circle since your high school days, volunteer. As you work with like-minded people, friendships will naturally unfold.

Play Guitar in an Hour

Countless rock, folk, and country songs are based on just three chords. Learn to strum G, C, and D, and hundreds of songs are within your reach, including "Knockin' on Heaven's Door," "Sweet Home Alabama," "Can't You See," "Stir It Up," "Twist and Shout," "Wild Thing," "Hang on Sloopy," "Free Fallin'," "Bad Moon Rising," and many more.

How to Build a Backyard Ice Rink

Leverage ice-cold temps to construct a private skating rink on your property. (Penalty box not included.)

Scope Your Turf

On a flat area, measure a 32 × 48-foot rectangle with string and pound a piece of rebar about 18 inches into the ground at each corner. Clear away any rocks or sticks.

Bracket the Rink

Run the fir 2 × 6s along the inside of the string, joining them with the 1-foot 2 × 6s and 2-inch deck screws.

Secure the Corners

At each corner, connect the boards with 3-inch deck screws—driven in at angles—to form a rectangle. Pound rebar outside each corner so that all the corners are braced by two pieces of rebar. Also, place two pieces of rebar at the joints along the length and width of the rink's frame.

WHAT YOU'LL NEED (EST. COST: $350)

Mason's string (at least 160')
20 24" rebar
10 16' Douglas fir 2 x 6s
6 1-foot 2 x 6s
2 lb 2" deck screws
2 lb 3" deck screws
1 40' x 100' spool 4-mm plastic liner

Lay Out a Liner

Plastic liner will compress your grass without killing it. Cover the box with plastic and push down at the edges to form a reservoir. Now trim the outside so the plastic overlaps your rink brace by a foot around the perimeter. Staple the plastic to the outside of the frame.

Fill 'Er Up

Fill your rink with 1 to $1^1/_2$ inches of water. Let it freeze overnight and add a second layer the next day. Let that sit for two nights. Filling in stages will ensure optimal results. Test to make sure the ice is solid before skating.

Smooth the Ice

Keep the Zamboni in the garage. If the ice is uneven, spray water on it and allow it to freeze. New ice!

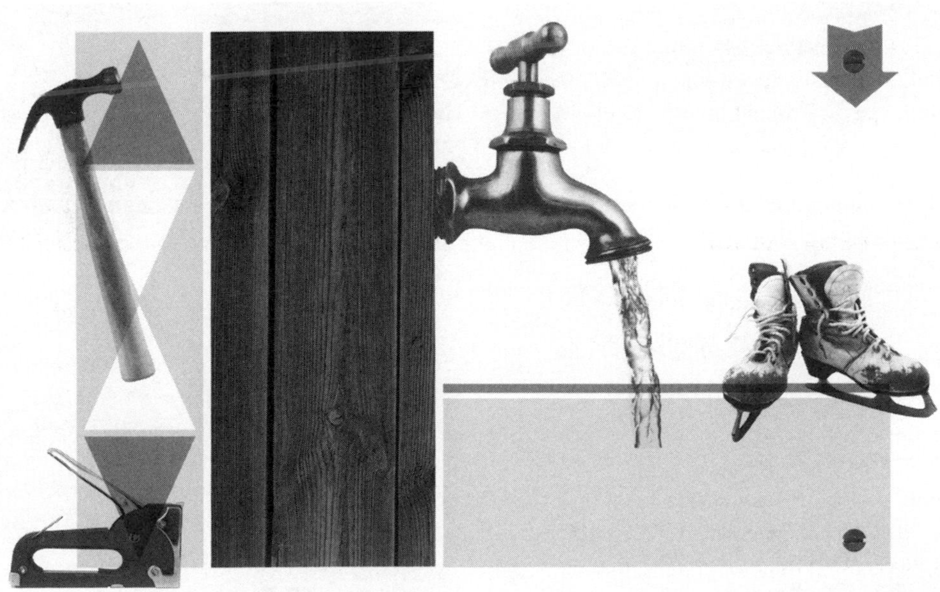

Scare the Bejesus out of
Trick-or-Treaters

Design a manor of mayhem with tips from Leonard Pickel, owner of Hauntrepreneurs, a haunted-house design firm.

Set a Scene

Aim for blood-pumping scares (surprises and startles) rather than brain-scarring terrors (gore and executions).

Fog Their View

Dry ice is dangerous and dissipates fast. Instead, rent a fog machine or buy a Chauvet 1300 ($220, froggysfog.com), which blows through ice cubes. Before using, wet the ground to help the fog linger.

Make Them Jump

Attach motion sensors (try a Parallax PIR sensor: $11, parallax.com) to a leaf blower you've hidden under a bush, or to a spotlight that illuminates a monster.

Take It Inside

Cover your foyer with dark curtains and install a black light. When kids approach, turn off the porch lights. Open the door wearing a white costume. You'll glow!

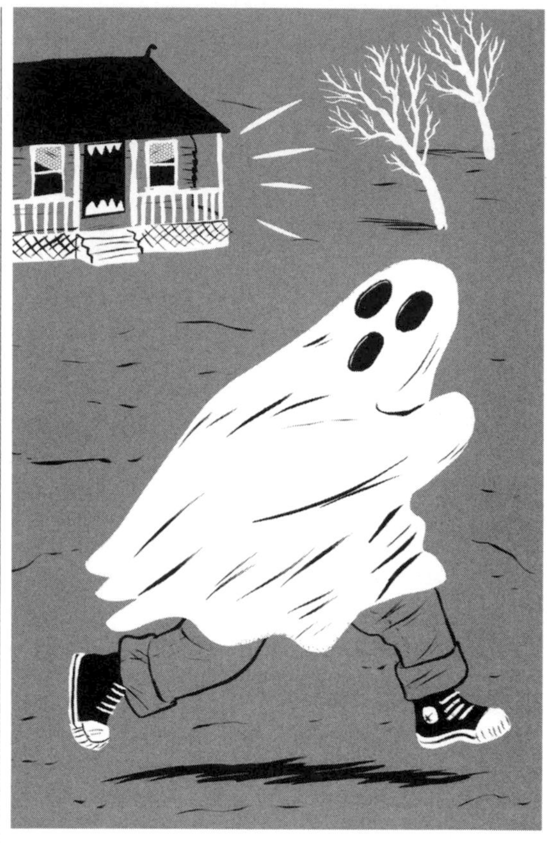

Send Them Running

Have a buddy dress up and sit in a porch chair. He stays still until the kids leave the porch, and then . . .

3 Best Albums for a Long Road Trip

1. Creedence Clearwater Revival: *Green River*
2. George Harrison: *All Things Must Pass*
3. Spiritualized: *Ladies and Gentlemen We Are Floating in Space*

RULE # 4

Take the day off on your kid's birthday. And keep him or her home from school. Tell your child that turning 5 or 8 is a real milestone and that you want to spend the day with him or her. Plan an event that will be memorable.

Look like Hell on HALLOWEEN

Create an authentic-looking bloody wound like the sickos on the set of *Saw VII*.

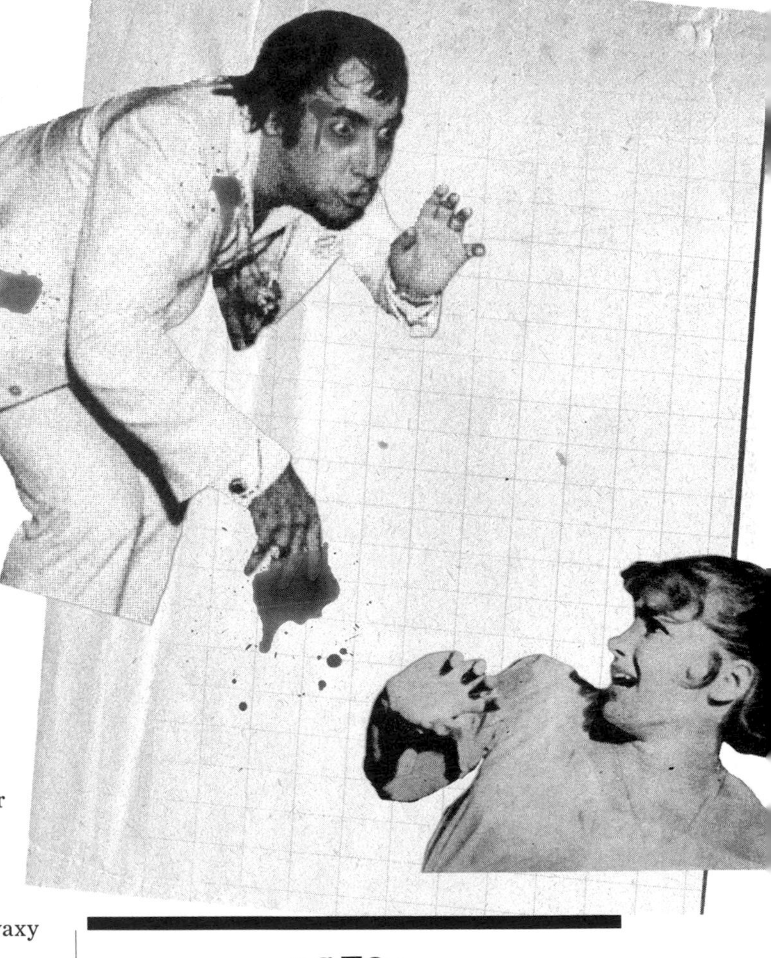

Prep Your Face

Use rubbing alcohol and cotton balls to remove the oils from your face so the makeup won't slide off.

Build Your Base

Roll a dime-size piece of scar wax (available at party stores) into a $1^1/_2$-inch-long cylinder, minimum. Press it onto your skin. It'll look best on a bony area, like your cheekbone, brow, or forehead.

Control the Border

Dip the tip of your finger in petroleum jelly and blend the wax's edges into your skin. Don't overspread the wax; leave a small lip for a realistic texture.

Make the Cut

Use a plastic knife to slice the middle of the waxy mound. For an incision-style cut, make one straight pass. For an impact wound, make jagged cuts.

Color

Dab red cream makeup over the wound, blending it into surrounding skin. Mix red and blue makeup and color the middle of the cut to create depth.

Bloody It Up

Squeeze stage blood into the top of the cut so that it drips down your face. Conceal any exposed waxy edges with a dot of blood. Commence moaning.

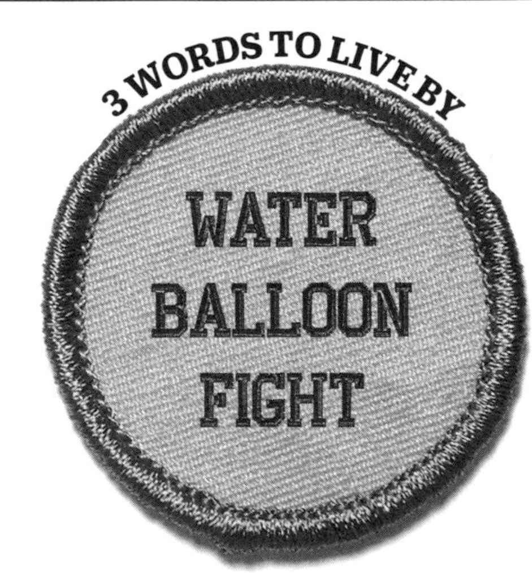
3 WORDS TO LIVE BY
WATER
BALLOON
FIGHT

Construct an Epic Last-Minute Costume

The only thing scary about store-bought Halloween costumes is that you might bore someone to death. Then there's the risk of mortification if someone shows up in the same outfit. Instead, customize your costume on the cheap and crank up your evil-genius mojo by harnessing your smartphone or tablet's

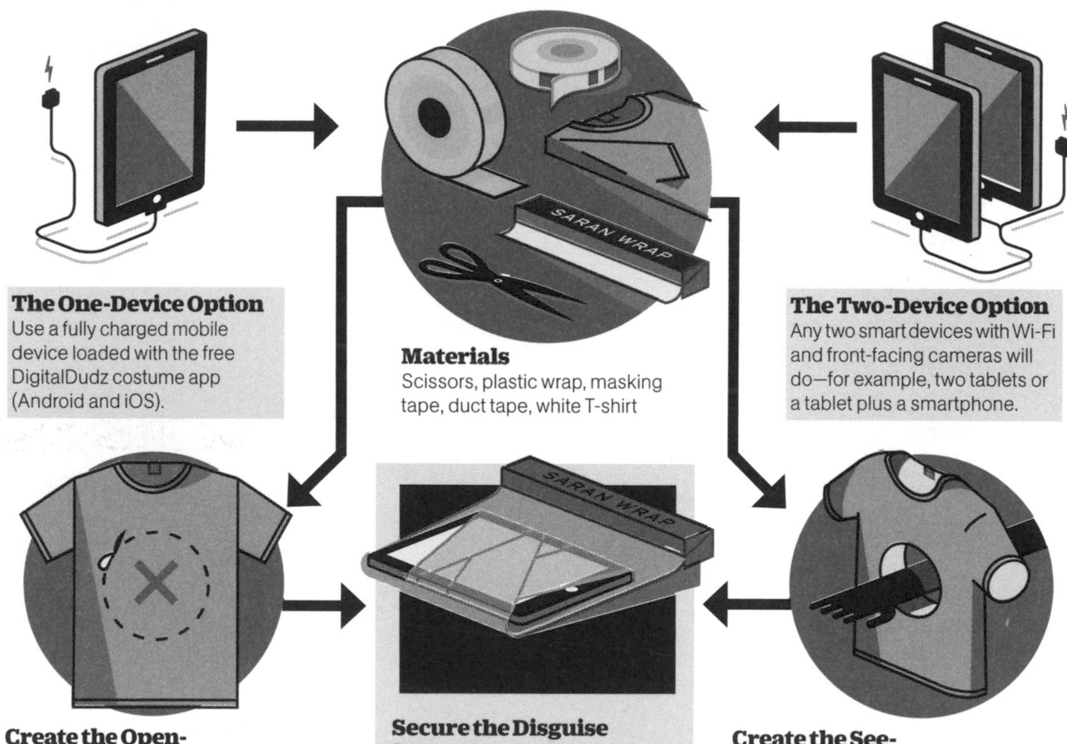

The One-Device Option
Use a fully charged mobile device loaded with the free DigitalDudz costume app (Android and iOS).

Materials
Scissors, plastic wrap, masking tape, duct tape, white T-shirt

The Two-Device Option
Any two smart devices with Wi-Fi and front-facing cameras will do—for example, two tablets or a tablet plus a smartphone.

Create the Open-Cavity Wound

1. Using your tablet as a measuring template, cut an X in the front of a shirt; the X should be slightly smaller than the screen. Trim away excess fabric to create a circle; this will be the viewing hole. Make the edges look torn and ragged.

2. Search your DigitalDudz apps and click "Flesh iWound" to choose the looping video that plays animation of a bloody beating heart. It's a close-up of the organ—complete with B-movie thriller music.

Secure the Disguise

1. To keep your device protected, encase it in plastic wrap.

2. Use masking tape to secure the wrap to the back of the device. Next cut four 6-inch strips of duct tape, and attach one end of each strip to the back of the wrapped device in all four corners.

3. Place the tablet inside the shirt—screen centered and visible through the hole—and press the free ends of the duct tape to the fabric. Aim for 2 inches of tape on the tablet and 4 on the shirt.

*If you're using two devices, repeat these steps with your second device on the back of the shirt.

Create the See-Through Wound

1. Cut a circle that's slightly smaller than your tablet's screen into the front of a shirt. Cut a same-size hole in the back of the shirt. (But if your second device is a smartphone, make it proportionately smaller.) Fray the holes' edges, making sure the front-facing cameras on both devices can see out.

2. Link the two tablets with FaceTime or another video chatting app. Whatever the back device broadcasts, the front screen will show. Zoom in to fix perspective.

built-in ghoulish potential. It'll take only a few minutes to make yourself look as if you have a gaping chest wound or as if someone blew a hole straight through you. Fraser Smeaton, the CEO of MorphCostumes, is the Dr. Frankenstein of gadget-inspired gore. He turns these creepy ideas into a monstrously good time.

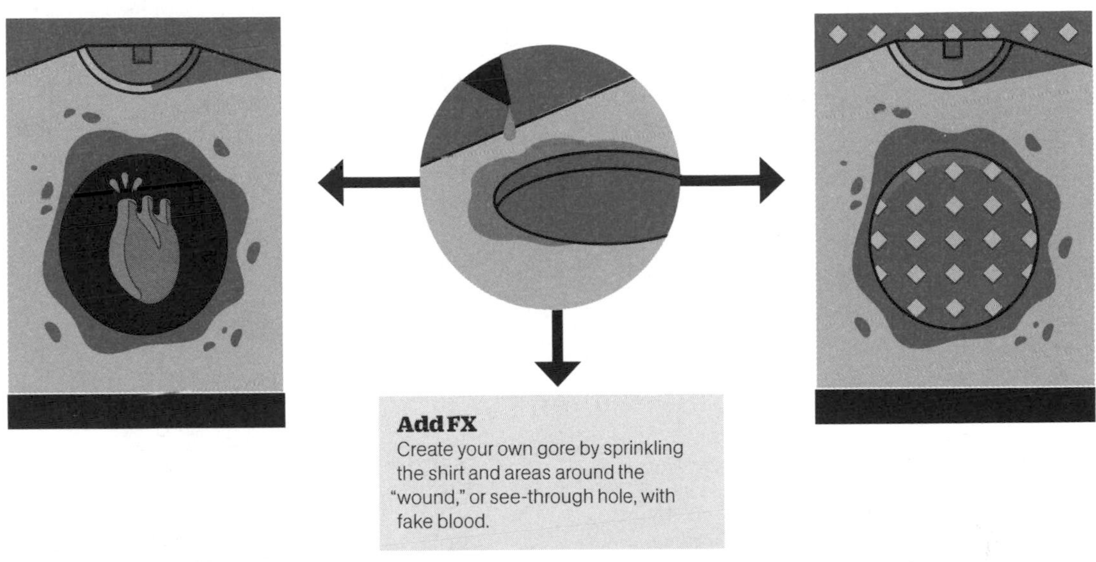

Add FX
Create your own gore by sprinkling the shirt and areas around the "wound," or see-through hole, with fake blood.

Throw an Outdoor Movie Party

Bring the big screen to your backyard with help from Randy Fisk, founder of backyardtheater.com, and Bob Deutsch, CEO of Outdoor Movies.

1. Pick Your Player

Look for an HD projector with at least 2,000 lumens of brightness, DLP or LCD display, and keystone correction. We like the portable Epson PowerLite Home Cinema 3010 1080P 3LCD Projector ($1,300, epson.com). For once-a-summer screenings, rent a rig from a party store or camera shop.

2. Repurpose Audio

A receiver and portable sound bar or old speakers will provide ample audio in a backyard. Place the speakers in front of the crowd for the best sound. Add a subwoofer for action-packed films and a center channel for clearer dialogue.

3. Hoist Your Screen

Any light surface that's wrinkle-free, taut, and unglossy will display a clear picture. Hang a bedsheet between two trees with the bottom 3 to 4 feet above the ground. Or impress the Joneses with the 12-foot Airblown Inflatable Widescreen Deluxe Outdoor Movie Screen ($195, target.com).

Carve an Ice Sculpture

1. Block It

Buy a square 4-gallon bucket from a home store ($11, lehmans.com). Fill it with distilled water, which will make clearer ice. If the bucket is too big for your freezer, take it outside (weather permitting). The water should freeze in 24 to 36 hours.

2. Extract the Ice

Remove the bucket from the freezer and let the ice sit at room temperature until it begins to melt. Don a pair of cotton gloves and place a wet towel on a large table. Slowly slide the block onto the towel. Still sticking? Pour cool water on top.

3. Assemble Your Tools

Sketch an outline on the ice using magic ink ($3, icecrafters.com); this is the choice of pro carvers because it doesn't run and the color fades. If you need to, use a stencil. Work with a small hand saw or drill to cut off larger chunks of the block.

Project #1: Star

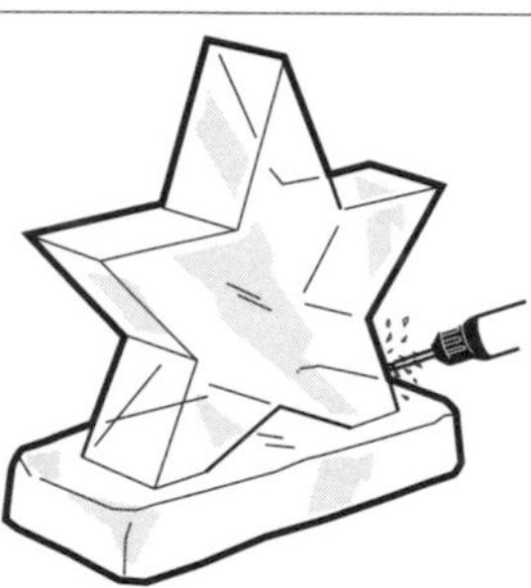

Fit your drill with a quarter-inch bit that's at least 5 inches long. Stencil a star on the side of the block. At one of the star's points, plunge the drill half an inch into the ice. Repeat along the stencil line, making holes at regular intervals. With each pass of the drill, go half an inch deeper, stopping occasionally to wipe the bit.

Project #2: Lantern

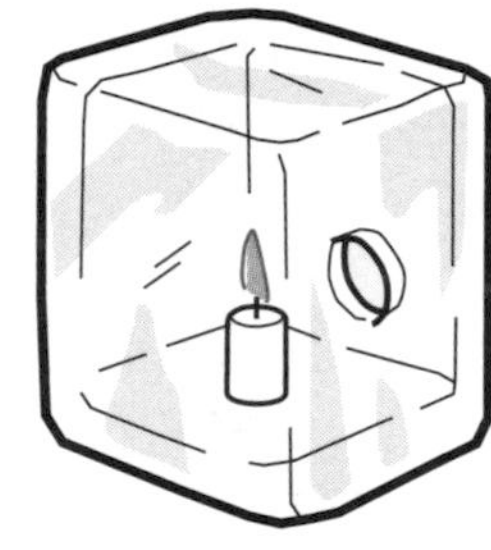

Use tap water this time; lanterns look best with cloudy ice. Eight to 10 hours into freezing, the block will form its frozen shell. Take it outside, drill a hole in its side, and pour the water out of its interior. Then bring the hollowed-out block indoors and carve a hole big enough to slide in a small tea light or LED.

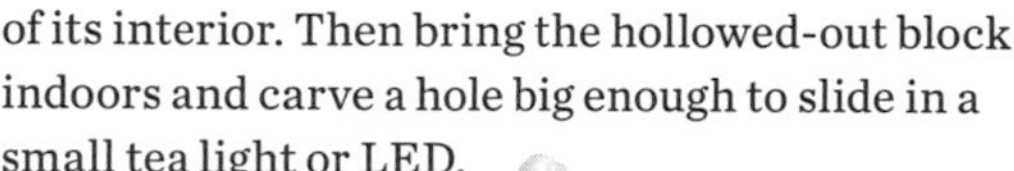

PADDLE A DRAGON BOAT

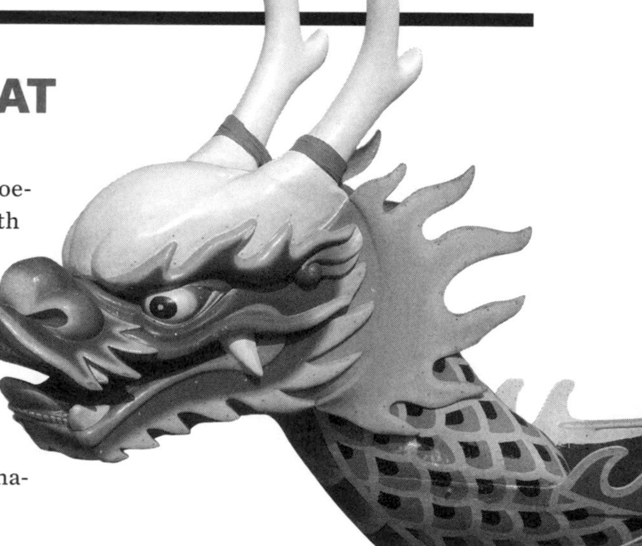

Dating back more than 2,000 years to ancient China, dragon boat racing has elements of both crew and canoeing. Races usually range from 250 to 1,000 meters, with seasoned crews cranking out 70 to 80 strokes per minute—no easy feat when you're propelling a dragon-headed craft with an oversize paddle that turns each pull into a strength and aerobic fitness challenge. Join a club and give it a shot, but first know what you'll be getting into by attending a race. Two of the top events are the Oklahoma Regatta Festival in Oklahoma City and the Philadelphia International Dragon Boat Festival, both held in the fall.

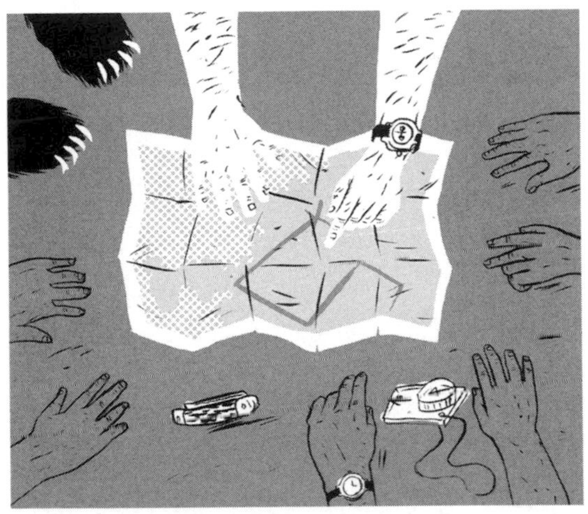

How to Hightail It Outta Town

Round up your adventurous buddies and organize a heart-pounding, snag-free trip with this advice from Shannon Stowell, president of the Adventure Travel Trade Association.

Save the Date

E-mail your friends at least 6 weeks in advance so they have time to clear their schedules. Pick a general focus (skiing in Vermont), but suggest some options (Stowe, Stratton) to encourage collaboration. Give everyone a week, max, to agree.

Stuff the Itinerary

Use PathWrangler or TripIt for Teams (tripit.com/teams) to prepare your budget, plans, and transportation. These link to social media tools, so you can also share photos during the trip.

Cash Out

As you plan, ask your friends to chip in on major expenses, such as the hotel and rental car. Then create a slush fund and have everyone throw in an equal amount of dough to cover miscellaneous costs like gas and beer. If cash is left over, divvy it up on the way home. Or make it the purse for whoever collects the most bug bites, bruises, or unread work e-mails.

Circle the Wagons

On the day of, add your buddies to a group text. If you're venturing off the grid, bring a mobile tracking device, like the Spot Satellite GPS Messenger ($120, findmespot.com), to alert emergency services of your location if you need to. Agree on a rendezvous point in case you split up and cell service is spotty.

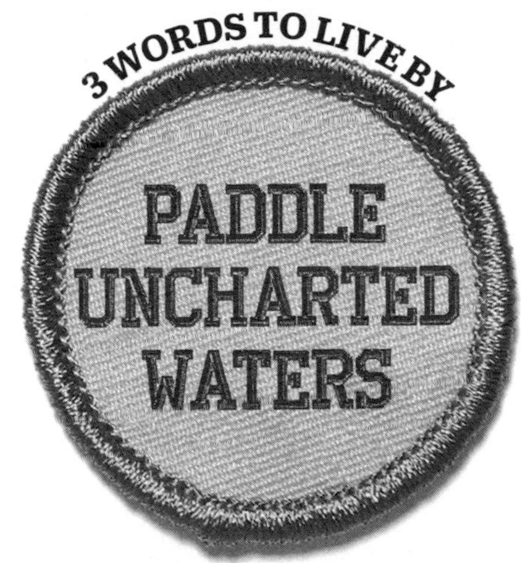
3 WORDS TO LIVE BY
PADDLE
UNCHARTED
WATERS

RULE # 5

Mondays are easier if you spent the weekend on a mountain or a river.

Dig a Legit
HORSESHOE PIT

Prep the pit, practice your ringers—and then beat all your buddies. Here's the how-to from Jerry LaBrosse, vice president of the National Horseshoe Pitchers Association.

Build the Frames

Nail the 2 × 4s into two 6 × 8-foot rectangular frames. These frames will house your sand, creating the pits you'll toss the horseshoes into.

Shape the Base

Place the frames 34 feet apart from front to front. (The center points will measure 40 feet apart.) Hammer a wood stake into the inside corners of each frame to secure the frames in place.

Anchor the Stakes

Set five patio blocks along the length of each frame. Fill the buckets with wet mortar and insert a steel stake into each bucket. As the mortar is setting, dig holes in the pits' centers deep enough for 15 inches of stake to surface.

Bury the Buckets

Drop in the buckets, aiming the two stakes toward each other at 12 degrees. Add enough sand so that the surface is level with the ground and 8 inches of stake sticks out. Game on!

WHAT YOU'LL NEED

Eight 2 × 4s (four 6', four 8')
16 nails/wood screws (16d size)
8 wood stakes (1 × 2 × 12")
20 cement patio blocks (18 × 18 × 3")
½ cubic yard mason sand
2 steel stakes (1" diameter, 3' long)
2 1-gallon buckets
1 bag mortar mix

Throw Ringers

Good balance helps horseshoes fly true. Stagger your feet, dominant foot forward, about 6 inches apart, placing the weight on your front foot and pointing your toes toward the stake for aim. Keeping your eyes fixed on the stake, take one step forward when you pitch to add control.

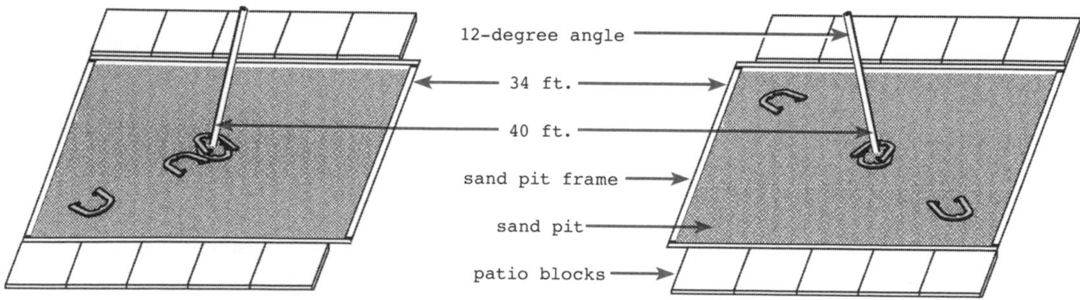

Shoot a Time-Lapse Movie

Send slow-moving scenes into overdrive—and rake in the YouTube views.

Choose Your Subject

Try scenes that unfold gradually and show clear progression, such as building a Lego kit or watching an arena fill.

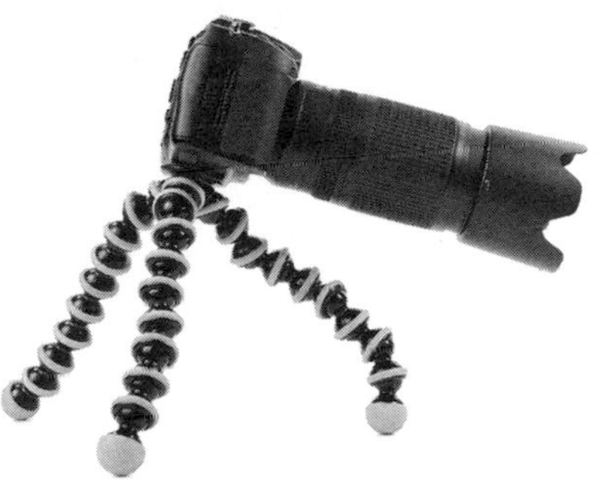

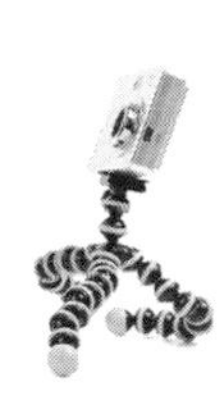

Gear Up

Your easiest option is to use an iPhone with the iTimeLapse Pro app ($2, iTunes) or an Android device with TimeLapse!. You can also use a digital SLR, such as GoPro HERO 2, 3, or 4. If your camera has no interval-shooting option, buy an intervalometer. Try Digital Timer Remote ($28, aliexpress.com).

Set Up

Optimal playback time is between 8 and 10 seconds with 240 photos. Try to predict how shadows and people will move throughout the shoot so you're not left with dark or empty scenes. For fast-moving subjects, adjust the interval to 1 second between shots. For slower ones, try 6 seconds. Manually lock the focus on the scene and let 'er rip.

Make Your Movie

The smartphone apps can create the movies for you, or import your sequences into QuickTime 7 Pro, which offers the easiest time-lapse function. For smooth motion, use 30 frames per second; then use video-editing software to add music and effects.

Serve Up Perfect *Watermelon*

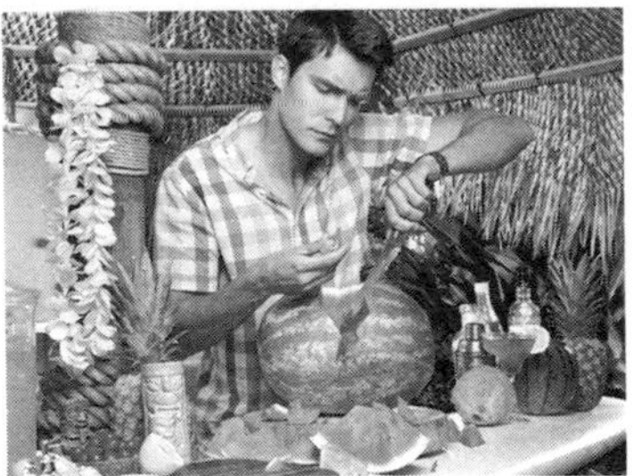

DECIPHER RIPENESS

Check the color, says Marcel Vigneron, star of *Marcel's Quantum Kitchen* on SyFy. "The melon should be dark green with a yellow area where it sat on the ground. If that area is white, then the melon hasn't matured." And give it a rap with your knuckles. If you hear a loud thud and the melon feels heavy, it's ripe.

SLICE WITH PRECISION

Use a large chef's knife to lop off the top and bottom of the watermelon so it sits flat on your cutting board. That's safer than trying to cut it as a wobbly whole. Now slice the melon into wedges. Or you can remove the rind with a smaller knife and then cut the flesh into cubes.

SERVE

Vigneron serves cubes of watermelon (drizzled with olive oil and sprinkled with sea salt) along with cherry tomatoes on a toothpick. "It sounds weird, but the acidity of the tomato and the sweetness of the watermelon go really well together," he says. Or try a side of watermelon with pork belly or duck—the sweetness contrasts nicely with fat.

How to Earn Your WINGS

Save about 15 grand on pilot's license instruction and take to the skies with a radio-controlled, prop-driven model airplane. Just stay out of those trees, Mav . . .

1. Avoid Toy-Store Junk

Choose a lightweight, hobby-grade, foam-built model that will bounce and resist breaking if it hits the ground. We like the prebuilt HobbyZone Champ RTF ($90, horizonhobby.com).

2. Start Off Hot

Take turns taxiing—use pavement or low grass as your runway—and doing some short hops to get used to the controls. When you take off (or hand-launch, if your plane is small enough), start at full throttle into the wind. (Altitude is mostly a function of motor speed.)

3. Go High

Stay at least 100 feet up—aka "two or three mistakes high." Set your throttle at about two-thirds (not too fast) and don't pitch the airplane's nose up without adding power—or you'll stall.

4. Flip Your Brain

When the plane is coming toward you, the controls feel reversed—moving your stick left will send the bird right. So if it starts to bank while coming at you, move the stick toward the dropping wing, as if you were propping it up.

5. Fly a Pattern

Don't fly randomly. Have a plan. Try a rectangle: Fly out, count to five, and turn right. Then do a two count and make another 90-degree turn. Repeat until you have the pattern down.

6. Bring It Home

Line up on your runway, reduce power, and keep the nose level or angled down a few degrees. When you're just a foot off the ground, level off and slide onto your strip. Now let her try.

Source: Gerry Yarish, flight instructor and senior technical editor at Model Airplane News

Fact: Roughly 4,200 men in the United States are propelled to the ER for firecracker-related injuries each year in the weeks around July Fourth.

Never drive on the beach without first letting some air out of your tires and bringing a shovel.

Turn an Empty Beer Bottle into Party Glassware

WARNING: This DIY project involves sharp edges, breaking glass, and fire (wear safety glasses). But if you're careful, it could also involve fun.

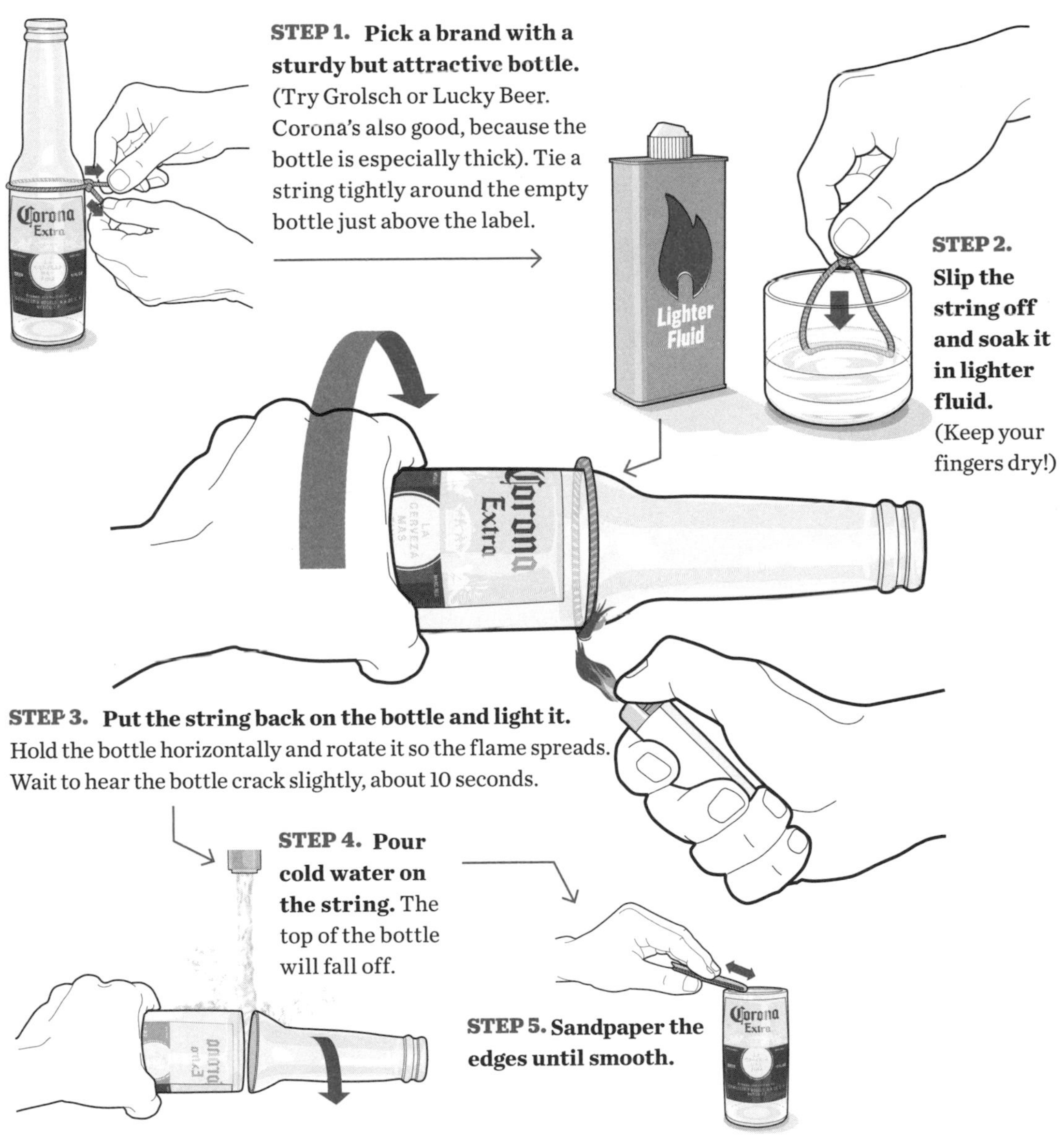

STEP 1. Pick a brand with a sturdy but attractive bottle. (Try Grolsch or Lucky Beer. Corona's also good, because the bottle is especially thick). Tie a string tightly around the empty bottle just above the label.

STEP 2. Slip the string off and soak it in lighter fluid. (Keep your fingers dry!)

STEP 3. Put the string back on the bottle and light it. Hold the bottle horizontally and rotate it so the flame spreads. Wait to hear the bottle crack slightly, about 10 seconds.

STEP 4. Pour cold water on the string. The top of the bottle will fall off.

STEP 5. Sandpaper the edges until smooth.

Shred the Terrain Park

Tear it up with snowboarding tips from Scotty Lago, 2010 Olympic bronze medalist in the half-pipe.

1. Grease a Butter Box

This long, elevated, rectangular feature in terrain parks is a good place for beginners to work on new tricks. Before you reach the ramp, position your board nose-first. Typically you'll slide onto the top of the box without having to jump. Keep your feet planted flat on the board and resist the urge to turn on the slick top. Wait until your board is completely off the box before you start carving snow again.

2. Catch Some Air

A jump is easier than it looks. Before your initial attempt, hang back and watch a few experienced riders launch. If possible, ask one of them if you can trail him or her off your first jump. Stay a safe distance behind, and mirror the person's speed and motions. Don't overthink the landing; just let the weight of the board help you hit the snow with your knees bent and body centered.

3. Be a Wingman

Chances are you won't be the only greenhorn in the park. If you see someone crash and "yard sale" (that's slang for when a rider's goggles, hat, and gloves fly off), block the top of the jump or rail and signal to the riders above to wait until the fallen rider is out of harm's way. You'll be saving a fellow rider from being crushed—and that's good karma, man.

4. Blend In

When you're practicing a trick the first few times, avoid any high-traffic areas. That way if you take a tumble, you're less likely to bring down another rider. Don't stand near the start or the landing of a jump, the rail, or the box. You'll hold up other riders and, worse, put yourself at risk of getting whacked.

5. Spin Out

The backside 180 (below) is one of the easier and flashier tricks, says Lago. Approach a jump riding your toe-side edge. At the lip of the jump, pop off and forcefully turn your head and shoulders backward; the rest of your body will follow. Look down as you rotate in the air, and once you can spot the landing, keep your eye on it to prevent overspinning. Land naturally.

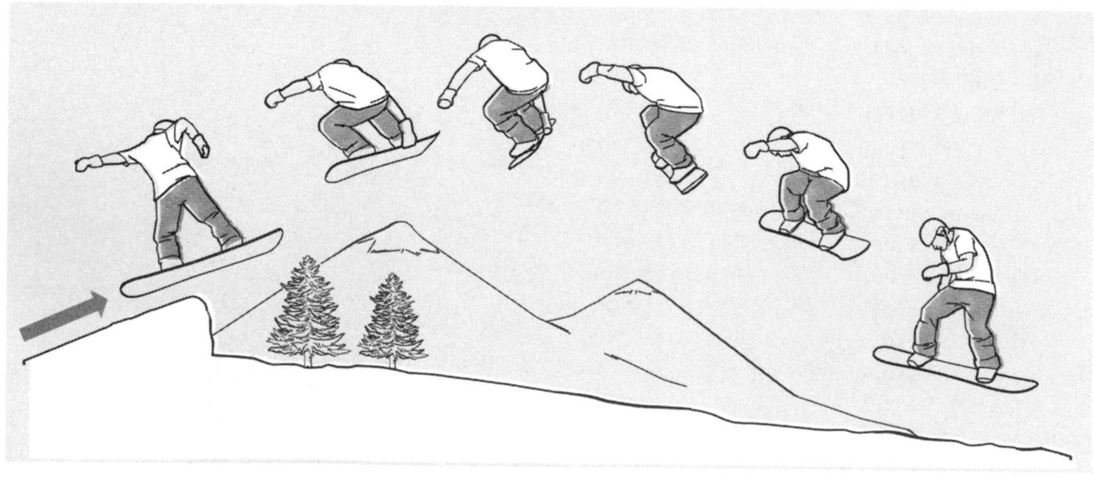

Hone Your Frisbee Accuracy

First off, ditch the cheap discs. They're often too rigid, small, and lightweight for stable flight. (They're also tougher to grip.) Look for a larger-diameter disc made from softer plastic, like the 10.5-inch, 160-gram Discraft Sky-Styler 160. $7, amazon.com

Use your whole body. To make sure one of you isn't always chasing discs tossed around by brisk headwinds, throw across the breeze to your partner. And don't rely on your arm for all the oomph—your power and accuracy will suffer. Instead, in one fluid motion, draw your arm across your body and toward your opposite shoulder. Then swing your arm back in the opposite direction, allowing your weight to shift from your back foot to your front foot to add power to the throw. When your arm is almost fully extended, release the disc with a flick of your wrist, to add spin and distance.

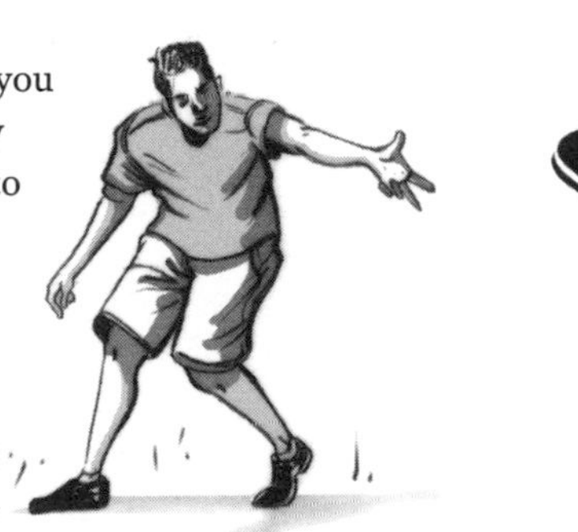

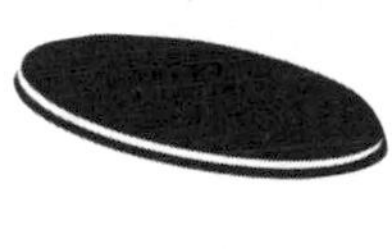

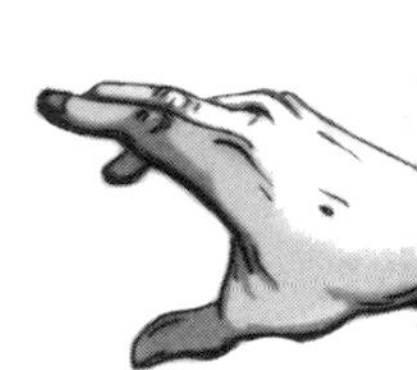

CRASH A HOTEL POOL

Pull off a caper that would make the *Entourage* crew proud, and give your gal an afternoon to remember. Our crafty insider: Toby Shuster, a Los Angeles social media manager and lifelong pool crasher.

Choose Your Target

Visit a user-review site like Yelp and look for a family-friendly spot.

"The staff will be worried about kids running around—not you," Shuster says. "Plus, they don't expect crashers at family-friendly luxury hotels." That said, avoid youth-oriented hotspots—they're on the watch for folks like you. And consider bad reviews a good thing: "If someone says the staff isn't helpful, that's your cue to go—employees are less likely to care," she says.

Time Your Crash

Go around 3 p.m., when it's neither too busy nor a ghost town. But don't bring your own beach towels—that's a dead giveaway. They'll have towels there. And look confident: No hotel employee will want to falsely accuse a guest of crashing. If you are confronted, simply say, "We're visiting a friend. I don't remember his room number." If they don't buy it, just leave. It's not like they're going to waterboard you.

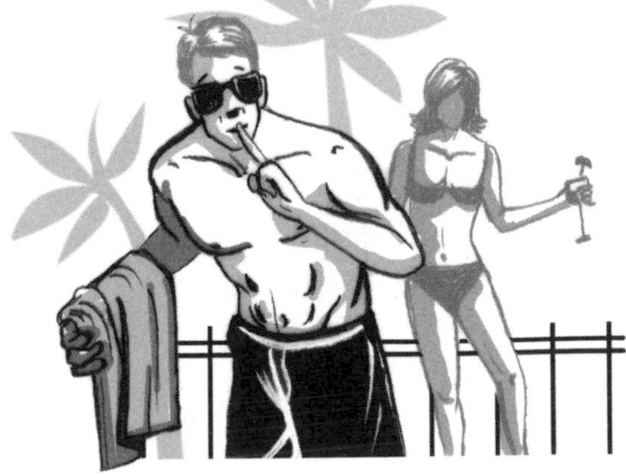

CLIMB ON BOARD

Four Ways to Enjoy a Wet and Wild Ride

Stand-Up Paddleboarding

"The first time you try stand-up paddleboarding, you'll feel it in your abs, your lats, your arches—everywhere. Sports like surfing require waves, wind. Stand-up paddleboarding requires only a board, a paddle, and water. It's the closest you'll ever come to walking on water. And let's face it: Everybody wants to walk on water."
—**Laird Hamilton,** surf legend considered the pioneer of stand-up paddleboarding

Rookie Mistake: Letting your arms do all the work. "You need to engage your abdominals," says pro paddleboarder Sean Poynter. Keep your arms extended and bend your elbows slightly, and with each stroke, rotate at your torso to generate more power.

Your First Move: Avoid the wind. Too many first-timers think strong gusts will help. They won't. "A beginner can be swept away by wind and strong currents," says Connor Baxter, a former world champion paddleboarder. Find a flat, calm area with as little wind as possible; work with an instructor to learn the basic techniques and ensure you can swim back to shore pulling your board behind you.

Surf Kayaking

"It's hard to describe the feeling you get from surfing a big wave. For me, it's about the pursuit of perfection. It takes training, experience, and an understanding of the ocean. When you do it right, it's immensely rewarding, and that's a feeling you just don't understand until you've had a 40-foot wave towering over your head."
—**Tao Berman,** former world champion kayaker and three-time world record holder

Rookie Mistake: Nervously sucking in your breath. "That's the last thing you want to do, and I see people do it all the time when they feel intimidated," Berman says. "You'll need more oxygen in your lungs if you get taken out, so focus on staying relaxed and breathing normally."

Your First Move: Focus on fit. "The kayak's size is important for performance and comfort," says instructor Ben Lawry, owner of Kayak Camp. Consider starting with an international-class kayak. It's longer and faster, and it picks up more waves. Then ask around about tide forecasts and reef spots. You don't want to hit coral in low tide.

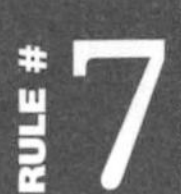

BOOK A HOUSEBOAT HOTEL

Some houseboats sleep more than a dozen people, making them great for bachelor parties or family reunions. Don't let the size intimidate you: Learning to operate a houseboat is relatively easy, says Ellen Hopkins of Discover Boating, a boating

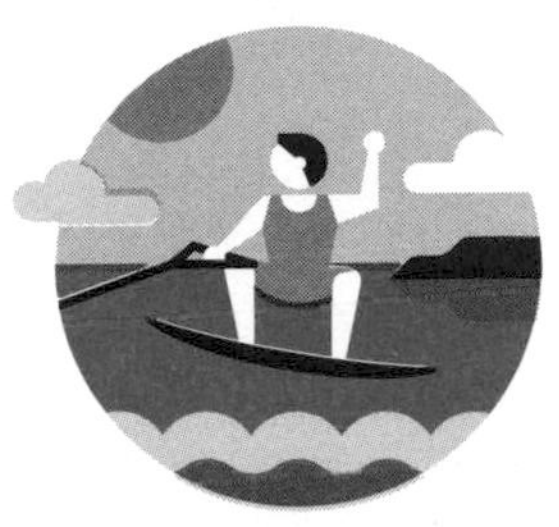

Wakeboarding

"There's a rhythm to the sport—a sort of pendulum effect, almost like a dance—that you don't get from other water sports. There's something about the moment the engine roars—10,000 pounds of weight pulling away all at once. The water displaces, you hit the wake and stand up sidewise, and it all just clicks for the first time."
—**Shaun Murray**, three-time world champion wakeboarder

Rookie Mistake: Trying to stand too early. "Let the boat pull you out of the water," says Tarah Mikacich, a professional wakeboarder and coach at Orlando's Freedom Wake Park. "Relax, straighten your arms, and bend your legs as much as possible. It's counterintuitive, but stay balled up and let the boat do the work." And ask the driver to pull you up slowly—hammering the throttle won't help.

Your First Move: Once you're on the wakeboard, don't face the boat. Instead, align your hips and shoulders with the length of the board. "That'll save you from a lot of hard falls," Mikacich says. And ask the driver to follow the same line as other boats—it's proper etiquette, and it'll cut down on the waves you'll encounter.

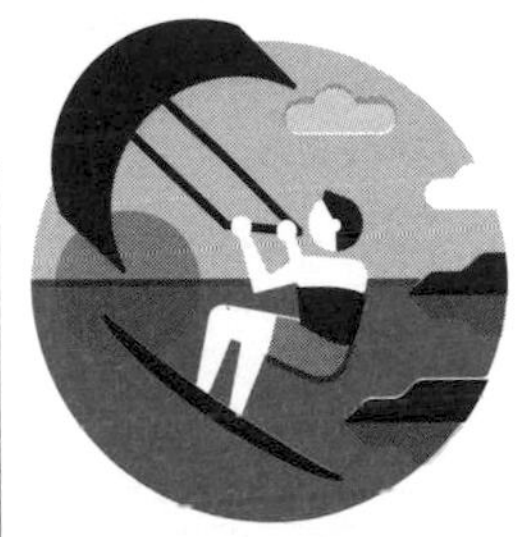

Kiteboarding

"It's the ultimate extreme sport. You can do it anywhere—flat water, waves, snow, dirt, ice, light winds, strong winds. There are no fuel costs, no lift tickets, no membership dues. You can jump higher than some buildings and travel faster than most speed limits, all while using nothing but wind and human power. That's pure freedom."
—**Rob Douglas**, professional sailor and kitesurfer who has held the world speed-sailing record

Rookie Mistake: Trying to outmuscle the kite. Control requires a light touch: "It's more like typing than a tug-of-war," says Karen Lang, an instructor at Aqua Sports Maui Kiteboarding School. "When the kite pulls forcefully, people tend to hold on tighter, which makes the kite gather even more force. Instead, let go of the bar and the kite will flutter down harmlessly."

Your First Move: Take lessons. But don't settle for any teacher. "Make sure the instructor is certified by the International Kiteboarding Organization and that you'll be followed in a chase boat or at least a jet ski," Douglas says. If you're hurt, fatigued, or stranded, the instructor can help. Douglas also recommends using a high-quality kite, such as one made by Cabrinha. Most cost more than $1,500, but a day rental runs $100 to $150.

advocacy nonprofit. The folks at the rental shop will show you how. Great houseboating waters to explore: Lake Powell has almost 2,000 miles of scenic shoreline, mostly in Utah; also try Lake of the Ozarks, Missouri; Shasta Lake, California; Captiva Island, Florida.

Thanks to Everyone In the Trenches

Many uncommonly clever and creative people contributed to the wisdom in this book. We are grateful to all those reporters, writers, editors, fact-checkers, interns, photographers, illustrators, designers, and photo and art directors who toiled in the trenches at *Men's Health* magazine to bring these useful tips, tools, and strategies to readers in the hopes of making good men even better men. Here are some of them:

Eric Adams, Lila Battis, Matt Bean, Nicole Beland, Mark Bricklin, Brian Boye, Denis Boyles, Steve Calechman, Adam Campbell, Sara Cann, Clint Carter, Jaclyn Colletti, Ben Court, Mike Darling, Kevin Donahue, Michael Easter, Jenny Everett, Jill Fanislaw, Jason Feifer, BJ Gaddour, Ron Geraci, Leisa Goins, Matt Goulding, Jeanne Graves, Greg Gutfeld, Mark Haddad, Madeline Haller, Jimmy the Bartender, Lisa Jones, George Karabotsos, Don Kinsella, Joe Kita, Paul Kita, Radnor Law, Anna Maltby, Nick Marino, Matt Marion, Tom McGrath, Jennifer Messimer, John McCarthy, Peter Moore, Thomas O'Quinn, Ben Paynter, Steve Perrine, Naomi Piercey, Bill Phillips, Eric Rinehimer, Laura Roberson, Joe Rodriguez, Amy Rushlow, Michael Schnaidt, Lou Schuler, Carol Ann Shaheen, Ted Spiker, Gregg Stebben, Julie Stewart, Bill Stieg, Trevor Thieme, Jim Thornton, Kyle Western, Mike Zimmerman, and David Zinczenko.

We owe much gratitude to our talented designer Joanna Williams, who built this jigsaw puzzle of amazing pages to be pleasing to the eye and fun to read. Also, many thanks go to those unsung heroes on the Rodale Books production team: Sean Sabo, Chris Krogermeier, Sara Cox, Jeff Batzli, Carol Angstadt, Brooke Myers, Keith Biery, Pat Burton, Wendy Hess Gable, Shannon Mushock, Gayle Diehl, and Jodi Schaffer.

The Boy Scout-y badges on the cover of this book were created by The Demerit Badge Company. You can order these and other fun patches at demeritwear.com.

Photo and Illustration Credits

(All left to right, top to bottom)

©Gregg Segal: page x

©Mitch Mandel/Rodale Images: pages 1 (round patch used throughout book), 51 (top 10), 176 (top, 3rd to 5th from top), 179 (4th from top), 190, 192 (bottom), 194, 196 (all except oatmeal), 244 (center and right)

©Public Domain: page 2 (top)

©iStockphoto: pages 2 (bottom), 5 (bottom), 6, 7 (top), 11, 23 (bottom), 26 (2), 27, 28 (top), 30 (bottom), 33, 34, 37 (top), 43 (bottom5), 45 (left), 46, 47 (top), 48, 54 (left), 55 (bottom), 57 (bottom), 58, 77 (right), 90-92, 93 (right 2), 94 (right), 96, 99 (top right), 100, 101 (top), 104 (sunglasses), 106-108, 114, 115 (top), 117 (right), 120, 122, 124, 133-135, 139 (left), 154 (bottom), 160, 163 (top), 165 (bottom), 167 (bottom), 169, 176 (2nd, 6th, 7th from top), 180 (top), 187 (top), 191, 197 (top 4), 197 (center), 197 (bottom-2nd, 3rd, 5th from left), 201 (top), 203 (bottom right), 211 (right), 219, 222, 223 (bottom), 225 (top), 229 (right), 231, 233, 236-237, 239 (bottom), 243, 244 (left and bottom), 245 (top), 251 (bottom), 254, 262 (bottom), 265 (bottom), 266, 267 (bottom), 274 (bottom)

©Jameson Simpson: pages 3, 18, 20, 47 (bottom), 66, 84, 112, 113 (bottom), 127, 150 (right), 164, 177 (right), 188, 203 (left), 209, 213, 215, 241-242, 246, 249, 250 (bottom), 251 (top)

©Toby Leigh: pages 4, 5 (top), 7 (bottom), 25, 49, 50, 60, 64, 74-75, 168 (left), 177 (left), 181, 185 (left), 187 (bottom), 193, 200, 206 (bottom), 211 (left), 216 (top), 223 (top), 229 (left), 235,250 (top), 253, 255, 261, 276, and 280

©Levi Brown: pages 8 (top), 99 (top left), 130, 238 (left), 239 (top)

©Matius Grieck/+ISM: pages 8 (bottom), 36, 43 (top 4), 59, 62 (top), 72, 147, 165 (top), 263, 279

©Claire Benoist: pages 10, 172, 247

©Jason Lee: pages 13, 16 (top), 42 (top), 67 (left), 77 (left), 136-137, 167 (top), 178 (top), 182 (top), 184, 202, 210, 212, 216 (bottom), 221, 225 (bottom), 232, 260 (top), 274 (top)

©Anthony Zinonos: pages 15, 23 (top), 271

©Jason Lee/Marek Haiduk: page 16 (bottom)

©Paul Blow: pages 17, 29, 98, 168 (right), 170, 252, 267 (top), 270, 275

©Richard Perez: pages 19, 132, 142, 152, 205, 224

©Comstock: pages 21, 39 (bottom), 71 (bottom)

©Michael Gellatly: page 24

©Arthur Mount: pages 28 (bottom), 82 (bottom)

©Beth Bischoff: pages 30 (top), 63 (bottom), 68-71 (top), 73, 83

©Si Maclennan: page 31

©Getty Images: pages 37 (bottom), 186 (top), 195, 197 (bottom-4th from left), 260 (bottom), 277 (top)

©Daniel R. Krovatin: pages 38, 39 (top)

©Rami Niemi: pages 40 (top), 228

©Bradley Hughes: pages 40 (bottom), 118, 182 (bottom), 183, 185 (right)

©clkr.com: page 41 (left)

©Tom MacDonald/Rodale Images: pages 41 (right), 65 (top), 71 (center), 126 (bottom)

©Dimitri Otis/Getty Images: page 42 (bottom)

©Browndogstudios/Getty Images: page 44 (left)

©Courtesy, Boy Scouts of America: pages 44 (right), 45 (right), and 55 (top 2)

©Nik Schulz: page 51 (bottom)

©Wikimedia Commons/Public Domain: pages 52 (all except bluegill) and 53 (4)

©Dept of Natural Resources-MD/Public Domain: pages 52 (bluegill), 53 (weakfish)

©Courtesy, Diane Rome Peebles/Florida Fish and Wildlife Conservation Commission, Division of MarineFisheries Management: page 53 (bluefish)

©Colin Newman/Getty Images: page 53 (billfish)

©Dorling Kindersley/Getty Images: page 53 (red drum and striped bass)

©Todd Detwiler: pages 54 (right), 186 (bottom), 217-218

©Courtesy of orvis.com: page 56 (6)

©Greg Manchess: page 57 (top)

©Joel Kimmel: page 62 (bottom)

©Nicholas Blechman: page 63 (top)

©Josh McKible: pages 65 (bottom), 105, 278

©Dustin Wallace: page 67 (bottom)

©Courtesy, ringside.com: page 76

©Trevor Reid: page 78 (top)

©Brown Bird Design: page 78 (bottom)

©Zander Dekker: page 79

©Sebastian Kaulitzki: page 82 (right)

©Bartholomew Cooke: page 86

©Joao Fazenda: page 89

©FoodCollection/Getty Images: page 93 (left)

©Inmagine: page 94 (left)

©Bob Dinetz: page 95

©Thinkstock/Getty Images: page 97

©Brad Muti: pages 99 (bottom), 149

©Digital Vision/Getty Images: page 101 (bottom)

©Dan Forbes/Trunk Archive: page 102

©Daniel Warren Johnson: pages 104 (except sunglasses), 110-111, 121 (top)

©Two Arms, Inc.: page 113 (top)

©Brooke Nipar: page 115 (bottom)

©Gio Pastori: pages 116 (top), 126 (top)

©Photodisc: pages 116 (bottom), 179 (top, 3rd from top), 197 (bottom left)

©Andrea Manzati: page 117 (left)

©Thomas and Erica Chadwick: page 119

©Julien Pacaud: page 121 (bottom)

©Charles Wilkin: pages 123, 206 (top)

©Rodale Images: page 125

©Andrew Tingle: page 128 (top)

©Scott Chambers: page 128 (bottom)

©Zach Graham: pages 138, 139 (right), 144

©Jennifer Robbins: page 140

©Miko Lim: page 141

©Masterfile: pages 143 (top), 238 (right)

©R. Kikuo Johnson: page 144

©Jonathan Barlett: pages 146, 281

©Mark Weaver: pages 148, 201 (bottom), 204

©Nicholas Blechman/Daniel Ting Chong: page 150 (left)

©Picdesk: page 153

©Hubert Tereszkiewicz: page 154 (top)

©Harry Campbell: page 155

©Dan Saelinger: page 156

©Ciara Phelan: page 158

©Jesse Lenz: pages 159, 173, 264, 265 (top)

©Tavis Coburn: pages 161, 166, 248

©Mario Wagner: pages 162, 262 (top)

©Matthew Hollister: page 163 (bottom)

©Elias Stein: page 171

©Grant Cornett: page 174

©Chris Philpot/Sidecar: page 178 (bottom)

©Stockbyte: page 179 (2nd from top)

©Kang Kim: page 179 (bottom)

©Michael Hoewler: page 180 (bottom)

©Jamie Chung: page 192 (top)

©Image Source: page 196 (oatmeal)

©Brand X: page 197 (bottom right)

©John Midgley: page 198

©Everette Collection: page 203 (top right)

©Courtesy, Warner Bros. Entertainment: page 206 (center left and center)

©Courtesy, RCA Music Group: page 206 (center right)

©Joshua Scott: page 207

©Marek Haiduk: pages 208, 214

©Mark Matcho: page 220 (2)

©Zmeel Photo/Getty Images: page 226

©Dogo: page 230 (top)

©Tim Ridley/Getty Images: page 230 (bottom)

©Greg Broom: pages 234, 256

©Anthony Calvert: page 245 (bottom)

©Joyce Lee: page 257

©Quinn Rooney/Getty Images Sport: page 258

©Travis Rathbone: page 268

©Cristiana Couceiro: page 269

©Mike McQuade: pages 272-273

©Jeff Minton: page 277 (bottom)

©DKNG Studios: pages 282-283

Index

Boldface page references indicate photographs and illustrations. Underscored references indicate shaded and boxed text, and charts.

A

Accessories. *See also* Ties
to avoid, 113, **113**
belts, 108, 111
cufflinks, 111
sunglasses, **104**, 109, **109**, 127, **127**
tie bars, 111, 115
watches, **104**, 109
Air guitar, 206, **206**
Air hockey, 204, **204**
Airplane
jet lag and, 164
model, flying, 278, **278**
seat on, reserving, 164, **164**
Alcohol. *See also* Beer; Wine
champagne, pouring, 14, **14**
driving after consuming, avoiding, 89
sangria, making, 190, **190**
signature drink, 10, **10**, 10
Altitude sickness, 58
Anger at work, avoiding, 172
Angry friend, calming, 15
Antiperspirant, 28, 124
Ants, 243
April Fools' pranks, 208
Arguments, 144, 150, 201
Arm wrestling, 203, **203**
Aspirin, 31, 92, 98, 101
Athlete's foot, 88
Ax head, tightening loose, 55

B

Baby, cradling, 5, **5**
Babysitting toddler, 6
Back massage, 137, **137**
Back pain, **71**, 71, 100
Bacon, cooking/eating, 179, 187
Bad breath, 123
Bad mood, 91
Bag, leather, **104**, 111
Ballpark food, **197**, 197
Banana, peeling, 177, **177**
Bar bet, winning, 206, **206**
Bar fight tactics, 4, **4**, 203
Baseball
curveball, throwing, 17
glove, breaking in/repairing, 2, 2
hat, breaking in, 112, **112**
hit by pitch in, 101
Basketball
arcade, 216, **216**
fast break scores, **201**, 201
March Madness bracket picks, 214
pickup, 222
running hook shot, **216**, 216
spinning ball on finger, 3, **3**
Bats (mammals), 245
Beach, driving on, 278
Beards and scruff, 147
Bears, avoiding/dealing with, 46, **46**
Beer. *See also* Alcohol
Black & Tan, pouring, **8**, 8
bottle
opening without opener, 2, **2**
as party glassware, 279, **279**
sticking to coaster, preventing, 6
chilling, fast, 190
dog fetching, 262, **262**
glass of, sliding down bar, 8, **8**
kegerator for, 233, **233**
weight gain and, 93
Bee stings, 43, **43**
Belts, 108, 111
Best man role, 29
Bike riding, 20, 225, **225**, 266
Billiards, 202, **202**, 203
Birds
identifying big, 58, **58**
removing from house, 245
Black eye, 98
Blackjack odds, 207
Blazers (coat), 31, **104**, 107
Blisters, 59
Blood sugar level and vinegar, 195
Blueberries, 194
Body language of women, 134, 151, 151
Body odor, 28, **28**, 122, 124
Boots, drying hiking, 37
Boss, managing, 158, 164
Bowling, 219
Boxing, 4, **4**, 65, **65**, 76, **76**, 76
Brain cancer, preventing, 99
Brainstorming, 164, 170
Branding self, 28
Bras, buying for woman, 141
Breaking into own home, 228
Broccoli, cooking/eating, 192, 195
Brown rice, 185
Brushing teeth, 89
Buffalo meat, 83
Burgers, cooking, 180, **180**
Burns, 88, 100, 101
Burrito, rolling perfect, 195, **195**

C

Calories burned by exercise, 63, 76
Campfires, 36–37, **36**, 37
Canker sores, 88
Canoeing, 38–39, **38–39**
Canoe parts, **39**, 39
Car
cleaning, 248, 249, **249**
diagnosing problems with, 14, 14
parking parallel, 7, **7**
speeding, cost of, 165
speeding ticket, beating, 204
Card playing, 207, 207
Carnival games, 210
Casino games. *See* Gambling tips
Ceiling, fixing drywall, 237
Cereal, 25, 187
Chainsaw, handling, 231, **231**
Champagne, pouring, 14, **14**
Charley horse, 88
Checkers, 211
Check, picking up, 3
Chelsea boots, 120, **120**
Chicken soup, making, 186, **186**

- Children. *See also* Fun, homegrown
  - babysitting toddler, 6
  - birthdays, celebrating, 270
  - coaching, 21
  - cradling baby, 5, **5**
  - science projects and, 224, 224
  - snot and, making simulated, 33
- Chili, making Texas-style, 191
- Chinos, **104**, 107
- Chocolate, dark, **99**, 99
- Chopping wood, 230, **230**
- Circadian clock, 37
- Circular saws, handling, 229
- Clams, cooking, 192, **192**
- Clay pigeon shooting, 209, **209**, 209
- Cliff, jumping from, 40, **40**
- Closets, clearing out, 107
- Clothing. *See also specific type*
  - color of, 113
  - essential, **104**, 105–11
  - fit of, 31
  - fixes, fast, 129
  - flattering, 122, 123
  - moths and, preventing, 114
  - patterns, 128, **128**
  - shopping for, 106
  - for thinner look, 122
  - underarm sweat stains, avoiding, 28, **28**
  - washing new, 108
- Coaching children, 21
- Coats, helping woman with, 136, **136**
- Cocktail sauce, making, 193
- Colds, 161
- Cold shower, 91
- Collars. *See also* Shirts
  - curling, fixing, 129
  - face shape and, 111, **111**
  - suits with, 128, **128**
  - tie knots with, 128, **128**
- Concert viewing, front-row, 217, **217**
- Conversation tips
  - greetings in foreign languages, 29
  - knowing versus not knowing subject matter, 27
  - at parties, 19
  - women and dating, 133
  - at work, 161
- Cooking. *See also* Diet; Grilling
  - bacon, 179
  - banana, peeling, 177, **177**
  - broccoli, 192, 195
  - burgers, 180, **180**
  - burrito, 195, **195**
  - chicken soup, 186, **186**
  - chili, Texas-style, 191
  - clams, 192, **192**
  - cocktail sauce, 193
  - dish washing tips, 191
  - dressings, making, 179
  - with eggs
    - cracking in one hand, **177**, 177
    - peeling quickly, 196
  - faster, tips for, 196
  - fish, buying fresh, 11, **178**, 178
  - flapjacks, flipping, 40
  - French toast, 176, **176**
  - garlic, mincing, 183, **183**
  - ginger, preserving, **186**, 186
  - with greens from salad bar, 196
  - guacamole, 197, **197**
  - heating serving dishes, 190
  - hummus, making, 187, **187**
  - knife sharpening, 7, **7**, 177
  - with leftovers, 185
  - lobster, 181, **181**
  - meat thermometer substitute, 185, **185**
  - men's skills at, 175
  - microwaving food in plastic, avoiding, 89, 193
  - nutcracker substitute, 176
  - on open fire, 55
  - oysters, 193, **193**, 193
  - pan-searing steak, 184, **184**
  - pasta, 182, **182**
  - popcorn, 194, **194**
  - potatoes, 196
  - protein shake, 81, 81
  - salsa
    - grilling ingredients to make, 237, **237**
    - growing ingredients for, 185, **185**
    - microbes in, 98
  - sangria, 190, **190**
  - shrimp cocktail, 192, **192**
  - smoky food without grilling, 189
  - smoothie cleanup tips, 184
  - substitute tools for, 176, **179**, 179
  - sushi, rolling own, 178, **178**
  - thawing food quickly, 196
  - trail mix, making, 37
  - tuna sandwich, 187
  - turkey
    - safety tips for deli, 181
    - in trash can, 188, **188**, 188
  - watermelon, serving perfect, 277, **277**
- Cramps, muscle, 80, 80
- Criticism at work, giving/taking, 168
- "C-tactile" nerve fibers, 137
- Cuddling, 155
- Cufflinks, 111
- Cursing, 19, 101
- Curveball, throwing, 17
- Cuts, minor skin, 101
- Cycling, 20, 225, **225**, 266

D

- Dancing tips, 147, **147**, 153
- Dark chocolate, **99**, 99
- Darts, pub, 210, **210**
- Dating. *See* Women and dating
- Dating sites, 143
- Deck, restoring, 244
- Degreasing hands, 27
- De-icing driveway, 238
- Deli turkey safety tips, 181
- Dental care, 89, 90, 117, 125
- Diet. *See also* Cooking; *specific food*
  - bacon, 187
  - ballpark food, **197**, 197
  - belly-filling food, 196, **196**
  - blueberries, 194
  - brown rice, 185
  - calories burned by exercise and, 76
  - cereal, 25, 187
  - dark chocolate, **99**, 99
  - flaxseed, 183
  - food combinations for health benefits, **100**, 100
  - food storage tip, 190
  - grapefruit, 81
  - maple syrup, 176
  - nutrient-dense food, 183
  - nuts, 83, 97
  - outdoor plants, edible, 45, **45**
  - pizza, 10
  - portion sizes, 11, 83
  - quinoa, 27
  - salsa, 98
  - soda, 63
  - vinegar, 195
  - weight gain and rigid, 63
- Dining out tips, 168
- Dinner toast, making, 11
- Dish washing tips, 191
- Diving off board, 223, **223**
- Doctor
  - DO versus MD, 92
  - selecting, 26
- Dogs
  - benefits of owning, 266
  - house for, building, 247, **247**
  - managing aggressive, while running, 26
  - photographing, 262, **262**
  - relationships and, effect on, 134
  - as running partners, **77**, 77
  - tricks for, teaching, 262, **262**, 267, **267**
- Door
  - kicking in, 25, **25**
  - replacing broken, 235, **235**
- Double Windsor tie knot, 128, **128**

Dragon boat, paddling, 274
Dressings, making, 179
Driveway, de-icing, 238
Drywall, fixing hole in, 243, 250, **250**

E

Earlobe heart test, 94
Eating contest, 212
Eggs
- cracking with one hand, **177**, 177
- peeling quickly, 196

Electronics, avoiding at bedtime, 89
Emotion, showing, 147
Engine light, checking car, 14, 14
Erections, 154
Etiquette, mastering, 152
Eulogy, delivering, 22
Exercise. *See also* Workouts
- abdominal crunch, avoiding, 84
- Bench Press, 67
- calories burned by, 63, 76
- Chest-Supported Incline Row, 70, **70**
- Drop Lunge, 62, **62**
- Dumbbell Bent-Over Row, 68, **68**
- Dumbbell Chest Press, 68, **68**
- Dumbbell Curve, 71, **71**
- Dumbbell Incline Press, 69, **69**
- Dumbbell Romanian Deadlift, 70, **70**
- Dumbbell Split Squat, 69, **69**
- Dumbbell Squat, 69, **69**
- Dumbbell Step-up, 70, **70**
- Dumbbell Swings, 70, **70**
- Glute Bridge, 62, **62**
- grip-strengthening, 65
- home gym for, building, 257
- Human Flag, 67, **67**
- with kettlebell, 78–79, **78**, **79**
- Lying Dumbbell Triceps Extension, 71, **71**
- Overhead Press, 82, **82**
- piriformis syndrome, 30, **30**
- pullup rings, making, 77, **77**
- Pushup, 62, **62**
- Pushup Jacks, 65, **65**
- resistance training, 71
- Rolling Plank, 62, **62**
- rope scaling, 64, **64**
- with sandbag, 72, **72**
- Single-Arm Standing Shoulder Press, 69, **69**
- Split Jump, 62, **62**
- stair-climbing machine, 64
- Standing Bent-Over Row, 83, **83**
- stretching, 66
- Superman, **71**, 71
- for tennis backhand, **62**, 62
- with tire, 75, **75**
- with towel, 74, **74**
- walking, 79, 99
- weight lifting, 63, **63**, 66, 71

Eyebrow care, 125
Eyeglasses, 37, 116, **116**
Eyes
- age-proofing, 127, **127**
- black, 98
- dark circles under, 119
- gaze directions of, 132
- grit in, clearing, 93
- itchy, 88
- sweat in, managing, 54

F

Face shape
- collars and, 111, **111**
- eyeglasses and, 116
- hair length and, 125
- sunglasses and, **109**, 109

Feet, sore, 89
Fighting, defensive, 4, **4**, 203
Financial goals, meeting, 28, 32
Firecracker-related injuries, 278
Fire, snuffing out small, 245, **245**
Fish
- buying fresh, 11, **178**, 178
- cleaning, 50, **50**
- freshwater, 52, **52**, 58
- lures, **51**, 51, **56**
- saltwater, 53, **53**, 58
- tossing back, 49

Fishing, 48–49, **49**, 49, 56–57, **57**
Fitness. *See* Exercise; Health and fitness
Flag, displaying, 26
Flapjacks, flipping, 40
Flaxseed, 183
Flirting, 28, 137, 141
Floor, fixing squeaky, 237
Flowers, giving to woman, 139, **139**
Fly fishing, 56–57, **57**
Food. *See* Diet; *specific type*
Foosball, 211
Football
- fantasy draft, 214
- flag, 200, **200**, 200
- punting tips, **207**, 207
- touch, 9, **9**
- winning tips, 9

Foreskin, penile, 94
Fractured bone, securing, 55, **55**
French kiss, delivering, 142
French toast, making, 176, **176**
Frenemy, outsmarting work, 163
Frisbee, 281, **281**
Frostbite, 100
Fungus, cleaning house, 238
Fun, homegrown. *See also* Social activities; Sports and games
- beach, driving on, 278
- beer bottle turned to party glassware, 279, **279**
- bike ride, 266
- birthdays, celebrating child's, 270
- dogs, 262, **262**, 266, **266**, 267, **267**
- dragon boat paddling, 274
- Frisbee throwing, 281, **281**
- guitar, learning to play, 268
- Halloween activities
  - costumes for, 272–73, **272–73**
  - pumpkin carving, 264, **264**
  - scaring trick-or-treaters, 270–71, **270**, **271**
- horseshoe pit, digging, 276, **276**
- hotel pool, crashing, 281
- houseboat, booking, 282–83
- ice rink, building backyard, 269
- ice sculpture, carving, 274, **274**
- kite flying, stunt, 265, **265**
- laddergolf, building/playing, 263, **263**
- list of activities, 259
- model airplane, flying, 278, **278**
- movies
  - outdoor party showing, 273
  - time-lapse, shooting, 277
- paddling watercraft, 282–83, **282–83**
- poker game, hosting, 268
- rope swing, rigging, 260, **260**
- snowboarding, 280, **280**
- trips, 267, 270, 275
- volunteering, 147, 268
- watermelon, serving perfect, 277, **277**
- water park, building backyard, 261, **261**

Furniture, moving, 251, **251**
Furniture scratches, covering, 251

G

Gambling tips, 17, 202, 207
Gameshow, getting spot on, 222
Games. *See* Sports and games
Garage, organizing, 248, 254
Garbage disposal, unjamming, 243
Garlic, mincing, 183, **183**
Geothermal heat pump, 249
Gifts, buying, 135, 154, **154**, 160
Ginger, preserving, **186**, 186
Glove, breaking in baseball, 2, 2

Gloves for home projects, wearing, 231
Go-kart track strategies, 215, **215**
Golf
chip shots, 211, **211**
drives, 220, **220**, 221
etiquette, 220
miniature, 212, **212**
putts, long, 211, 221, **221**
strokes, cutting, 221
Grapefruit, 81
Grass, playing blade of, 5, **5**
Greetings, foreign language, 29
Grilling
cleaning grill, 189, 236
meat sticking to grill, preventing, 183
propane gas in, gauging, 183
salsa ingredients, 237, **237**
smoky food without, 189
temperature of grill, guesstimating, 182, **182**
Grime, cleaning, 252, 252
Groin, blows to, 92, **92**
Grooming and style. *See also* Clothing; Hair
bad breath, 123
beards and scruff, 147
body odor, 28, **28**, 122, 124
details and, 103
eyebrow care, 125
eyes, age-proofing, 127, **127**
hands, degreasing/washing, 27, 90, 170
nail care, 88, 98, 125
nose hairs, trimming, 114
pillowcase, washing, 123
razor blades, changing, 126
shaving tips, 126, 129, 138
sheets, washing, 144
skin care, 114, 122, 126
sonic scrubbers, 122
whitening teeth, 117, 125
Group dates, 135
Guacamole, making, 197, **197**
Guitar, learning to play, 268
Gun safety tips, 209

H

Hair
bad haircut, outgrowing, 124
face shape and length of, 125
sideburns, 124, **124**
thinning, 33, 118
washing, 125
for younger look, 118
Half Windsor tie knot, 116, **116**, 128, **128**
Halitosis, 123
Halloween activities
costumes for, 272–73, **272–73**
pumpkin carving, 264, **264**
scaring trick-or-treaters, 270–71, **270**, **271**
Hammering nail, 16, 90
Hammock, hanging, 239, **239**
Handshake grip, 30
Hand washing, 27, 90, 170
Harmonica, playing, 4
Hat, breaking in baseball, 112, **112**
Health and fitness. *See also* Mental acuity; Sleep; Weight loss
altitude sickness, 58
athlete's foot, 88
back pain, **71**, 71, 100
bad breath, 123
bad mood, 91
blisters, 59
body odor, 28, **28**, 122, 124
burns, 88, 100, 101
canker sore, 88
charley horse, 88
colds, 161
cuts, minor skin, 101
doctor, selecting, 26
earlobe heart test, 94
effort in improving, 61
eyes
black, 98
clearing grit from, 93
dark circles under, 119
itchy, 88
firecracker-related injuries, 278
food combinations for, **100**, 100
fractured bone, securing, 55, **55**
frostbite, 100
gender differences and, 87
groin, blows to, 92, **92**
heart attack, 31, 172
heartburn, 88
Heimlich maneuver, 96
hiccups, 96
hoarseness, 88
hypertension, 187, 194
hypothermia, 42
indigestion, 88
ingrown toenail, 88, 98
jet lag, 164
kidney stones, 88
massages, 75, 137, **137**
mishaps, sudden, 101
mistakes, daily, 89
muscle cramps, 80, 80
nosebleed, 89
out-of-date/used objects, tossing, 97
pain scale, **95**, 95
pelvic flexibility, 94, **94**
periformis syndrome, 30
pillows, bed, 91
rashes, 89
refrigerator safety tips, 97
sarcopenia, 99
scratching, 94
skin cancer, 92
smashed thumb, 90
smoking, avoiding, 97
sore feet, 89
sponge safety tips, 97, **97**
stretching, 91, **91**
sunburn, 89
testicle care, 31
walking, 79, 99
Heart attack, 31, 172
Heartbeat, average male, 91
Heartburn, 88
Heat pump, geothermal, 249
Heimlich maneuver, 96
Hiccups, managing, 96
High blood pressure, 187, 194
Hiking
blisters from, 59
boots, drying, 37
shoes, selecting, 46
stick, selecting, 41, **41**
sweat in eyes and, managing, 54
technique, 46
Hoarseness, 88
Holiday party, planning work, 160
Home gym, building, 257
Home heating, 249
Home projects and repair. *See also* Pests
breaking into own home, 228, **228**
car, cleaning, 248, 249, **249**
ceiling, fixing drywall, 237
chainsaw, handling, 12, 231, **231**
challenges of, 227
circular saw, handling, 229
closets, clearing out, 107
deck, restoring, 244
doghouse, building, 247, **247**
door, replacing broken, 235, **235**
driveway de-icing, 238
drywall, fixing hole in, 243, 250, **250**
fire, snuffing out small, 245, **245**
floor, fixing squeaky, 237
furniture, moving, 251, **251**
furniture scratches, covering, 251
garage, organizing, 248, 254
garbage disposal, unjamming, 243
gloves for, 231
grill, cleaning, 189, 236
grime, cleaning, 252, 252
gym, building home, 257

Home projects and repair. *(cont.)*
- hammering nail, 16, 90
- hammock, hanging, 239, **239**
- kegerator, building, 233, **233**
- ladder safety tips, 253
- lawn care, 230, 232, 249, 252
- lightbulb, removing smashed, 243
- measuring items, 234, 243
- mold/fungus, removing, 238
- mower, tuning, 230, **230**
- mowing lawn, 230, 232, 249
- painting tips, 234, 234, 251
- patio chair, making, 255, **255**
- picture, hanging on brick wall, 250, **250**
- power drill/driver, 256, **256**
- screw, pulling stripped, 243
- security tips, 253, **253**
- selling house, 254
- showerhead, fixing leaky, 229
- sink clog, clearing, 238
- snow shoveling, 237
- spark plugs, changing, 13, **13**
- studs, finding, 228
- tile, laying, 232
- toilet bowl, cleaning, **239**, 239
- tree house, building, 240–42, **241**, **242**
- trees
  - felling, 12, **12**
  - planting, 253
  - pruning, 231
- water pipe, thawing frozen, 254
- weeds, killing, 249
- windows, cleaning second-story, **244**, 244
- wood
  - chopping, 230, **230**
  - stacking, 232, **232**
- workbench, building, 229, **229**

Hormones, female, 155
Horseback riding, 20, **20**
Horseshoe pit, digging, 276, **276**
Horshoes tip, 276
Hotel pool, crashing, 281
Hotel room upgrade, receiving, 166
Houseboat, booking, 282–83
Hummus, making, 187, **187**
Humor, sense of, 151
Hydration, 101
Hygiene. *See* Grooming and styling
Hypertension, 187, 194
Hypothermia, 42

I

Ice, boiling water before making, 190
Ice rink, building backyard, 269
Ice sculpture, carving, 274, **274**
Ice skating backward, 16, **16**
Indigestion, 88
Ingrown toenail, 88, 98
Injuries and illness. *See specific type*
Insects, biting/stinging, **43**, 43, 236, **236**
Intimacy levels of women, 133

J

Jacket, leather, **104**, 106
Jeans, **104**, 107, **107**, 118, 129
Jet lag, 164
Jokes, avoiding long, 22
Judgment, good, 167

K

Karaoke, 218, **218**, 218
Kayaking, 42, **42**, 282, **282**
Kegerator, building, 233, **233**
Kettlebell, exercising with, 78–79, **78**, **79**
Kidney stones, 88
Kissing, 142, 143
Kiteboarding, 283, **283**
Kite, flying stunt, 265, **265**
Knife, sharpening, 7, **7**, 177
Knots, tying. *See also* Ties
- bowline, 41, **41**
- clinch, improved, **51**, 51
- clove hitch, 41, **41**
- reef, 41, **41**
- square, 41, **41**
- trucker's hitch, 24, **24**
- two half hitches, 41, **41**

L

Laddergolf, building/playing, 263, **263**
Ladder safety tips, 253
Laughing, 77
Lawn care, 230, 232, 249, 252
Lawn mower, tuning, 230, **230**
Leather bag, **104**, 111
Leather jacket, **104**, 106
Leftovers, livening up, 185
Life jacket, pants as, **55**, 55
Light bulb, removing smashed, 243
Lightning strikes, 54
Linen, washing bed, 123, 144
Lingerie, buying for woman, 140, **140**, 140
Linked-In profile, 138, 169
Lip balm, mentholated, 101
Loafers, 120, **120**, 122
Lobster, cooking, 181, **181**
Longevity, 79, 93
Love letter, writing, 138
Luggage check-in tips, 165, **165**

M

Magic tricks
- Dime-Drop Deception, 206, **206**
- rabbit/duck drawing, **143**, 143

Maple syrup, 176
Marathon, running first, 80
Marriage, benefits of, 142
Massage oil, 146
Massages, 75, 137, **137**
Meat. *See also* Turkey
- buffalo, 83
- burgers, cooking, 180, **180**
- fish, buying fresh, 11, **178**, 178
- pan-searing steak, 184, **184**
- sticking to grill, preventing, 183
- temperature of, gauging, 185, **185**

Meat thermometer substitute, 185, **185**
Medicine ball, **62**, 62, 66, **66**
Memory tips, 21, 96
Men's knowledge, stereotypical, 1. *See also specific type*
Men's room tips, work, 158, 164
Mental acuity
- memory tips, 21, 96
- phone numbers, remembering, 21
- tips for improving, 92, 96
- weight lifting and, 66

Mental health day, taking, 162
Mentoring at work, 170
Menu, looking at, 168
Metabolism, 71
Mice, 233, 246, **246**, 246
Microwaving food in plastic, avoiding, 89, 193
Miniature golf, 212, **212**
Model airplane, flying, 278, **278**
Mold, cleaning house, 238
Moles and skin cancer, 92
Money, measuring with, 243
Money-saving strategies, 28, 32, 153
Mood, overcoming bad, 91
Mosquitoes, killing, 236
Moths, preventing clothing, 114
Mountain biking, 225, **225**
Mouth. *See also* Dental care
- burns on roof of, 88
- objects to avoid putting in, 90

Movies
- outdoor party showing, 273
- time-lapse, shooting, 277

Mower, tuning, 230, **230**
Mowing lawn, 230, 232, 249

Muscle cramps, 80, 80
Music
  Air guitar and, 206
  for Halloween costume, 272
  for mood improvement, 91
  party, 2, 268
  for poker game, 268
  for road trip, 270
  for time-lapse movie, 277
  for wedding, 29
Musical instrument, learning to play, 92, 268

N

Nail care, 88, 98, 125
North, finding without compass, 44, **44**
Nose
  bleeding, 89
  clearing stuffy, 90
  hairs, trimming, 114
Nutcracker substitute, 176
Nuts, 83, 97

O

Objects
  finding small, 234
  tossing out-of-date/used, 97
One-night stand, reading possibility of, 134, 153
Online profiles, 138, 169
Outdoor plants, edible, 45, **45**
Outdoor survival. *See also specific activity*
  ax head, tightening loose, 55
  bears, 46, **46**
  bee stings, 43, **43**
  birds, identifying big, 58, **58**
  boots, drying hiking, 37
  campfires, 36–37, **36**, 37
  canoeing, 38–39, **38–39**
  challenges of, 35
  cliff, jumping from, 40, **40**
  fractured bone, securing, 55, **55**
  frostbite, 100
  hiking stick, selecting, 41, **41**
  hypothermia, 42
  kayaking, 42, **42**
  knots, tying, 41, **41**
  lightning strikes, 54
  north, finding, 44, **44**
  plans, 42, 46
  plants, edible outdoor, 45, **45**
  rip currents, 47, **47**
  rock climbing, 54, **54**
  shark attacks, 23, 47
  shitting in woods, 46
  sleeping bag tips, 44, 44
  snake, catching, 27
  SPEAR acronym and, 42
  survival kit, homemade, 45
  tent, pitching, 59
  tick removal, 59, **59**
  whitewater safety tips, 38, 39
  wind speed, guesstimating, 44
Out-of-date/used objects, tossing, 97
Oxford shoes, 120, **120**
Oysters, identifying and shucking, 193, **193**, 193

P

Paddleboarding, stand-up, 282, **282**
Paddling watercraft, 38–39, **38–39**, 282–83, **282–83**
Pain scale, **95**, 95
Pain. *See specific ailment*
Painting tips, 234, 234, 251
Pancakes, flipping, 40
Pan-searing steak, 184, **184**
Pants
  Chinos, **104**, 107
  cleaning, 129
  dress, **104**, 108
  fit of, 117, **117**
  jeans, 107, **107**, 118, 129
  as life jacket, **55**, 55
  socks with, 124
Parking car, parallel, 7, **7**
Pasta, cooking, 182, **182**
Patio chair, making, 255, **255**
Pelvic flexibility, 94, **94**
Penis size, 31, 97
Pen, spinning in hand, 167, **167**
Periformis syndrome, 30
Pests
  ants, 243
  bats, 245
  birds, 245
  insects, biting/stinging, **43**, 43, 236, **236**
  mice, 233, 246, **246**, 246
  roaches, 239
  slugs/snails, 236
  squirrels, 245
Pets. *See* Dogs
Pheromones, 136
Phone numbers, remembering, 21
"Picking up" women, 132, 135, 138, 147, 148, 149
Picture, hanging on brick wall, 250, **250**
Pillowcase, washing, 123
Pillows, bed, 91
Ping Pong, 213
Piriformis syndrome, 30, **30**
Pizza, 10
Pocket square, folding, 118, **118**
Poker game, hosting, 268
Pool (table), 202, **202**, 203
Popcorn, making, 194, **194**
Portion sizes, 11, 83
Potatoes, 196, 243
Power drill/driver, 256, **256**
Pranks, 208
Presentation, giving work, 159
Promotion, earning work, 169
Propane gas in grill, gauging, 183
Protein shake, making, 81, 81
Pullup rings, making, 77, **77**
Pumpkin, carving, 264, **264**
Punting football, **207**, 207

Q

Quinoa, 27

R

Raise, asking for, 160–61
Rashes, 89
Razor blades, changing, 126
Reciprocal inhibition (RI), 80
Recommendation, writing work, 163
Refrigerator
  for beer, building, 233, **233**
  cleaning, 252
  safety tips, 97
Relationships
  arguments in, 144, 150, 201
  dogs and, effect on, 134
  flowchart for troubleshooting problems in, **145**
  good, 150
  spontaneity in, 138, 147
Resistance training, 71
Respect, earning, 14
Retirement savings, 173, **173**
Rip currents, 47, **47**
Risk taking, summer as time for, 265
Roaches, 239
Road trip tips, 267, 270
Rock climbing, 54, **54**
Rock, Paper, Scissors game, 205
Romance. *See* Women and dating
Rope scaling, 64, **64**
Rope swing, rigging, 260, **260**
Roulette, 17, 207
Running
  barefoot, 84
  distance, increasing, 207
  dogs as running partners, **77**, 77
  dogs chasing you while, 26

Running *(cont.)*
- form, 79
- marathon, first, 80
- sweat in eyes and, 54
- time, being last, 212

S

Salmon, buying, **178**, 178
Salsa
- grilling ingredients to make, 237, **237**
- growing ingredients for, 185, **185**
- microbes in, 98

Sandbag exercises, 72, **72**
Sandbag, making, **73**, 73
Sangria, making, 190, **190**
Sarcopenia, 99
Saving-money strategies, 28, 32, 153
Sazerac drink, The, 10, **10**, 10
"Scarecrow technique," 42
Science projects, children's, 224, 224
Scrabble (game), 205
Scratching, 94
Screw, pulling stripped, 243
Secret Santa gifts, buying, 160
Security tips for home, 253, **253**
Selling house, 254
Serving dishes, heating, 190
Sexual attraction, 134, 149, 153
Shark attacks, 23, 47
Shaving tips, 126, 129, 138
Sheets, washing, 144
Shirts. *See also* Collars
- dress, **104**, 105, **105**, 105, 106
- fit of, 117, **117**
- folding, **105**, 105
- length of, 108
- nipples showing underneath, 129
- pink, 112
- polo, **104**, 105
- sport, **104**, 106
- stains on white, **121**, 121
- suits with, 110, 112
- ties with, 117, 129
- T-shirts, **104**, 105, 107

Shitting in woods, 46
Shoes
- belt and, matching, 108
- Chelsea boots, 120, **120**
- dress, **104**, 108, **108**
- essential, 120, **120**
- fit of, 108
- hiking, 46
- loafers, 120, **120**, 122
- Oxfords, 120, **120**
- protecting when traveling, 165
- shining, 113, 129
- sneakers, **104**, 108
- storing, 121, 129
- with suits, 117, **117**
- wet, restoring, 121, **121**

Shoe trees, 121
Shotgun parts, 6, **6**
Showerhead, fixing leaky, 229
Shrimp cocktail, making, 192, **192**
Shuffleboard, 223, **223**
Signature drink, 10, **10**, 10
Sink clog, clearing, 238
Skeet shooting, 209, **209**, 209
Skin
- burns, 101
- cancer, 92
- care, 114, 122, 126
- cuts, minor, 101
- rashes, 89
- sunburn, 89

Sky watching, 146
Sleep
- electronics and, avoiding at bedtime, 89
- eyes and, age-proofing, 127
- outdoors, 37
- snoring and, 100
- socks and, wearing, 101
- "spooning" during, 150, **150**
- weight gain and lack of, 63

Sleeping bag tips, 44, 44
Slugs, 236
Smartphone tip, 167
Smells and timed tests, 219
Smiling, 83, 162
Smoky food without grilling, 189
Smoking, avoiding, 97
Smoothie cleanup tips, 184
Snails, 236
Snake, catching, 27
Sneakers, **104**, 108
Sneezing, 93
Snoring, 100
Snot, making simulated, 33
Snot rocket, launching, **16**, 16
Snowboarding, 280, **280**
Snow shoveling, 237
Social activities. *See also* Conversation tips; Fun, homegrown; Sports and games; Women and dating
- angry friend, calming, 15
- best man role, 29
- check, picking up, 3
- dancing tips, 147, **147**, 153
- dinner toast, making, 11
- eulogy, delivering, 22
- handshake grip, 30
- jokes, avoiding long, 22
- thank-you note, writing, 22
- tipping for service, 4, 23
- work-related, tips for, 173

Socks
- with pants, 124
- sleeping with, 101

Sonic scrubbers, 122
Spark plugs, changing, 13, **13**
SPEAR acronym, 42
Speed bag, punching, 65, **65**
Speeding, cost of, 165
Speeding ticket, beating, 204
Sperm production, 31, 89
Splint from magazine/newspaper, 55, **55**
Sponge safety tips, 97, **97**
Spontaneity in relationship, 138, 147
"Spooning" in bed, 150, **150**
Sports and games. *See also* Fun, homegrown; Social activities; *specific sport*
- Air guitar, 206, **206**
- air hockey, 204, **204**
- April Fools' pranks, 208
- arm wrestling, 203, **203**
- bar bet, 206, **206**
- bar fight tactics, 4, **4**, 203
- bike riding, 20, 225, **225**, 266
- billiards, 202, **202**, 203
- bowling, 219
- canoeing, 38–39, **38–39**
- card playing, 207, 207
- carnival games, 210
- checkers, 211
- clay pigeon shooting, 209, **209**, 209
- coaching kids, 21
- concert viewing, front-row, 217, **217**
- darts, pub, 210, **210**
- Dime-Drop Deception trick, 206, **206**
- eating contest, 212
- fantasy football draft, 214
- foosball, 211
- Frisbee, 281, **281**
- gambling tips, 17, 202, 207
- gameshow, getting spot on, 222
- go-kart track strategies, 215, **215**
- grass, playing blade of, 5, **5**
- harmonica, playing, 4
- horseback riding, 20, **20**
- ice skating backward, 16, **16**
- karaoke, 218, **218**, 218
- kayaking, 42, **42**, 282, **282**
- laddergolf, 263, **263**
- March Madness bracket picks, 214
- miniature golf, 212, **212**
- paddling watercraft, 282–83, **282–83**

  Ping Pong, 213
  pranks, 208
  rock climbing, 54, **54**
  Rock, Paper, Scissors, 205
  rope scaling, 64, **64**
  science projects, 224, 224
  Scrabble, 205
  self-talk and, 200
  shotgun, parts of, 6, **6**
  shuffleboard, 223, **223**
  skeet shooting, 209, **209**, 209
  snowboarding, 280, **280**
  table tennis, 213
  winning and, 199
  wishbone, splitting, 201, **201**
Squirrels, 245
Stains on white shirts, cleaning, **121**, 121
Stair-climbing machine, 64
Steak, pan-searing, 184, **184**
Stocks, selecting winning, 225
Storm, weathering, 57
Strength training. *See* Weight lifting
Stress at work, avoiding, 172
Stretching, 66, 91, **91**
Studs, finding without stud finder, 228
Style. *See* Clothing; Grooming and style
Suits
  bottom button on, 119
  collars with, 128, **128**
  fit of, **110**, 110, 117, **117**, 119, **119**, 126, 126
  height of man and, 110, **110**
  navy blue, **104**, 110
  pocket square and, folding, 118, **118**
  shirts with, 110, 112
  shoes with, 117, **117**
Sunburn, 89
Sunglasses, **104**, 109, **109**, 127, **127**
Sunlight and appearance, 149
Surf kayaking, 282, **282**
Survival kit, homemade, 45
Sushi, rolling own, 178, **178**
Sweaters, **104**, 106, 107, 114, 114
Sweat in eyes, managing, 54
Swimming
  flip dive, 223, **223**
  flip turn, **84**, 84
  in hotel pool, 281
  jumping from cliff and, 40, **40**
  rip currents and, 47, **47**
  shark attacks and, 23
  whitewater safety tips, 38, 39

T

Table tennis, 213
Tennis
  backhand, exercise for, **62**, 62
  grunting when hitting ball, 213
  serve, 213, **213**
Tent, pitching, 59
Terrarium, creating office, 171, **171**
Testicle care, 31
Testicular torsion, 95
Test, scoring better on timed, 219
Thank-you note, writing, 22
Thawing food quickly, 196
Theft in locker rooms, preventing, 66
Thin look, quick, 84, 122
Thumb, soothing smashed, 90
Tick removal, 59, **59**
Tie bars, 111, 115
Ties
  casual, 109, 115, **115**
  collars and knots of, 128, **128**
  color of, 115
  dimpling, 115, **115**
  double Windsor knot, 128, **128**
  floral, 109
  half Windsor knot, 116, **116**, 128, **128**
  knots for, 128, **128**
  length of, 113, 129
  polka dot, 109
  power, 109
  seer-sucker, 109
  shirts with, 117, 129
  silk, black, 109
  size of, 117, **117**
  skinny, 109
  solid, 109
  texture of, 107, 115
  uncreasing, 129
  Windsor knot, 128, **128**
  wool blend, 109
Tile, laying, 232
Tipping for service, 4, 23
Tire, exercising with, 75, **75**
Toenail, ingrown, 88, 98
Toilet bowl, cleaning, **239**, 239
Tongue, burn on, 100
Tooth care, 89, 90, 117, 125
Touch and women, 137, 151, 151. *See also* Massage
Touch-football plays, 9, **9**
Towel, exercising with, 74, **74**
Trail mix, making, 37
Travel for work, 164–66
Tree house, building, 240–42, **241**, **242**
Trees
  felling, 12, **12**
  planting, 253
  pruning, 231
Trips, 267, 270, 275. *See also* Work, travel for
Trucker's hitch, tying, 24, **24**
T-shirts, **104**, 105, 107
Tuna sandwich, making, 187
Turkey
  cooking in trash can, 188, **188**, 188
  safety tips for deli, 181
Twitter and dating, 149

U

Unconscious person, dragging to safety, 2

V

Vacations with women, 143
Valentine's Day date, 139
Vinegar and blood sugar level, 195
Voicemail, landing job via, 167
Volunteering, 147, 268

W

Wakeboarding, 283, **283**
Walking, 79, 99, 146
Washing hands, 27, 90, 170
Watches, **104**, 109
Watercraft, paddling different types of, 38–39, **38–39**, 282–83, **282–83**
Water intake, 101
Watermelon, serving perfect, 277, **277**
Water park, building backyard, 261, **261**
Water pipe, thawing frozen, 254
Wedding
  attending alone, 148
  best man role for, 29
  music for, 29
Weeds, killing, 249
Weight gain causes, 63, 93
Weight lifting, 63, **63**, 66, 71
Weight loss
  knees and, 78
  thin, look and, quick, 84, 122
  31-day plan, 85
  tips, 30, 33, 73, 83
  water intake and, 101
Weight maintenance, 88
Whistling with two fingers, 15, **15**
Whitening teeth, 117, 125
Whitewater safety tips, 38, 39
Windows, cleaning second-story, **244**, 244
Windsor Tie knot, 128, **128**
Wind speed, guesstimating, 44

Wine. *See also* Alcohol
cork, broken, 190
decanting, 190
suggestions, 18
Wishbone, splitting, 201, **201**
Women and dating
arguments, 144
beards and scruff, 147
body language of woman, 134, 151, **151**
bras, buying for woman, 141
challenges of, 131
check, picking up, 3
coat, helping woman with, 136, **136**
conversation tips, 133
cuddling, 155
dancing tips, 147, **147**, 153
dates to remember, 144
dating sites, 143
emotion and, showing, 147
etiquette, mastering, 152
first move, making, 143
flirting, 28, 137, 141
flowers for woman, giving, 139, **139**
foods with shells and, avoiding, 12
French kiss, delivering, 142
gaze directions of woman, 132
gifts for woman, 135, 154, **154**
group dates, 135
hormones of woman, 155
intimacy levels of woman, 133
kissing, 142, 143
language, understanding woman's, 154
lingerie, buying for woman, 140, **140**, 140
love letters, writing, 138
lowering your voice, 138
magic trick to make woman smile, **143**, 143
marriage, benefits of, 142
massages, 137, **137**
meeting women, 132
naked women, things to never say to, 141
name of woman, forgetting, 134
one-night stand, reading possibility of, 153
online profiles and, 138
out of your league, 133
party bore, rescuing woman from, 152
pets and, 134
pheromones and, 136
"picking up" women, 132, 135, 138, 147, 148, 149
picture taking and, 148
in room full of women, 11
scary movies, 151
sense of humor, 151
sexual attraction, 134, 149, 153
shaving and, 138
sky watching, 146
spontaneity and, 138, 147
"spooning" in bed, 150, **150**
touch and, 137, 151, 151
Twitter and, 149
vacations, 143
Valentine's Day date, 139
Wood
chopping, 230, **230**
stacking, 232, **232**
Work
anger at, avoiding, 172
boss, managing, 158, 164
brainstorming at, 164, 170
branding self, 28
challenges of, 157
conversation tips at, 161
criticism at, giving/taking, 168
day off after boss's day off, taking, 260
dining out tip, 168
drinking with boss, 168
frenemy at, 163
graduating from college to, things lost, 159
holiday party for, planning, 160
Linked-In profile, 169
men's room tips, 158, 164
mental health day, taking, 162
mentoring at, 170
mistakes at, 162, 172
pen, spinning in hand, 167, **167**
presentation, giving, 159
promotion, earning, 169
raise, asking for, 160–61
recommendation, writing, 163
retirement savings and, 173, **173**
Secret Santa gifts, buying, 160
silence at, 166
small talk at, 161
smartphone tip, 167
social activities related to, tips for, 173, **173**
stress, avoiding, 172
terrarium in office, creating, 171, **171**
travel for, tips, 164–66
voicemail, landing job via, 167
washing hands at, 170
worry at, avoiding, 172
Workbench, building, 229, **229**
Workouts. *See also* Exercise
boxing, 76, **76**, 76
enjoyable exercises first, doing, 283
fast muscle, 68–71, **68–71**
high-intensity, 20
kettlebell, 78–79, **78**, 78, **79**
in morning, 85
opposing muscle groups and, 83
skipping, 67
Worry at work, avoiding, 172
Wounds, minor skin, 101

Z

Zippers, unsticking, 106, **106**